Novel Medical and General Hebrew Terminology from the Middle Ages

Novel Medical and General Hebrew Terminology from the Middle Ages

VOLUME 6

By

Gerrit Bos

BRILL

LEIDEN | BOSTON

Cover illustration: Nathan ha-Me'ati's Hebrew translation of: *Canon medicinae Avicennae*, Biblioteca Universitaria di Bologna, Ms.2197 c.7r.

Library of Congress Cataloging-in-Publication Data

Names: Bos, Gerrit, 1948- author.
Title: Novel medical and general Hebrew terminology from the Middle Ages. volume 6 / by Gerrit Bos.
Description: Leiden ; Boston : Brill, [2023]. | Includes bibliographical references and index.
Identifiers: LCCN 2023002045 (print) | LCCN 2023002046 (ebook) | ISBN 9789004534407 (hardback) | ISBN 9789004534421 (ebook)
Subjects: LCSH: Medicine, Medieval–Dictionaries–Hebrew. | Hebrew language–Dictionaries–English. | Hebrew language, Medieval–Glossaries, vocabularies, etc. | Jews–Medicine–History–To 1500–Sources.
Classification: LCC R123 .B6684 2023 (print) | LCC R123 (ebook) | DDC 610.1/4–dc23/eng/20230118
LC record available at https://lccn.loc.gov/2023002045
LC ebook record available at https://lccn.loc.gov/2023002046

Typeface for the Latin, Greek, and Cyrillic scripts: "Brill". See and download: brill.com/brill-typeface.

ISBN 978-90-04-53440-7 (hardback)
ISBN 978-90-04-53442-1 (e-book)

This book is printed on acid-free paper and produced in a sustainable manner.

Contents

Sigla, Sources, and Abbreviations VII

Introduction 1

List of Terms 11

Bibliography 225
Used Hebrew Sources 227
Corrections to NM 1–5 and BCD 229
Index of Greek Terms 231
Index of Arabic/Persian Terms 232
Index of Latin/Romance Terms 242

Sigla, Sources, and Abbreviations

Sigla

a	Arabic text.
AMP	Arnaldus de Villa Nova, *Opera Medica Omnia*, vol. 6.1: *Medicationis parabole/Pirqei Arnavṭ de-Vila Nova*, ed. by E. Feliu, L. Ferre, and J.A. Paniagua (Barcelona 1990).
BCD	G. Bos, *A Concise Dictionary of Novel Medical and General Hebrew Terminology from the Middle Ages* (Leiden 2019).
BDB	F. Brown, S.R. Driver, and C.A. Briggs, *A Hebrew and English Lexicon of the Old Testament: With an Appendix Containing the Biblical Aramaic, Based on the Lexicon of William Gesenius as Translated by Edward Robinson* (Repr., Oxford 1978).
BIJS	G. Bos (ed. and trans.), *Ibn al-Jazzār on Sexual Diseases and Their Treatment* (London 1997).
BLS	C. Brockelmann, *Lexicon Syriacum*, 2nd ed. (Halle 1928).
BM	E. Ben Yehuda, *Millon ha-Lashon ha-Ivrit: Thesaurus Totius Hebraitatis et Veteris et Recentioris*, 17 vols. (Repr., Tel Aviv 1948–1959).
BMA 1	Maimonides, *On Asthma: A Parallel Arabic–English Text Edited, Translated, and Annotated*, ed. and trans. by G. Bos (Provo, UT 2002).
BMA 2	Maimonides, *On Asthma*, vol. 2: *Critical Editions of Medieval Hebrew* (ed. by G. Bos) *and Latin Translations* (ed. by M.R. McVaugh) (Provo, UT 2008).
BMCH	Maimonides. *Commentary on Hippocrates'* Aphorisms: *A New Parallel Arabic-English Edition and Translation, with Critical Editions of the Medieval Hebrew Translations*, ed. and trans. by G. Bos, 2 vols. (Leiden 2020).
BMMG	Maimonides, *Medical Aphorisms: Glossary & Indexes*, ed. by G. Bos (Leiden 2021).
BMMN	Maimonides, *Medical Aphorisms: Hebrew Translation by Nathan ha-Me'ati*, ed. by G. Bos (Leiden 2020).
BMMZ	Maimonides, *Medical Aphorisms: Hebrew Translation by Zeraḥyah ben Isaac ben She'altiel Ḥen*, ed. by G. Bos (Leiden 2020).
BMR	Maimonides, *On the Regimen of Health: A New Parallel Arabic-English Translation, with Critical Editions of Medieval Hebrew Translations* (ed. by G. Bos) *and Latin Translations* (ed. by M.R. McVaugh) (Leiden 2019).
BMW	Maimonides, *The Medical Works of Moses Maimonides: New English Translations Based on the Critical Editions of the Arabic Manuscripts*, trans. by G. Bos (Leiden 2022).
BMZ	G. Bos, G. Mensching, and J. Zwink (eds.), *Medical Glossaries in the Hebrew*

Tradition: Shem Tov ben Isaac, Sefer Almansur, *with a Supplement on the Romance and Latin Terminology* (Leiden 2017).

BnF Bibliothèque nationale de France (Paris).

CD D.J.A. Clines, *The Dictionary of Classical Hebrew*, 9 vols. (Sheffield 1993–2016).

CN C. Caballero-Navas, *The Book of Women's Love: Sefer Ahavat Nashim* (London 2004).

D R. Dozy, *Supplément aux dictionnaires Arabes*. 2 vls. (Paris 1927).

DAN G.H. Dalman, *Aramäisch-Neuhebräisches Handwörterbuch zu Targum, Talmud und Midrasch*, 2nd ed. (Frankfurt am Main 1922).

DiTMAO G. Bos, M.S. Corradini, G. Mensching (eds.), *Dictionnaire des termes médico-botaniques de l'ancien occitan*, in cooperation with the Institute for Computational Linguistics "A. Zampolli" (ILC-CNR), Pisa (Database, in preparation).

DKT P. De Koning, *Trois traités d'anatomie arabes*, ed. by F. Sezgin (Repr., Frankfurt am Main 1986).

DMLBS R.E. Latham, D.R. Howlett, and R.K. Ashdowne (eds.), *The Dictionary of Medieval Latin from British Sources*, 3 vols. (London 1975–2013).

DT *Dioscurides Triumphans: Ein anonymer arabischer Kommentar* (*Ende 12. Jahrh. n. Chr.*) *zur Materia medica*, vol. 2, trans. by A. Dietrich (Göttingen 1988).

EM A. Even-Shoshan, *Ha-Millon he-Ḥadash* (Repr., 7 vols., Jerusalem 1983).

EP I. Efros, *Philosophical Terms in the* Moreh Nebukim (New York 1966).

FAQ I. Fellmann, *Das Aqrābāḏīn al-Qalānisī: Quellenkritische und begriffsanalytische Untersuchung zur arabisch-pharmazeutischen Literatur* (Beirut 1986).

FEW W. von Wartburg, *Französisches Etymologisches Wörterbuch*, 25 vols. (Bonn 1922–).

FL G.W. Freytag, *Lexicon Arabico-Latinum*, vols. 1–4 (Halis Saxonum 1830–1837).

GL A.M. Goichon, *Lexique de la langue philosophique d'Ibn Sīnā* (*Avicenne*) (Paris 1938).

HCD A. Heschel, *A Concise Dictionary of Hebrew Philosophical Terms* (Cincinnati 1941).

HIM W. Hinz, *Islamische Maße und Gewichte umgerechnet ins metrische System* (Repr., Leiden 1970).

HLA J. Hirschberg and J. Lippert (trans.), *Die Augenheilkunde des Ibn Sina* (Leipzig 1902).

HM S. Heymans, *Ha-Millim ha-She'ulot mi-Yewanit u-mi-Latinit ba-Mishnah: Leksikon we-Torat Hegeh* (PhD diss., Tel Aviv 2013).

IBF	Ibn al-Bayṭār, *Traité des simples*, trans. by L. Leclerc, 3 vols. (Paris 1877–1883).
IJZ 1–2	G. Bos and F. Käs (eds. and trans.), *Ibn al-Jazzār's* Zād al-musāfir wa-qūt al-ḥāḍir (*Provisions for the Traveller and Nourishment for the Sedentary*), *Books I and II: Diseases of the Head and the Face, with the Medieval Hebrew translations* (ed. by G. Bos) *and the Medieval Latin translation* (ed. by M.R. McVaugh) (Leiden 2022).
IJZ 7	G. Bos (ed. and trans.), *Ibn al-Jazzār's* Zād al-musāfir wa-qūt al-ḥāḍir (*Provisions for the Traveller and Nourishment for the Sedentary*), *Book 7 (7–30), with Moses ibn Tibbon's Hebrew translation* (Ṣedat ha-Derakhim) (Leiden 2015).
KA	A. Kohut, *Arukh shalem: Aruch Completum* (vols. 1–8), and S. Krauss, *Tosefet he-Arukh: Additamenta* (vol. 9) (Repr., Tel Aviv 1970).
KB	L. Koehler and W. Baumgartner, *The Hebrew and Aramaic Lexicon of the Old Testament*, subsequently revised by W. Baumgartner and J.J. Stamm, with assistance from B. Hartmann, Z. Ben-Hayyim, E.Y. Kutscher, and Ph. Reymond, ed. and trans. under the supervision of M.E.J. Richardson, 5 vols. (Leiden 1994–2000).
KDS	D. Kaufmann, *Die Sinne*: *Beiträge zur Geschichte der Physiologie und Psychologie im Mittelalter aus hebräischen und arabischen Quellen*; repr. in: idem, *Die Spuren al-Baṭaljûsi's* (Budapest 1880), and *Studien über Salomon Ibn Gabirol* (Budapest 1899), and *Die Sinne* (Budapest 1884), with an introduction by L. Jacobs (Farnborough 1972).
KM	F. Käs, *Die Mineralien in der arabischen Pharmakognosie: Eine Konkordanz zur mineralischen Materia medica der klassischen arabischen Heilmittelkunde nebst überlieferungsgeschichtlichen Studien*, 2 vols. (Wiesbaden 2010).
KTP	J. Klatzkin, *Thesaurus Philosophicus linguae hebraicae et veteris et recentioris* (Repr., 4 pts. in 2 vols., New York 1968).
L	Latin text.
Lane	E.W. Lane, *Arabic-English Lexicon*, 8 vols. (London 1863–1879).
LF	I. Löw, *Die Flora der Juden*, 4 vols. (Repr., Hildesheim 1967).
Low	A. Lowinger, 'Register of Hebrew and Aramaic Terms, translated and edited by S. Paley,' in: J. Preuss, *Biblisch-talmudische Medizin: Beiträge zur Geschichte der Heilkunde und der Kultur überhaupt* (Repr., New York 1971).
LSG	H.G. Liddell and R. Scott, *A Greek English Lexicon*: *Revised and Augmented Throughout* by H.S. Jones, a.o., with a supplement (Repr., Oxford 1989).
LW	J. Levy, *Wörterbuch über die Talmudim und Midraschim*, nebst Beiträgen von H. Leberecht Fleischer, 2nd. ed., mit Nachträgen und Berichtigungen von L. Goldschmidt, 4 vols. (Berlin/Vienna, 1924).

MIG — Marwān ibn Janāḥ, *On the Nomenclature of Medicinal Drugs* (*Kitāb al-Talkhīṣ*): *Edition, Translation, and Commentary with Special Reference to the Ibero-Romance Terminology*, ed. by G. Bos, F. Käs, M. Lübke, and G. Mensching, 2 vols. (Leiden 2020).

MMT — M. Meyerhof, *The Book of the Ten Treatises on the Eye Ascribed to Humain Ibn Isḥāq* (*808–877 A.D.*); repr. in: *Augenheilkunde im Islam: Texte, Studien und Übersetzungen*, vol. 2: *Werke von Hunain b. Isḥāq und Muhammad al-Ġāfiqī*, ed. by F. Sezgin (Frankfurt am Main 1986).

MSh — Maimonides, *Sharḥ asmā' al-ʿuqqār: Un glossaire de matière médicale composé par Maïmonide*, ed. by M. Meyerhof (Cairo 1940); repr. in: *Islamic Medicine*, vol. 63, ed. by F. Sezgin (Frankfurt am Main 1996).

NA — N. Nasrallah (trans.), *Annals of the Caliphs' Kitchens: Ibn Sayyār al-Warrāq's Tenth-Century Baghdadi Cookbook*, with introduction and glossary (Leiden 2007).

ND — J. Norri, *Dictionary of Medical Vocabulary in English, 1375–1550: Body Parts, Sicknesses, Instruments, and Medicinal Preparations*, 2 vols. (London 2016).

NM 1 — G. Bos, *Novel Medical and General Hebrew Terminology from the 13th Century*: *Translations by Hillel ben Samuel of Verona, Moses ben Samuel Ibn Tibbon, Shem Tov ben Isaac of Tortosa, and Zeraḥyah ben Isaac ben She'altiel Ḥen*, = *Journal of Semitic Studies*, suppl. 27 (Oxford 2011).

NM 2 — G. Bos, *Novel Medical and General Hebr. Terminology from the 13th Century*, vol. 2, = *Journal of Semitic Studies*, suppl. 30 (Oxford 2013).

NM 3 — G. Bos, *Novel Medical and General Hebrew Terminology: Hippocrates' Aphorisms in the Hebrew Tradition*, = *Journal of Semitic Studies*, suppl. 37 (Oxford 2016).

NM 4 — G. Bos, *Novel Medical and General Hebrew Terminology from the 13th Century*, vol. 4 (Leiden 2019).

NM 5 — G. Bos, *Novel Medical and General Hebrew Terminology from the Middle Ages*, vol. 5 (Leiden 2022).

NTT — N. Nasrallah (trans.), *Treasure Trove of Benefits and Variety at the Table: A Fourteenth-Century Egyptian Cookbook*, with introduction and glossary (Leiden 2018).

PAE — Paul of Aegina, *Epitomes iatrikes biblia hepta* (*Medical Compendium in Seven Books*), vol. 1 (bks. I–IV), ed. by J.L. Heiberg, CMG IX.1 (Leipzig-Berlin 1921–1924).

PESHAT — *Premodern Philosophic and Scientific Hebrew Terminology* ("PESHAT") *in Context: An Online Thesaurus*, ed. by R. Leicht and G. Veltri (Database: https://www.peshat.org).

RL — Fr. Raynouard, *Lexique roman: Ou dictionnaire de la langue des troubadours comparée avec les autres langues de l'Europe latine*, 5 vols. (Heidelberg 1970).

RMA R. Mielck, *Terminologie und Technologie der Müller und Bäcker im islamischen Mittelalter* (Ing. diss., Glückstadt 1914).

RSA G. Bos, M. McVaugh, and J. Shatzmiller (eds.), *The* Regimen Sanitatis *of 'Avenzoar': Stages in the Production of a Medieval Translation* (Leiden 2019).

S J. Derenbourg, J. (ed.), *Targum Ḥamishah Ḥumshei Torah be-Lashon 'Aravit le-Rabbeinu Sa'adyah Ga'on Ben Yoseph ha-Fayyumi* (*Version arabe du Pentateuque de R. Saadia ben Iosef al-Fayyoûmî*) (Repr. Hildesheim 1979).

SCP F. Steingass, *A Comprehensive Persian-English Dictionary* (Repr., London 1984).

SD M. Sokoloff, *A Dictionary of Jewish Palestinian Aramaicof the Byzantine Period* (Ramat Gan 1990).

SDA M. Sokoloff, *A Dictionary of Jewish Babylonian Aramaic of the Talmudic and Geonic Period*, 2nd ed. (Ramat Gan 2020).

ShMM A.O. Shemesh, *Ḥomrei Marpe: Medical Materials in Medieval and Modern Jewish Literature. Pharmacology, History and Halakha* (Ramat Gan 2013).

SHS 1 G. Bos, M. Hussein, G. Mensching, and F. Savelsberg (eds.), *Medical Synonym Lists from Medieval Provence*: *Shem Tov ben Isaac of Tortosa,* Sefer ha-Shimmush, *Book 29—Part 1: Edition and Commentary of List 1* (*Hebrew-Arabic-Romance/Latin*) (Leiden 2011).

SHS 2 G. Bos, J. Kley, G. Mensching, and J. Zwink (eds.), *Medical Synonym Lists from Medieval Provence: Shem Tov ben Isaac of Tortosa,* Sefer ha-Shimmush, *Book 29—Part 2: Edition and Commentary of List 2* (*Romance/Latin-Hebrew-Arabic*) (forthcoming).

SN D. Sontheimer, 'Nachricht von einer arabisch-medicinischen Handschrift, vermutlich des Ibn-Dschezla,' *Janus* 2 (1847): 246–272; repr. in: *Beiträge zur Geschichte der arabisch-islamischen Medizin: Aufsätze*, vol. 1 (1819–1869), ed. by F. Sezgin, in collaboration with M. Amawi, D. Bischoff, and E. Neubauer, 92–128 (Frankfurt am Main 1987).

UW M. Ullmann, *Wörterbuch zu den griechisch-arabischen Übersetzungen des neunten Jahrhunderts* (Wiesbaden 2002).

UWS 1 Ullmann, M., *Wörterbuch zu den griechisch-arabischen Übersetzungen des neunten Jahrhunderts*, suppl. 1: *A–O* (Wiesbaden 2006).

UWS 2 Ullmann, M., *Wörterbuch zu den griechisch-arabischen Übersetzungen des neunten Jahrhunderts*, suppl. 2: *Π–Ω* (Wiesbaden 2007).

VL I.A. Vullers, *Lexicon Persico-Latinum Etymologicum*, 2 vols. (Repr., Graz 1962).

WKAS *Wörterbuch der klassischen arabischen Sprache*, ed. by Deutsche Morgenländische Gesellschaft (Wiesbaden 1957–).

Biblical Sources

Deut	Deuteronomy
Ex	Exodus
Ez	Ezekiel
Is	Isaiah
Ju	Judges
Lam	Lamentations
Lev	Leviticus
Num	Numbers

Rabbinic Sources

bShab	*Babylonian Talmud*, Tractate Shabbat
mPes	*Mishna*, Tractate Pesaḥim

Abbreviations

a.o.	among others
abbr.	abbreviation
Acc.	accusative case
add.	added
Adj.	adjective
Arab.	Arabic
Aram.	Aramaic
Bibl. Hebr.	Biblical Hebrew
conj./conjs.	conjugation(s)
corr.	correction
corresp.	corresponding
Det.	determinative
e.g.	for example (*exempli gratia*)
ed.	edition
emend. ed.	emendation editor
esp.	especially
f.	feminine
fol./fols.	folio(s)
foll.	following
Gen.	genitive case

Gr.	Greek
h.l.	here (*hoc loco*)
Hebr.	Hebrew
i.e.	that is (*id est*)
Inf.	infinitive
intr.	introduction
intrans.	intransitive
l./ll.	line(s)
L. Lat.	Late Latin
Lat.	Latin
lit.	literally
m.	masculine
M. Fr.	Middle French
M. Ir.	Middle Iranian
M. Lat.	Middle Latin
Mod. Cat.	Modern Catalan
Mod. Occ.	Modern Occitan
Mod. Sp.	Modern Spanish
Ms/Mss	manuscript(s)
N.	noun
N. Pers.	New Persian
O. Cat.	Old Catalan
O. Fr.	Old French
o.l.	other language
O. Occ.	Old Occitan
Part.	participle
Pass.	passive
perh.	perhaps
Pers.	Persian
Plur.	plural
poss.	possibly
Rabb.	Rabbinic
re	as related to
resp.	respectively
Rom.	Romance
s.v.	under the word (*sub voce*)
sc.	namely (*scilicet*)
Sing.	singular
trans.	translation
var./vars.	variant(s)
vol./vols.	volume(s)

Introduction

The current volume[1] is part of a wider project aiming at mapping the novel[2] Hebrew[3] technical medical and general terminology as it features in medieval Hebrew medical works translated both from Arabic and Latin.[4] It is my hope that this volume, just like the earlier ones, will facilitate the consultation of medical works and the identification of translators whose identity is unknown or uncertain. An example is the *Sefer ha-Mezonot*, a Hebrew translation of Abu Marwan ʿAbd al-Malik ibn Zuhr, *K. al-Aghdhiya*. My analysis of the technical terminology of the *Sefer ha-Mezonot* and comparison with that featuring in Nathan ha-Meʾati's *Sefer ha-Peraqim* (*Pirqei Moshe*), i.e., his translation of Maimonides, *K. al-Fuṣūl fī al-ṭibb* (*Medical Aphorisms*), confirms the supposition that Nathan is also the translator of this treatise (see below). And in another case, namely that of the translation of Ibn Sīnā, *K. al-Qānūn fī al-ṭibb* II, my research casts doubt on certain assumed identities and calls for a new investigation into all the material at hand (see below).

The main texts consulted are:

1. *Sefer Ṣedat ha-Derakhim*; i.e., Moses ben Samuel ben Judah ibn Tibbon's translation of Ibn al-Jazzār, *Zād al-musāfir wa-qūt al-ḥādir* (*Provisions for*

1 I thank Felix Hedderich for proofreading the manuscript.

2 With 'novel,' I mean those terms that do not feature in the current dictionaries of the Hebrew language at all or that feature in these dictionaries either without proper explanation or in a later period only. Occasionally, I include terms that have already been mentioned in the first five volumes (NM 1–5) dealing with novel Hebrew medical terminology in order to show the wider distribution of a certain term; this is especially the case with terms that appear in earlier sources than those mentioned in previous volumes.

3 In addition to the Hebrew terms, the list below also includes (common) loan words from Latin and Romance.

4 Earlier volumes published are: NM 1 = *Novel Medical and General Hebrew Terminology from the 13th Century: Translations by Hillel ben Samuel of Verona, Moses ben Samuel Ibn Tibbon, Shem Tov ben Isaac of Tortosa, and Zeraḥyah ben Isaac ben She'altiel Ḥen*, = *Journal of Semitic Studies*, suppl. 27 (Oxford 2011); NM 2 = *Novel Medical and General Hebrew Terminology from the 13th Century*, vol. 2, = *Journal of Semitic Studies*, suppl. 30 (Oxford 2013); NM 3 = *Novel Medical and General Hebrew Terminology: Hippocrates'* Aphorisms *in the Hebrew Tradition*, = *Journal of Semitic Studies*, suppl. 37 (Oxford 2016); NM 4 = *Novel Medical and General Hebrew Terminology from the 13th Century*, vol. 4 (Leiden 2019); NM 5 = *Novel Medical and General Hebrew Terminology from the Middle Ages*, vol. 5 (Leiden 2022). The terms listed in NM 1–4 feature also in an alphabetical arrangement in: BCD = *A Concise Dictionary of Novel Medical and General Hebrew Terminology from the Middle Ages* (Leiden 2020) and PESHAT = *Premodern Philosophic and Scientific Hebrew Terminology* ("PESHAT") in *Context: An Online Thesaurus* (https://www.peshat.org).

 | DOI:10.1163/9789004534421_002

the Traveller and the Nourishment for the Sedentary), bks. IV–VII.[5] The terms selected are derived from the forthcoming critical edition of bks. IV–VII.[6] The basic Hebrew manuscript consulted for the edition is Ms Oxford, Bodleian Library, Poc. 353, Uri Heb. 314 (Neubauer 2111).

2. *Sefer Ya'ir Netiv*; a translation made from Constantinus Africanus, *Viaticum peregrinantis*.[7] It was done by an anonymous author living in the Midi who, after his conversion to Christianity, called himself Do'eg ha-Edomi.[8] Between 1197 and 1199 he allegedly translated a corpus of twenty-four medical texts, both practical and theoretical, from Latin into Hebrew. These texts were the first complete Hebrew translations of works by non-Jewish authors on secular subjects. The terms selected are derived from the forthcoming critical edition of bks. IV–VII. The basic manuscript is Ms London, British Library, Add. 18969. In the case of corruptions, omissions, or variant readings, I consulted Ms Moscow, Russian State Library, Guenzburg 1481, or Ms Parma, Biblioteca Palatina, Cod. Parm. 2474. The parallel Latin terms from Constantine's translation are derived from the forthcoming critical edition.
3. *Sefer Ṣedah la-Oreḥim*, bk. VI; an incomplete translation made from the original Arabic text of Ibn al-Jazzār's *Zād al-musāfir wa-qūt al-ḥādir*, prepared by the otherwise unknown Abraham ben Isaac. The terms selected are derived from the forthcoming critical edition. The basic manuscript I consulted is Ms Florence, Biblioteca Medicina Laurenziana, Plut. 88.37, and in the case of corruptions Ms Jerusalem, National Library of Israel, Fr. 95.[9]
4. *Ha-Ma'amar ha-Teshiʿi le-Sefer ha-Mansuri le-Razi*, Ms. Munich, Bayerische Staatsbibliothek, Cod. hebr. 296, copied in the year 1395. It concerns the Hebrew translation by Abraham Avigdor (1351–1402)[10] of *Prac-*

5 For Moses ibn Tibbon's translation, possibly hailing from the year 1259, cf. the intr. to IJZ 1–2:429–437.

6 For the Arabic terms derived from bk. 6, I consulted BIJS; for those derived from bk. 7, chs. 1–6, I consulted G. Bos (ed. and trans.), *Ibn al-Jazzār on Fevers* (London 2000); and for the Arabic as well as the Hebrew terms from Moses ibn Tibbon's translation (*Sefer Ṣedat ha-Derakhim*), derived from bk. 7, chs. 7–30, I consulted IJZ 7.

7 I.e., his Latin translation of Ibn al-Jazzār's *Zād al-musāfir wa-qūt al-ḥāḍir*. The Hebrew translator attributed the text to Ibn al-Jazzār's teacher, Isaac Israeli.

8 For Do'eg ha-Edomi's translation, possibly prepared between 1197 and 1199, cf. IJZ 1–2:595–600; NM 3:3; and also the recent article by G. Freudenthal, M.R. McVaugh, and K. Mesler, 'Twelfth-Century Latin Medicine in Hebrew Garb: Doeg the Edomite as a Cultural Intermediary,' *Medieval Encounters* 26 (2020): 226–284.

9 For Abraham ben Isaac's translation, see IJZ 1–2:525–537; and NM 5:2–3.

10 On Abraham Avigdor (1351–1402), the first Provençal Jew to state explicitly that he studied

tica super nono Almansoris, i.e., Gerard de Solo's commentary on the *Liber nonus ad Almansorem*, i.e., the Latin translation of the *K. al-Manṣūrī fī al-ṭibb* by Abū Bakr Muḥammad ibn Zakarīyā al-Rāzī (Lat. Rhazes), known under the name *Liber ad Almansorem* in the translation of Gerard de Cremona in 1175. Several names of different illnesses employed by Abraham Avigdor have close parallels to those featuring in Moses ibn Tibbon's *Sefer Ṣedat ha-Derakhim*, and in Shem Tov ben Isaac's *Sefer Almansur*. His familiarity with the *Sefer Ṣedat ha-Derakhim* is also borne out by an explicit quotation from it in the chapter on leeches: 'The author of the *Sefer Ṣedat ha-Derakhim* (i.e., Moses ibn Tibbon) said that it is beneficial to gargle with a decoction of lupines, garlic, and colocynth.' The different illnesses featuring in *Ha-Ma'amar ha-Teshi'i* are discussed twice, once under a Hebrew heading and a second time under a Latin heading (in Hebrew transcription). For instance, the illness of spasms is discussed under שער עשירי בחולי הכויצה as well as under שער עשירי דֵי אֶשפַּשמוֹ (fol. 38[a]). The consulted Latin original of *Practica super nono Almansoris* is that printed in Lyon 1504.

5. *Sefer Almansur*; i.e., Shem Tov ben Isaac's translation of al-Rāzī, *K. al-Manṣūrī fī al-ṭibb*, possibly hailing from the year 1264.[11] The manuscript consulted is Ms Vatican, Vatican Library, Urb. Ebr. 50, which was copied in the fifteenth century.[12] The consulted Arabic original manuscript is Ms London, British Library, Or. 5316, dated Mashhad, 1 Ramaḍān 1000 (11 June 1592). For the Latin translation by Gerard de Cremona, entitled *Liber ad Almansorem*, I consulted the edition Venice 1497.
6. *Sefer ha-Refu'ot le-Ḥakham Qoṣṭa'ntin* (ספר הרפואות לחכם קוצטאנתין); a compilation of texts on illnesses from head to toe derived from a Hebrew translation of Constantinus Africanus, *Viaticum peregrinantis*, with relevant quotations from Platearius, Alexander of Tralles, and Orpheus (fol. 131[b]), sometimes with the author's own opinion (cf. fol. 139[b]: ואני אומר), and recipes the author received orally (cf. fols. 129[a], 151[a], 162[a]: שמעתי). The text is extant in Ms Munich, Bayerische Staatsbibliothek, Cod. hebr. 275,

---

at the University of Montpellier, see J. Shatzmiller, *Jews, Medicine, and Medieval Society* (Berkeley 1994), 29–30; L. Ferre, *Práctica de Johannes de Parma: Un tratado farmacologico en sus versiones hebreas y catalana* (Granada 2002), 18–20; and G. Bos, S. Hajek, and G. Mensching, 'A Fragment of Abraham Avigdor's Translation of Gerard de Solo's *Practica* from the Cairo Genizah: Edition and Analysis with Special Regard to the Old Occitan Elements', *Aleph* 21, no. 2 (2021): 309–357.

11 Cf. M. Steinschneider, *Die hebräischen Übersetzungen des Mittelalters und die Juden als Dolmetscher* (Berlin 1893); BMZ 4–6; and SHS 1:10–11.

12 Cf. B. Richler, *Hebrew Manuscripts in the Vatican Library: Catalogue* (Vatican 2008), 632.

fols. 116ª–230ª und was copied in a Sephardic cursive script in the year 1483.[13]

7. *Shinnui ha-Shemot ha-Niqra'im Synonimi* (Ms Florence, Bibliotheca Laurenziana, Or. 17). The Ms is a medical miscellany copied by Abraham ben Moses in Anagni in the year 1464. It contains a.o., an extensive list of 1.749 entries of medical synonyms (fols. 68ª–92ᵇ),[14] and an alphabetical list of substitute drugs, belonging to the genre of *quid pro quo* (substitute drugs) (fols. 10ª–15ᵇ).[15]
8. *Ma'amar ʿal ha-Qaṣeret*;[16] Hebrew translation of Maimonides, *Maqāla fī al-rabw* (*Treatise on Asthma*), ascribed to Samuel Benveniste, who was possibly the physician by that name who lived in Tarragona and Saragossa, served Don Manuel, the brother of King Peter IV of Aragon, and died sometime after 1356.[17]
9. *Ma'amar ʿal ha-Qaṣeret*; Hebrew translation of Maimonides, *On Asthma*, by Joshua Shatibi of Xátiva.[18] Shatibi, called "the scholar in every science, especially medicine," allegedly translated the text for the referendary Fernán Díaz of Toledo at the court of King John II of Castile.
10. *Sefer ha-Qaṣeret*; anonymous Hebrew translation of Maimonides, *On Asthma*.[19] The translation is incomplete, as it stops at XIII.34. An analysis of the Hebrew terminology used by the author shows that he was not familiar with the standard medieval technical (medical) terminology as it was coined by the Tibbonides and other translators. But in spite of this lack of familiarity and the uncommon, often inadequate vocabulary used by the author, he clearly understood the text at hand. The problem was that he did not have adequate tools to deal with it. An indication for a correct understanding of the text and familiarity with its contents is the

13 Cf. M. Steinschneider, *Die hebräischen Handschriften der K. Hof- und Staatsbibliothek in München*, 2nd ed. (Munich 1895); Ktiv: The International Collection of Digitized Hebrew Manuscripts, The National Library of Israel (https://www.nli.org.il/en/discover/manuscripts/hebrew-manuscripts).

14 This list is currently being edited with support of the DFG by a team consisting of G. Bos, F. Hedderich, F. Käs, J. Kley, S. Lauschus, G. Mensching, and F. Savelsberg. For a detailed description, see NM 5:6–7.

15 For a discussion of the genre of *quid pro quo* in medieval Hebrew medical literature, see M. Steinschneider, 'Eine medicinische hebräische Handschrift,' *Magazin für die Wissenschaft des Judentums* 12 (1885): 182–216; and G. Bos, S. Lauschus, and F. Savelsberg, 'Substitute Drugs in the Hebrew Tradition' (forthcoming).

16 For the edition of the Arab. text, see BMA 1.

17 Cf. BMA 2:lii–lviii (introd.), 241–316 (ed.).

18 Cf. BMA 2:lviii–lix (intr.), 319–385 (ed.).

19 Cf. BMA 2:lix–lxii (intr.), 387–448 (ed.).

fact that the names of medicines have generally been transcribed or translated correctly.[20]

11. *Sefer ha-Mezonot*; Hebrew translation of Abu Marwan ʿAbd al-Malik ibn Zuhr, *K. al-Aghdhiya*, Ms Munich, Bayerische Staatsbibliothek, Cod. hebr. 220, fols. 2^a–33^b, copied in a Sephardic semi-cursive script in the fourteenth/fifteenth century.[21] The treatise was translated by a certain "[…] ben Eliezer called *Me'ah Liṭrin*" (אמר ⟨...⟩ בן אלעזר המכונה מאה ליטרין). Moritz Steinschneider suggests that the term *Me'ah Liṭrin* is the name of a place, and remarks that according to Gross, the translator might be identical with Nathan (ben Eliezer) ha-Me'ati, wo hailed from Cento.[22] My analysis of the technical terminology of the *Sefer ha-Mezonot* and comparison with that featuring in his *Sefer ha-Peraqim* (*Pirqei Moshe*) confirms the supposition that Nathan is indeed the translator of this treatise. For the Arabic text of the *K. al-Aghdhiya*, I consulted the edition and translation into Spanish by Expiración García Sánchez.[23]

12. *Sefer ha-Qanun*; Hebrew translation of Ibn Sīnā, *K. al-Qānūn fī al-ṭibb* II, by Nathan ha-Me'ati, Ms Oxford, Bodleian Library, Can. Or. 88, on medical substances, copied in the fourteenth/fifteenth century in a Sephardic semi-cursive script.[24] In case of corruptions, I consulted Ms Paris, BnF, héb. 1136, which was copied in a Sephardic semi-cursive script in Villalón de Campos (Spain) in 1487.[25] Nathan ha-Me'ati's translation of the *K. al-Qānūn fī al-ṭibb* is probably one of the first translations of many Arabic medical works he took upon himself. It has several non-standard, odd, and unprecise expressions, which he corrected in later translations of other medical works,[26] e.g., in his *Sefer ha-Peraqim* (*Pirqei Moshe*).[27] A fur-

20 In case the translations of Maimonides' *On Asthma* have identical terminology, the basic information about the term in question will be part of the entry of the oldest translation that is known.

21 Cf. Steinschneider, *Hebräische Handschriften in München*.

22 On Nathan ha-Me'ati and his translations, see Bos in BMMN 1–4.

23 Madrid 1992.

24 Cf. A. Neubauer, *Catalogue of the Hebrew Manuscripts in the Bodleian Library* (Repr., Oxford 1994), no. 2101.

25 Cf. H. Zotenberg (ed.), *Catalogues des manuscrits hébreux et samaritains de la Bibliothèque Impériale* (Paris 1866), 212; Ktiv (https://www.nli.org.il/en/discover/manuscripts/hebrew-manuscripts). The Arabic edition consulted is that printed in Bulaq 1876 (Repr. in 3 vols.).

26 These non-standard terms are not peculiar to Ms Oxford, Bodleian Library, Can. Or. 88, they also feature in the same quotations in Ms Paris, BnF, héb. 1136.

27 Some examples are: the term עבי for Arab. خشونة ('roughness'), subsequently replaced by

ther indication for an early dating of the translation of the *K. al-Qānūn fī al-ṭibb* can be found in its preface where he explicitly states that he only started his translating enterprise from Arabic into Hebrew once he had acquired sufficient knowledge of both languages to undertake this difficult task.[28]

13. *Sefer ha-Qanun*; Hebrew translation by Zeraḥyah Ḥen, Ms Oxford, Bodleian Library, Opp. Add. Fol. 12, copied in a semi-cursive Sephardic script in the fourteenth/fifteenth century.[29] The terminology featuring in this translation is that recurring in other translations from his hand, notably in his *Sefer ha-Peraqim* (*Pirqei Moshe*).
14. *Sefer ha-Qanun*; anonymous Hebrew translation, Ms Paris, BnF, héb. 1142. This translation is ascribed to Zeraḥyah Ḥen in Ktiv[30] and also in Benjamin Richler's list of manuscripts of the Hebrew translations of the *K. al-Qānūn fī al-ṭibb*;[31] Zotenberg however ascribed the translation to Nathan ha-Meʾati.[32] This discrepancy hails from the technical terminology used by the translator and/or adapter, which partly agrees with Nathan ha-

---

נחירות (BMMG no. 1359 (VI.37, 41; VII.67; XXV.8)); the expression הכשיר ריח הפה for Arab. طيب النكهة ('to improve the smell of the mouth'), replaced by ייטיב ריח הפה (BMMN 217, l. 19 (XXII.68)); the term ספחת for Arab. سعفة ('cradle cap'), replaced by נתק (BMMN 225, l. 15 (XXIII.54)); the term צפד for Arab. غراء ('glue'), replaced by דבק (BMMG no. 3657 (IX.123)); the term קנקן for Arab. حقنة ('enema'), replaced by חוקן (BMMG no. 1021 (IX.47, 48; XIII.35, 37, 40)); or the term סמנים for Arab. بثور ('pustules'), replaced by צמחים (BMMG no. 179 (XXIII.40)).

28 Cf. BMMN 1: 'I have learned the tongues of these foreign nations among which I have dwelt. Until now I have lingered; till I have acquired distinct speech and the tongue of the learned, lovely and pleasant, Hebrew and Arabic joined together. I have kept them in my heart and they have become united in my hand.' If one accepts the supposition that the translation of the *K. al-Qānūn fī al-ṭibb*, completed in 1279, is one of his earlier endeavors, if not the earliest, it would also mean that the translation of the *Medical Aphorisms* must have been completed at some time after that date, and not shortly after 1277 as supposed by Steinschneider (cf. Steinschneider, *Hebräische Übersetzungen des Mittelalters*, 766).

29 Cf. Neubauer, *Catalogue of Hebrew Manuscripts*, no. 2099. According to Mauro Zonta, the manuscript is the archetype copied from a lost autograph, see 'Zeraḥyah: Philosopher and Translator and his Role in 13th Century Rome' (Paper read in Jerusalem, January 1, 2007).

30 https://www.nli.org.il/en/discover/manuscripts/hebrew-manuscripts/itempage?docId=PNX_MANUSCRIPTS990001316280205171&vid=MANUSCRIPTS&SearchTxt=paris%201142.

31 See B. Richler, 'Manuscripts of Avicenna's *Kanon* in Hebrew Translation: A Revised and Up-to-Date List,' *Korot* 30, no. 8 (1982): 163, no. 77.

32 Zotenberg, *Catalogues des manuscrits hébreux*, 212.

Me'ati[33] and partly with Zeraḥyah Ḥen[34] but is also partly different from that used by both translators.[35] For this reason, I have omitted the name of the translator. The uncertain identity of the translator not only concerns this particular manuscript, but also two others, namely (1) Ms Jerusalem, National Library of Israel, Fr. 122 (abbr. J122) that was copied in a Sephardic script in the fourteenth century in Provence,[36] and (2) Ms Parma, Biblioteca Palatina, Cod. Parm. 2920 (abbr. P2920) that was copied in a Sephardic script in Lecce in 1473.[37] My conclusion is based on a comparison of the main subentries describing the different properties of the plants listed in eleven manuscripts accessible online.[38] Both

33 Some examples are: בקיעים ('cracks,' see entry בָּקִיעַ); זוז ('measure of weight; *dirham*'); טֶרִי ('bleeding (of a wound)'); הסם הממרק ('detergent drug'); הסם המתיך ('dissolving drug,' see entry סַם). In some cases, the terminology is identical or nearly identical to that featuring in other works translated by Nathan ha-Me'ati, such as in his *Sefer ha-Peraqim* (*Pirqei Moshe*): התיצבות הנשימה ('orthopnea,' see entry הַצָּבָה; cf. הִתְיַצְּבוּת in BCD 75; NM 2:42; BMMG no. 5143 (XXIV.38)); מתיחה ('spasm; cramp; convulsion,' see entry הִשְׁתַּטְּחוּת; cf. BMMG no. 4732 (IX.91)); חלב בקר מסוכסך ('buttermilk,' see entry: חֶמְאָה; cf. החלב המשוכשך in BCD 94; NM 2:63; BMMG no. 4719 (XXIII.107)); הפשט המעיים ('[intestinal] abrasion,' see entry נֶגַע; cf. הֶפְשֵׁט in BCD 71; NM 2:40–41); הניח למטה ('to apply in a suppository,' see entry סָבַל; cf. BCD 171; NM 2:65–66; BMMG no. 1183 (XVI.18)); צמחים ('pimples,' see entry סִמָּן; cf. BMMG no. 179 (XXIII.40)); מרוק ('deterging property,' entry תַּמְרוּק; cf. BMMG no. 667 (XIII.6)); יגיעה ('fatigue,' see entry עַצְלָה; cf. BMMG no. 3599).

34 Some examples are: גבניות ('cheese-like substance,' see entry גִּבּוּן); חושים ('senses,' see entry הַרְגָּשָׁה); קצף ('foam,' see entry זַעַף); שטות ('mania; madness,' see entry טִפְּשׁוּת); מותרות ('superfluities,' see entry יִתְרוֹן); פעולות ('[healing] effects,' see entry מִפְעָל); נחירות הקול ('hoarseness,' see entry נְחוּר); נתק ('scurf; dandruff; favus,' see entry סַפַּחַת); רַעַשׁ ('trembling; tremor').

35 Some examples are: הגרב המשתחן ('ulcerating scabies,' see entry גָּרָב); כמינת הדם ('dark grey color,' see entry הַטְמָנָה); החום הטבעי ('the innate heat,' see entry חֹם); הניח הנחה חמה ('to foment,' see entry [חתל]); עדשי הפנים ('freckles,' see entry כֶּתֶם); לקוה ('paralysis of the facial nerve,' see entry לָקוּת); זכאם ('rheum,' see entry מִלּוּי); הנתק הנקר׳ סעפה ('scurf; dandruff; favus,' see entry מִסְפַּחַת); סמור ('shivering fit; rigor,' see entry נְעִירָה).

36 Data derived from Ktiv (https://www.nli.org.il/en/discover/manuscripts/hebrew-manuscripts).

37 Cf. B. Richler, *Hebrew Manuscripts in the Biblioteca Palatina in Parma: Catalogue* (Jerusalem 2001), 443 (no. 1507).

38 These manuscripts are: (1) Ms Jerusalem, National Library of Israel, Fr. 122; (2) Jerusalem, National Library of Israel, Heb. 4°607; (3) Paris, BN, héb. 1136; (4) Paris, BnF, héb. 1137; (5) Paris, BnF, héb. 1141; (6) Ms Paris, BnF, héb. 1142; (7) Ms Paris, BnF, héb. 1145; (8) Parma, Biblioteca Palatina, Cod. Parm. 2920; (9) Moscow, Russian State Library, Guenzburg 573; (10) Ms Oxford, Bodleian Library, Opp. Add. fol. 12; and (11) Ms London, British Library, Add. 21967. Not part of this list is Ms Paris, BnF, héb. 1146 (copied in an Ashkenazi script in the fourteenth century), because it is not a straightforward translation but a severely abbreviated version, as already noted by Zotenberg, *Catalogues des manuscrits hébreux*, 212.

manuscripts (J122 and P2920) are ascribed to Nathan ha-Me'ati in Ktiv but share characteristic terms of the subentries with Ms Paris, BnF, héb. 1142 (abbr. P1142), ascribed to Zeraḥyah Ḥen in Ktiv. These subentries and their Hebrew translations are:

(1) 'identity (what is it?)' (الماهية): המהות (both Nathan and Zeraḥyah); מהות (J122; P2920; and P1142);
(2) 'choice' (الاختيار): המבחר (Nathan); המובחר (Zeraḥyah); הבחירה (J122; P2920; and P1142)
(3) 'nature (temperament)' (الطبع): הטבע (both Nathan and Zeraḥyah); הטבע (J122; P2920 and P1142)
(4) 'actions and specific properties' (الأفعال والخواصّ): המפעלים והסגולות (Nathan); הפעולות והסגולות (Zeraḥyah); הפעולות והסגולות (J122; P2920; and P1142)

These four general entries are followed by more specific ones, detailing the healing properties of the plant in question for different skin afflictions and organs of the body:

(5) 'cosmetics' (الزينة): העדי (Nathan); היפוי (Zeraḥyah); הקשוט (J122; P2920; and P1142)
(6) 'swellings (tumors) and pimples' (الأورام والبثور): המורסות והסימנים (Nathan); המורסות והבתור (Zeraḥyah); הצמחים והמורסות (J122; P2920; and P1142)
(7) 'wounds and ulcers' (الجراح والقروح): המכות והנגעים (Nathan); החבלות והנגעים (Zeraḥyah); החבורות והשחינים (J122; P2920; and P1142)
(8) 'organs of the head' (أعضاء الرأس): א(י)ברי הראש (Nathan); א(י)ברי הראש (Zeraḥyah); איברי הראש (J122; P2920; and P1142)
(9) 'parts of the eye' (أعضاء العين): א(י)ברי העין (Nathan); א(י)ברי העין (Zeraḥyah); איברי העין (J122; P2920; and P1142)
(10) 'excretory organs' (أعضاء النفض): איברי הנעירה (Nathan); איברי הנקיון (Zeraḥyah); איברי הנפוץ (J122; P2920; and P1142)

The following table of the first entry dealing with the 'identity' (המהות; see entry מָהוּת below) of the plant melilot may be further indication of how the three manuscripts J122, P2920, and P1142 form a distinct group within the translations of the *K. al-Qānūn fī al-ṭibb* and cannot simply be ascribed to either Nathan ha-Me'ati or Zeraḥyah Ḥen, but possibly represent an adaptation or even independant translation. Further research may throw more light upon this complicated question.

Nathan, Ms Oxford, Bodleian Library, Can. Or. 88, fol. 61[a]	Zeraḥyah, Ms Oxford, Bodleian Library, Opp. Add. Fol. 12, fol. 166[a]	J122, fol. 181[a]	P2920, fol. 14[a]	P1142, fol. 22[a]
אכליל אלמלך:	**אִכְלִיל אַלְמַלִךְ:** מַלִילוֹטָה.	**אכליל אלמלך:** כלומר נזר המלך ונקרא בלשונם מלילוט.	**אכליל אלמלך:** כלומ׳ נזר המלך ונק׳ בלשונם מלילוט.	**אכליל אלמלך:** כלו׳ נזר המלך ונקר׳ בלשונם מלילוט.
חמהות הוא ציץ צמח תבניי הגוון עגול כתכונת הלבנה יש בו עם הרוך קושי כל שהוא ויש ממנו מכורכם.	**חמהות** הוא פרח עשב מראהו כמראה התבן צורתה כמו הירח יש בו עם רפיונו קושי ויהיה ממנו לבן ויהיה ממנו צִיטְרִינוֹ.	**מהות** הוא פרח צמח תבניי המראה ירחיי בתבנית יש בו עם רפיונו איזה קושי ויש ממנו לבן ויש ממנו כרכומי.	**מהות** הוא פרח צמח תבניי המראה ירחיי כתבנית יש בו טעם עם רפיונו איזה קושי ויש ממנו לבן ויש ממנו כרכומי.	**מהות** הוא פרח צמח תבניי המראה ירחיי בתבנית יש בו עם רפיונו איזה קושי ויש ממנו לבן ויש ממנו כרכומי.

In addition to the primary sources listed above, occasional reference will be made to secondary ones that have not been searched systematically and will only be named as part of a specific entry.

List of Terms

א

אִבּוּן • אבון הפרקים • stiffness of the joints (ankylosis): Arab. حجر المفاصل · Ibn Sīnā, *K. al-Qānūn fī al-ṭibb* · trans. Nathan ha-Me'ati, *Sefer ha-Qanun*, fol. 75[b]: גבן הוא הגבנה ... ישחקו הישן ממנו עם זית או במי כרעי חזיר ויעשו ממנו תחבשת לאבון הפרקים (Cheese: ... Old cheese, pounded with olive oil or water of pig's trotters, is used as a plaster for stiffness of the joints). Hebr. אבון הפרקים is not attested in the current dictionaries. Zeraḥyah Ḥen translates Arab. حجر المفاصل as קושי הפרקים and Anonymous renders Arab. حجر المفاصل as התאבנות הפרקים (see entry הִתְאַבְּנוּת).

אֶבֶן • אבן הלבנה • moonstone (selenite): Arab. حجر القمر (Gr. λίθος σεληνίτης) · [*Synonima*], Ms Vatican, Biblioteca Apostolica, ebr. 550, fol. 120[b]: חגר אלקמר הוא אבן הלבונה (הלבנה*) ([Arab.] *ḥajar al-qamar*; i.e., [Hebr.] *even ha-levanah*). In the sense of 'moonstone (selenite),' Hebr. אבן הלבנה is a non-attested calque of Arab. حجر القمر.

• אבן הרחים • (lit., 'millstone'); a hard formation in a woman's womb: Arab. حجر الرحى, after Gr. μύλη (cf. Maimonides, *K. al-Fuṣūl fī al-ṭibb* (*Medical Aphorisms*) XXIII.97) · [*Synonima*], Ms Vatican, Biblioteca Apostolica, ebr. 550,[1] fol. 120[b]: חגר אלרחא הוא אבן הרחיים ([Arab.] *ḥajar al-raḥā* (lit., 'millstone'); i.e., [Hebr.] *even ha-reḥayim*). Hebr. אבן הרחים is a non-attested calque of Arab. حجر الرحى. For רחים on its own and in the same sense, see entry רֵחַיִם.

• אבן שיש • (lit., 'marble stone'); a pounding stone (mortar): Arab. صَلاَّيَة (cf. FL 2:517: 'lapis, in quo teruntur odoramenta' (from Pers. صلاّية; cf. VL 2:516: 'lapis manualis in quo medicamenta teruntur')) · Ibn al-Jazzār, *Zād al-musāfir wa-qūt al-ḥāḍir* · trans. Moses ibn Tibbon, *Sefer Ṣedat ha-Derakhim* VI.6: ואחר ישתדל במורסא בטיחות כמו שיקח עלי ארן[2] וינגבם וישרפם ויקח אפרם וישחקהו בשמן ורדים על אבן שיש ויטוח בו המורסא (Then one should look after the tumor and treat it with plasters. Take, e.g., boxthorn/buckthorn leaves, dry and burn them, take the ashes and pound them with rose oil in a mortar and rub this on the tumor). Hebr. אבן שיש is not attested in the current dictionaries.

אָבָק • אבק הברזל • iron slag; scoria: Lat. *ferrugo* (cf. DMLBS 1177) (Arab. خبث الحديد; cf. KM 1:545–548) · Constantinus Africanus, *Viaticum peregrinantis* · trans. Do'eg ha-Edomi, *Sefer Ya'ir Netiv* IV.19: ונשמור שלא נתן לו כבוס מחודד כמו אלואין אשקמוניא קולוקונטידא ונתן לו טריפרא הגדולה והקטנה וריקוח העשוי עם אבק הברזל (We should be careful not to give him [i.e., someone suffering from hemorrhoids] a sharp purgative such as aloe, scammony, colocynth, but we should give him the large and small tryphera[3] and the remedy prepared with iron slag). Hebr. אבק הברזל does not fea-

1 For the list featuring on fols. 113[b]–131[a] and for the Ms copied in the early fourteenth century, cf. Richler, *Hebrew Manuscripts Vatican*, 466.

2 ארן: عوسج a.

3 'tryphera': A generic drug name, lent to certain compound preparations that were considered

ture in this sense in the current dictionaries. Moses ibn Tibbon translates Arab. خبث الحديد as סיג הברזל.

אֵבֶר • איברי הנעירה · **excretory organs:** Arab. أعضاء النفض · Ibn Sīnā, *K. al-Qānūn fī al-ṭibb* · trans. Nathan ha-Me'ati, *Sefer ha-Qanun* II, fol. 61[b] (Ms Paris, BnF, héb. 1136, fol. 63[a]): אפסנתין ... איברי נעירה: משלשל השתן ודם הוסת שלשול חזק וקל וחומר כשעושין ממנו תשומות עם דבש וישלשל המרה האדומה (Absinth wormwood ... Excretory organs: It acts as a strong diuretic or emmenagogue, especially when used as a vaginal suppository (pessary) with honey and acts as a purgative for the yellow bile). Hebr. איברי הנעירה is not attested in the current dictionaries. Zeraḥyah Ḥen translates Arab. أعضاء النفض as איברי הנקיון and Anonymous renders Arab. أعضاء النفض as איברי הנפוץ (see next entry).

• **איברי הנפוץ** · **excretory organs**: Arab. أعضاء النفض · Ibn Sīnā, *K. al-Qānūn fī al-ṭibb* · Anonymous, *Sefer ha-Qanun* II, fols. 23[a]–24[b]: אפסנתין[4] הוא אבשנסי ... איברי הנפוץ מגיר השתן והנדות בחוזק וכל שכן פתילה עם הדבש ומשלשל האדומה (Absinth wormwood, i.e., [Rom.] ʾBŠNSY ... Excretory organs: It acts as a strong diuretic or emmenagogue, especially when used as a vaginal suppository (pessary) with honey and acts as a purgative for the yellow bile). Hebr. איברי הנפוץ is not attested in the current dictionaries. The term נִפּוּץ on its own features in BM 3717 in the sense of 'dispersal; scattering; shattering.' Nathan ha-Me'ati translates Arab. أعضاء النفض as איברי הנעירה (see previous entry) and Zeraḥyah Ḥen as איברי הנקיון.

• *Plur.* **אברים • עזר האברים** → עֵזֶר.

• **רפיון האיברים** → רִפְיוֹן.

אַבְרָהָם • אילן אברהם → אִילָן.

אֲגֻדָּה · **swelling; inflammation:** Lat. *nodus* · Gerard de Solo, *Practica super nono Almansoris* · trans. Abraham Avigdor, *Ha-Ma'amar ha-Teshi'i le-Sefer ha-Mansuri le-Razi*, fol. 97[b]: שער באגודה אשר תתקשר תחת הלשון ותקרא צפרדע (Chapter on a swelling arising beneath the tongue that is called 'frog' [i.e., Lat. *ranula*]). In the sense of 'swelling,' Hebr. אֲגֻדָּה features in BM 41 in an attestation from the *Sefer Asaph ha-Rofe*. Shem Tov ben Isaac translates the parallel Arab. term غدّة as צְפַרְדֵּעַ (see entry).

אגודה → אֲגֻדָּה.

אדום → אָדֹם.

אדומה → אֲדָמָה.

אָדֹם · **bilious; choleric:** Lat. *colericus* (Arab. صفراوي) · Constantinus Africanus, *Viaticum peregrinantis* · trans. Do'eg ha-Edomi, *Sefer Ya'ir Netiv* IV.17: וסבת החולי הוא בשבעה ענינים. הראשון הוא כאשר החום האשי והאדום נוסף על התוצאות ובסבה הזאת לחות

to be 'based' on myrobalans and often further split into types of 'smaller' or 'larger' complexity and strength; cf. O. Kahl, *The Sanskrit, Syriac, and Persian Sources in the* Comprehensive Book *of Rhazes* (Leiden 2015), 123–124.

4 אפסנתין: אבשנסו Ms[1]

התוצאות יבש ונתקשה ועל כן לא יצאו (This illness [i.e., a colic] is caused by [one of] seven matters. The first is when the fiery, choleric heat increases over the feces and consequently the moisture of the feces dries up [and they] become hard and cannot be passed). Hebr. אֹדֶם does not feature in this sense in the current dictionaries. Moses ibn Tibbon translates Arab. صفراوي as כַּרְכֻּמִי (see entry).

אֹדֶם • אודם ביצים · **egg yolk**: Lat. *vitellus ovorum* (Arab. صفر البيض) · Constantinus Africanus, *Viaticum peregrinantis* · trans. Do'eg ha-Edomi, *Sefer Ya'ir Netiv* IV.14: ונאכילהו תרנוגלים קטנים פרדיץ פאיין[5] עם אודם ביצים (We give him to eat young chickens, partridge, and pheasant with egg yolk). Hebr. אודם ביצים is attested as אודם הביצה in BCD 18 (NM 1:128) in a later attestation from Zeraḥyah Ḥen, *Sefer ha-Peraqim* (*Pirqei Moshe*) (corr.) II.3 (cf. BMMZ 28, l. 2; BMMZ no. 2897). Moses ibn Tibbon translates the parallel Arab. term صفر البيض as חלמון ביצה.

אֲדֻמָּה · **red (yellow) bile**: Lat. *colera rubea* (Arab. المرّة الصفراء) · Constantinus Africanus, *Viaticum peregrinantis* · trans. Do'eg ha-Edomi, *Sefer Ya'ir Netiv* IV.6: ואם הצמאון יהיה מהאדומה נסגרת באסטומכא יכובס עם פרמסיא ועם וומיט (Thirst caused by red (yellow) bile that is enclosed in the stomach should be purged with PRMSY' [i.e., Lat. *farmacie* ('remedies')] and with WWMYṬ [i.e., Lat. *vomitu* ('vomiting')]). In the sense of 'red (yellow) bile,' Hebr. אֲדֻמָּה features in BM 54, s.v. אדומה, in later attestations, a.o., from the *Sefer ha-Qanun* (cf. also BCD 17–18 (NM 2:166) for an attestation from David Caslari, *Sefer Ro'a Mezeg Mitḥallef* IV.3). Moses ibn Tibbon translates Arab. المرّة الصفراء as מרה כרכומית.

אודם → אֹדֶם.

אוזן → אֹזֶן.

אֲוִיר • *Plur.* **אוירים** · **vapors**: Arab. أبخرة · Maimonides, *Maqāla fī al-rabw* (*On Asthma*) · trans. Samuel Benveniste, *Ma'amar 'al ha-Qaṣeret* XIII.1 (cf. BMA 2:297, ll. 4–6): הראוי להשגיח תחלה בתקון האויר ואחר כן בתקון המים ואחר כן בתקון המסעדים. והוא כי מה שיקראו הרופאים רוחות הם אוירים קלים נמצאים בגוף החי (One should first pay attention to the improvement of the air, then to the improvement of the water, and then to the improvement of the foods [we take]. This is so because what the physicians call 'pneumas' are fine vapors found in the bodies of living creatures). Hebr. אֲוִיר, *Plur.* אוירים, does not feature in this sense in the current dictionaries. Joshua Shatibi and Anonymous both render Arab. أبخرة as אדים.

אוֹכֵל (*Part.*) → אָכַל.

אונגלון • בקיעות הקורה מן האונגלון → בְּקִיעָה.

אופל → אֹפֶל.

אֹזֶן • מורסות שרשי האזן → מֻרְסָה.

• **צליל באוזן** → צְלִיל.

• **הקול הנשמע באוזן** → קוֹל.

---

5 פאיין: פאישון Ms Parma, Biblioteca Palatina, Cod. Parm. 2474 *fasianum* L.

אַחֲרוֹן • החלקים האחרונים → חֵלֶק.

אֲטִימוּת · **dullness of understanding**: Arab. بلادة فهم · Maimonides, *Maqāla fī al-rabw* (*On Asthma*) · trans. Samuel Benveniste, *Ma'amar 'al ha-Qaṣeret* XIII.3 (cf. BMA 2:297, ll. 15–17): ועל כן תמצא רבים מבני אדם ירגישו בחסרון פעולות⟨יה⟩ם הנפשיות בחסרון האויר ר״ל שיתחדש להם אטימות וקצר השגה וחסרון זכרנות (Therefore, one sees that many people notice a deterioration in their psychical functions with the corruption of the air—that is to say that they suffer from dullness of understanding, lack of comprehension, and loss of memory). Hebr. אֲטִימוּת features in BM 168 in a later attestation from Joseph Albo, *Sefer ha-Iqqarim* in the sense of 'stupidity' and in PESHAT[6] as 'difficulty in comprehension' with an additional attestation from Menahem Bonafos, *Sefer ha-Gedarim*; cf. EM 48. Joshua Shatibi translates Arab. بلادة فهم as עצלת ההבנה and Anonymous has נמהרות הבנה.

אֵיכוּת • *Plur.* איכויות · **conditions**: Lat. *qualitas* (Arab. أحوال) · Constantinus Africanus, *Viaticum peregrinantis* · trans. Do'eg ha-Edomi, *Sefer Ya'ir Netiv* V.3: כפי שיתראה כח החולי ואיכויות החולה ונערב יחד מהרפואה המורכבת המועילה אל הצמח החם (According to our observation of the severity of the illness and the conditions of the patient, we mix [the aforementioned ingredients] with a compound medicine that is beneficial for a hot tumor). Hebr. אֵיכוּת features in medieval philosophical and scientific literature in the sense of 'category of quality' and in mathematical literature in the sense of 'denominator; number below the line in a fraction, divisor of the numerator; positional value; value of the rank in the positional decimal system' (cf. PESHAT[7]). Moses ibn Tibbon translates Arab. أحوال as ענינים.

אֵיכְיוּת · **quality**: Arab. كيفية · Ibn al-Jazzār, *Zād al-musāfir wa-qūt al-ḥādir* · trans. Abraham ben Isaac, *Sefer Ṣedah la-Oreḥim* VI.10: ותהיה הירידה או מחמת כמיותה או מחמת אכיותיה ([Loss of blood occurring to women] can be caused either by its quantity or by its quality). Hebr. אֵיכְיוּת is a non-attested var. of אֵיכוּת, which is used by Moses ibn Tibbon and also by Do'eg ha-Edomi for the parallel Lat. term *qualitas*.

אִילָן • אילן אברהם · **(lit., 'Abraham's tree'); chaste tree [*Vitex agnus-castus* L.]**: Lat. *agnus castus* · [*Synonima*], Ms. Oxford, Bodleian Library, Opp. 180 (Neubauer 2134),[8] fol. 149b: א⟨נ⟩גנוש קשטוש אילן ופירי הנולד אצל הים אילן אברהם ([Lat.] *agnus castus*; the tree and its fruit, growing near the sea; [Hebr.] *ilan Avraham*). Hebr. אילן אברהם is not attested in the current dictionaries. It also features in Shem Tov ben Isaac, *Sefer ha-Shimmush* XXIX, list 1 (SHS 1:114 (Alef 30)). The synonyms עץ אברהם and העץ הצנוע are mentioned by Löw (cf. LF 3:491–492).

---

6 https://peshat.org/display/peshat_lemmas_00000152 (accessed March 24, 2022).

7 https://peshat.org/display/peshat_lemmas_00000157 (accessed March 24, 2022).

8 The manuscript is a medical miscellany that was copied in the beginning of the fourteenth century in an Ashkenazic semi-cursive script. The synonyms are in Latin-German, with occasional Hebrew.

אימוץ → אִמּוּץ.

אַיִן • האין בשול · **bad digestion; lack of digestion**: Lat. *indigestibilitas* (Arab. سوء الهضم) · Constantinus Africanus, *Viaticum peregrinantis* · trans. Do'eg ha-Edomi, *Sefer Ya'ir Netiv* v.5: דיאברברום זה יועיל לאפיסת הכבד ולסתימתו ואל רוח הקרבים ואל האין בשול (*Diabarbarum* [i.e., a rhubarb compound]: It is beneficial for weakness and obstruction of the liver, wind in the intestines, and bad digestion). Hebr. האין בשול is not attested in the current dictionaries. Moses ibn Tibbon translates Arab. سوء الهضم as רוע הבשול (for his use of this term for Arab. تخمة ('indigestion') in *Sefer Ṣedat ha-Derakhim* iv.9, see entry רֹעַ).

אִינְדִּי • לוז אינדי → לוז.

איפיטימא · **poultice**: Lat. *epithema* (from Gr. ἐπίθεμα) (Arab. ضمّد) · Constantinus Africanus, *Viaticum peregrinantis* · trans. Do'eg ha-Edomi, *Sefer Ya'ir Netiv* v.3: ונעשה לו איפיטימא משמן נרדי ומשמן אירין ומשמן קשטור ומשמן משטיק ודומיהם (We should prepare a poultice for him [i.e., someone suffering from a hard liver or spleen] made from nard oil, lily oil, castor oil, mastic oil, and the like). Hebr. איפיטימא is a non-attested loan word from Lat. *epithema*. Moses ibn Tibbon translates Arab. ضمّد as חבש.

אָכַל • *Part.* **אוֹכֵל** · **corrosive**: Arab. أكّال · Ibn Sīnā, *K. al-Qānūn fī al-ṭibb* · trans. Nathan ha-Me'ati, *Sefer ha-Qanun* ii, fol. 82b: זנגאר ... הוא ממרק אוכל הבשר הקשה והרך יחד והוא חד (Verdigris: ... It is detergent and pungent and corrosive both for hard and soft flesh). In the sense of 'to corrode,' Hebr. אָכַל features in BM 212, a.o., in a later attestation from Abraham Portaleone, *Shiltei ha-Gibborim*. For *Part. Hitpa'el* מִתְאַכֵּל in the same sense, cf. BCD 21 (NM 4:16) for an attestation from Abraham Avigdor, *Pirqei Arnavṭ de-Vila Nova* v.96 (AMP 110).

• *Pi'el* **אִכֵּל** · **to digest**: Arab. استمرأ · Maimonides, *Maqāla fī al-rabw* (*On Asthma*) · trans. Anonymous, *Sefer ha-Qaṣeret* ii.2 (cf. BMA 2:393, ll. 24–26): ואמר בפרק אחר מאמר זה לשונו: ולפיכך איעץ לכל בני אדם שימנעו מכל המאכלים המולידים הלחות הרעות ואפילו שהאדם יאכלם בקלות ומהירות אל יסתכן[9] בזה שבאורך הימים יתקבץ מהן בגידיו והוא לא ירגיש [ש]לחה רעה (In another chapter, he [i.e., Galen] said the following: Therefore, I advise everyone to abstain from all the foodstuffs that produce bad humors; even if someone digests them easily and quickly, he should not be deluded[10] by this, for in the process of time one of these bad humors will collect in his veins while he does not notice it). In the sense of 'to digest,' Hebr. אִכֵּל is not attested in the current dictionaries. Samuel Benveniste and Joshua Shatibi both translate Arab. استمرأ as עִכֵּל.

אֲלוּם • אלום לבן · **white alum**: Arab. شبّ أبيض · Ibn al-Jazzār, *Zād al-musāfir wa-qūt al-ḥādir* · trans. Moses ibn Tibbon, *Sefer Ṣedat ha-Derakhim* iv.15: תואר עוגות אחרות

---

9 יסתכן: بغترّ a.

10 'deluded': Trans. after a.

מארסיניקום ואורופימנט יועילו כמו אשר לפניהם והם חזקות מנוסות ערובם: יקח ארסיניקום ואורופימינט ושמרי חומץ יין מנוגב שרוף ואכסיא וגומא ארביקא מ״א שקל וסיד בלתי מכובה וכאגד שרוף מ״א ב׳ דר׳ אלום לבן דר׳ אופי חצי דר׳ יודקו הסמים וינופו ויולשו ביין אדום ריחני ויעשה עוגות ויגגבם בצל וירגילם (A recipe for other pastilles with red and yellow arsenic that are beneficial just like the ones [mentioned] before and that are strong and tested: Take one *sheqel*[11] each of red and yellow arsenic, of dried, burned vinegar sediment, of acacia gum, and of gum Arabic, two *dirhams* each of quicklime and burned papyrus, one *dirham* of white alum, half a *dirham* of opium. Pound the ingredients, sieve them, knead them with red wine, make pastilles, dry them in the shade and apply them). The term אלום לבן is a non-attested mixed term, consisting of Rom. (O. Occ. or O. Cat.) *alum*; i.e., 'alum' (cf. SHS 1:308 (Mem 210)) and Hebr. *lavan* ('white'). Do'eg ha-Edomi renders the parallel Lat. term *alumen* as אלום.

אֵם • מציקת האם → מְצוּקָה.

אַמָּה • זקיפת האמה ברוב → זְקִיפָה.

אִמּוּץ • I. **retention [of food] (constipation)**: Arab. احتباس (Gr. ἐπίσχεσις/ἐποχή; cf. UW1:390, 395) · Maimonides, *Maqāla fī al-rabw* (*On Asthma*) · trans. Anonymous, *Sefer ha-Qaṣeret* N.4 (cf. BMA 2:389, l. 10): הפרק הט׳ בהנהגת האימוץ והשלשול (Chapter nine: On the [proper] regimen for retention and evacuation). Hebr. אִמּוּץ does not feature in this sense in the current dictionaries. Samuel Benveniste translates Arab. احتباس as הַעֲמָדָה (see entry) and Joshua Shatibi has העצר.

· II. **astringency**: Arab. قبض · Maimonides, *Maqāla fī al-rabw* (*On Asthma*) · trans. Anonymous, *Sefer ha-Qaṣeret* V.4 (cf. BMA 2:404, ll. 7–8): וכמו כן יקדים מה שיש בו שלשול ויאחר מה שיש בו אימוץ לפי כל[12] דעת (Similarly, one should first [eat] that which has a diluting effect and then [eat] that which is astringent, according to the opinion of all[13] [physicians]). Hebr. אִמּוּץ does not feature in this sense in the current dictionaries. Samuel Benveniste renders Arab. قبض as חבישה and Joshua Shatibi has קביצות.

[אמן] • *Part. Nif'al* **נֶאֱמָן** · **chronic**: Arab. مزمن · Maimonides, *Maqāla fī al-rabw* (*On Asthma*) · trans. Samuel Benveniste, *Ma'amar 'al ha-Qaṣeret* XIII.36 (cf. BMA 2:311, ll. 1–2): ויצורים רבים הגיעו לחלי נאמן מפני שכחם נמק וחלש מרב ההרקה (Many people fell victim to a chronic illness because they lost their strength as a result of excessive bleeding). In the sense of 'chronic,' Hebr. נֶאֱמָן features in BCD 23 (NM 4:110) in an attestation from Judah ben Jacob, *Hanhagat ha-Beri'ut*. Joshua Shatibi translates Arab. مزمن as נמשך, which features in the sense of 'lasting' in medieval philosophical literature (cf. BM 3378; KTP 3:43; PESHAT[14]).

11 Hebr. *sheqel* stands for Arab. *mithqāl*. One *mithqāl* equals 4.46 grams; cf. HIM 4–7.

12 كل :بعض a.

13 'all': 'some' a.

14 https://peshat.org/display/peshat_lemmas_00003140 (accessed March 24, 2022).

[אמץ] • *Nitpaʿel* **נִתְאַמֵּץ** · **to be dry [of one's stools], suffer from constipation**: Arab. يبس · Maimonides, *Maqāla fī al-rabw* (*On Asthma*) · trans. Samuel Benveniste, *Maʾamar ʿal ha-Qaṣeret* IX.1 (cf. BMA 2:271, ll. 2–4): מן ההנהגה הטובה לכל בני אדם וכל שכן למי שיתקבצו בגופו הלחות שיהיה טבעו רפה לעולם או קרוב מן הרפיון. ואם נתאמץ בקצת העתים ועמד בזה ימים ירפה עצמו (A good regimen for all people—and especially for someone in whose body [bad] humors have accumulated—is that the stools always be soft or nearly soft. When [the stools] are dry at a certain moment and stay like that for some days, one should soften them). In the sense of 'to suffer form constipation,' Hebr. נִתְאַמֵּץ features in BM 289 in an attestation from Maimonides, *Mishneh Torah: Hilkhot Deʿot*. Joshua Shatibi and Anonymous render Arab. يبس as נתייבש.

אָמַר · **to prescribe**: Arab. وصف · Ibn al-Jazzār, *Zād al-musāfir wa-qūt al-ḥādir* · trans. Abraham ben Isaac, *Sefer Ṣedah la-Oreḥim* VI.6: וזו משיחה אמר אותה אצחק בן סלימאן לפלגמוני שבשתי הביצים הבא מחמת רוח חמה וכבר נסיתיה (This is the composition of a plaster (salve) prescribed by Isḥāq ibn Sulaymān for a tumor of the testicles caused by a hot flatulence. I have tested it). In the sense of 'to prescribe,' Hebr. אָמַר is not attested in the current dictionaries. Moses ibn Tibbon translates Arab. وصف as *Piʿel* סִפֵּר (see entry [ספר]).

אנידא · **duck**: Arab. بط · Ibn al-Jazzār, *Zād al-musāfir wa-qūt al-ḥādir* · trans. Moses ibn Tibbon, *Sefer Ṣedat ha-Derakhim* IV.19: אם יהיה בפי הטבעת סדיקה והחדוד והכאב הטוב לו מכל הדברים ריר זרע חבושים או ריר דרגגן או שומן תרנגולת או אנידא (If there is a fissure in the anus and a sharp pain, the best [medication] is mucilage of quince seed or of gum tragacanth or fat of a chicken or duck ...). Hebr. אנידא is a non-attested calque of O. Occ. or O. Cat. *aneda* ('little duck; female duck,' < Lat. *anas*; see FEW 24:523a).

אִסְטוֹמְכָא • **דפי האסטומכא** → **דַּף**

אִסְטְנִיסוּת · **indigestion**: Lat. *fastidium* (Arab. تخمة; Gr. ἀπέψια) · Constantinus Africanus, *Viaticum peregrinantis* · trans. Doʾeg ha-Edomi, *Sefer Yaʾir Netiv* IV.9: והמדוים הנולדים מהאסטניסות הם ארבעה (Indigestion causes four [different] illnesses). In the sense of 'indigestion,' Hebr. אִסְטְנִיסוּת is not attested in the current dictionaries. Moses ibn Tibbon translates Arab. تخمة as רוע הבשול (see entry רֹעַ). Hebr. אִסְטְנִיסוּת features also in the sense of 'want of appetite' in *Sefer Yaʾir Netiv* III.6 (cf. NM 5:21); see also BCD 24 (NM 3:26) for an attestation from Hillel ben Samuel, *Aphorismi* IV.17. • **עורר אסטניסות** → [עור].

[אסף] • *Part. Piʿel* **מְאַסֵּף** · **coagulating**: Lat. *coagulo* (Arab. جمّد) · Constantinus Africanus, *Viaticum peregrinantis* · trans. Doʾeg ha-Edomi, *Sefer Yaʾir Netiv* IV.1: כי כל דבר מקרר מחזק החפץ ודבר המחמם יעשה ההפך כי הקרירות מאסף ומקבץ חלקי הדם המפוזרים במקורות האסטומכא (All cooling things strengthen the appetite and all heating things have the opposite effect. The reason is that cold coagulates and congeals the blood that is in the veins of the stomach). In the sense of 'to coagulate,' Hebr. *Piʿel* אִסֵּף is not attested in the current dictionaries. Moses ibn Tibbon translates Arab. جمّد as *Piʿel* קִבֵּץ (see entry [קבץ]).

אַף • **הוטף באף** → [נטף].

אֲפִיסָה • אפיסת הדם · **blood clot:** Lat. *sanguis coagulata* (Arab. علق) · Constantinus Africanus, *Viaticum peregrinantis* · trans. Do'eg ha-Edomi, *Sefer Ya'ir Netiv* v.20: עצור הדרך מאשר יוצא השתן מהמקוה יקרה בסתימת האבן ואפיסת הדם או הליחות הגסות או הבלוי או מאיזה דבר שנולד שם כמו ורוגא או בשר עודף (An obstruction in the passage through which the urine passes from the bladder occurs when it is blocked by a stone or by a blood clot or by coarse humors or by pus or by whatever grows there such as a wart or fleshy excrescence). Hebr. אפיסת הדם is not attested in the current dictionaries. Moses ibn Tibbon translates Arab. علق as דם קרוש (see entry דָּם).

• אפיסת דם נידות · **amenorrhea:** Arab. احتباس الطمث · Ibn al-Jazzār, *Zād al-musāfir wa-qūt al-ḥāḍir* · trans. Abraham ben Isaac, *Sefer Ṣedah la-Oreḥim* VI.9: אפיסת דם נידות יהיה על שני מינים (Amenorrhea occurs in two ways). Hebr. אפיסת דם נידות is not attested in the current dictionaries. In addition to אפיסת דם נידות, Abraham ben Isaac translates Arab. احتباس الطمث as עכוב דם הנדות (see entry עִכּוּב). Moses ibn Tibbon translates Arab. احتباس الطمث as העצר הנדות (see entry עֶצֶר) and Do'eg ha-Edomi translates the parallel Lat. term *ablatio* as הַעֲדָרָה (see also next entry).

אֲפִיסוּת • אפיסות והפסקה · **retention:** Arab. احتباس · Ibn al-Jazzār, *Zād al-musāfir wa-qūt al-ḥāḍir* · trans. Abraham ben Isaac, *Sefer Ṣedah la-Oreḥim* VI.12: ויש שיוולד מחמת מכה ויש שיוולד מחמת אפיסות והפסקת דם הנידות (Sometimes it [i.e., a tumor in the uterus] is caused by an injury and sometimes by retention of the menstruation). Hebr. אֲפִיסוּת is not attested in medical literature in the current dictionaries; cf. BM 346. Moses ibn Tibbon translates Arab. احتباس as עצירה. Do'eg ha-Edomi translates the parallel Lat. term *ablatio* as הַעֲדָרָה (see entry).

אֲפִיקוֹמָן • אפיקימון · **aftermeal entertainment; dessert:** Arab. التنقّل · Maimonides, *Maqāla fī al-rabw* (*On Asthma*) · trans. Anonymous, *Sefer ha-Qaṣeret* III.8 (cf. BMA 2:398, ll. 16–18): ויסמך באפיקימון של פסתק והשקדים ובלבד המרים מהן יערב אותן עם המתוקים עד שירגיל אכלם שהם רפואה גדולה לזה החלי מדקקין הלחות מפתח לכל האטמים מנקים הריאה מסייעים להריק הלחות עם הרוק שימם בדעתך (And for dessert one should take pistachio nuts and almonds, especially the bitter [nuts], which one may mix with sweet [nuts] until one becomes accustomed to eating them. For [this] is an excellent remedy for this disease, because it thins the humors, opens all the obstructions, cleans the lungs, and helps expectoration. Keep it in mind). In the sense of 'aftermeal entertainment; dessert,' Hebr. אֲפִיקוֹמָן features in Rabb. literature; cf. JD 104; BM 348–349; HM 56–59. Samuel Benveniste translates Arab. التنقّل as היותו מפטיר (see entry [פטר]) and Joshua Shatibi has אכול אחר האכילה.

אפיקימון → אֲפִיקוֹמָן.

אֹפֶל · **night blindness (nyctalopia):** Arab. عشا (cf. MMT 253[15]) · Gerard de Solo, *Practica super nono Almansoris* · trans. Abraham Avigdor, *Ha-Ma'amar ha-Teshi'i le-Sefer ha-Mansuri le-Razi*, fol. 79b: שער באופל והוא אלעשא (Chapter: On nightblindness; i.e.

15 The Arabic term can also refer to the opposite of night blindness, i.e., hemeralopia (cf. IJZ 1–2:273, n. 429).

[Arab.] *al-ʿashā*ʾ). Hebr. אֹפֶל does not feature in this sense in the current dictionaries. It features in the sense of 'dullness [of sight]' (Gr. ἀμβλυωπία) in BCD 26 (NM 4:20) in an attestation from Moses ibn Tibbon, *Sefer Ṣedat ha-Derakhim* II.6.0 (IJZ 1–2:492). See also entries לִילִית and סַנְוֵר.

אָפֵס • to become weak: Lat. *deficio* (Arab. ضعف) · Constantinus Africanus, *Viaticum peregrinantis* · trans. Do'eg ha-Edomi, *Sefer Ya'ir Netiv* IV.17: השביעי הוא כאשר אפס הרגש המעי ואינו מרגיש היזק התוצאות ועל כן נשארו במעי ולא יצאו (The seventh [cause of a colic] is [the condition] when the sensitivity of the intestines weakens so that they do not feel the harm caused by the feces; consequently they [i.e., the feces] remain in the intestines and are not passed). Hebr. אָפֵס features in BM 354 in the sense of 'to cease, fail,' a.o., in an attestation from Meir Aldabi, *Shevilei Emunah*: ויקרה לנשים חכוך ברחם ומצוקת האם ובו יאפס הכח מהם ומתדלדלות תמיד ורזות. Moses ibn Tibbon translates Arab. ضعف as חלש. For the noun אֲפִיסָה in the sense of 'weakness' as it features in *Sefer Ya'ir Netiv* I.25.1, cf. NM 5:21–22; IJZ 1–2:631.

• *Inf. Nifʿal* **הֵאָפֵס • weakening:** Lat. *deficior* (Arab. ضعف) · Constantinus Africanus, *Viaticum peregrinantis* · trans. Do'eg ha-Edomi, *Sefer Ya'ir Netiv* V.13: ועל כן יאות כי בסבות ובאותות הצמחים אשר בכליות נחוש לרפאתם כי הכליות קשות לעזור וכח הרפואה לא יבא שם בהאפסו באריכות הדרך (Therefore, once we see the causes and symptoms of kidney ulcers we should hasten to treat them since it is hard to cure the kidneys and the medicine does not reach it with its full strength but only in a weakened form because it has such a long way to go before getting to [the kidneys]). In the sense of 'weakening,' Hebr. *Inf. Nifʿal* הֵאָפֵס is not attested in the current dictionaries. For *Part. Nifʿal* נֶאֱפָס in the sense of 'losing,' see NM 5:22 for an attestation from Abraham ben Isaac, *Sefer Ṣedah la-Oreḥim* I.22.2 (cf. IJZ 1–2:574). Moses ibn Tibbon translates Arab. ضعف as נחלש.

אֶצְבַּע • המקור שהוא בין הגודל והאצבע → מָקוֹר.

• **העורק אשר על הכף בין האצבע הקטן ושכנו** → עֹרֶק.

• *Plur.* **אצבעות • מורסות ראשי האצבעות** → מֻרְסָה.

אִצְטוֹמְכָה • גלדי האצטומכה → גֶּלֶד.

• **רפיון האצטומכה** → רִפְיוֹן.

אַרְבָּעִים וְאַרְבַּע • בעל ארבעים וארבע רגלים → בַּעַל.

ארגליון • clyster; tube [for injecting medecines into internal parts]: Arab. حقن (Gr. ἐργαλεῖον; Lat. *ergalium*; M. Lat. *argalia*) · Ibn al-Jazzār, *Zād al-musāfir wa-qūt al-ḥādir* · trans. Abraham ben Isaac, *Sefer Ṣedah la-Oreḥim* VI.13: או קח לובן ביצה וחלב אשה מינקת נקבה ומי פרפחינים ושמן זרע דלעת מכל א׳ חלק וערב הכל ועשה ארגליון ברחם (Or take egg white, milk of a woman who is nursing a girl, common purslane juice, oil of gourd seed; of each one part, mix everything, and inject it with a tube into the uterus). Hebr. ארגליון is a non-attested calque of Gr. ἐργαλεῖον.[16] Moses ibn Tibbon

16 For the occurrence of Greek loan words in Abraham ben Isaac's *Sefer Ṣedah la-Oreḥim*, cf. IJZ 1–2: 528–531.

translates Arab. حقن as קלח (cf. BCD 243 (NM 4:104), s.v. [קלח], *Part. Pi'el* מְקַלֵּחַ for an attestation from *Sefer Ṣedat ha-Derakhim* I.23.4 (IJZ 1–2:477)).

אֵשׁ • האש הפרסי · **carbuncle; furuncle**: Arab. النار الفارسي (Gr. ἄνθραξ; cf. UW 112) · Ibn Sīnā, *K. al-Qānūn fī al-ṭibb* · trans. Nathan ha-Me'ati, *Sefer ha-Qanun* II, fol. 74[a]: ... גואשיר עקרו יכשר לרפואת העצמות[17] ועם הדבש יועיל לנגעים הישנים[18] והאש הפרסי ובערבי נאר[19] פרסי (Opopanax: ... Its root is suitable for the treatment of loss[20] of flesh covering the bones and, if applied with honey, it cures chronic ulcers and carbuncles). Hebr. האש הפרסי, lit., 'Persian fire,' a calque of Arab. النار الفارسي, features in BCD 28 (NM 4:22) in the sense of 'erysipelas' (for Lat. *ignis sacer*) in an attestation from Abraham Avigdor, *Pirqei Arnavṭ de-Vila Nova* V.102 (AMP 112). The Arab. term can mean both 'erysipelas' and 'carbuncle,' as attested by Ibn Sīnā, *K. al-Qānūn fī al-ṭibb* III.118: 'Chapter on حمرة and النار الفارسية and other [afflictions]: These two names are sometimes applied to every corrosive, burning hot, blistering pustule that makes eschars, just like fire and cautering, and sometimes the term النار الفارسية is applied to a pustule that is of the kind of the corrosive, burning, blistering shingles ...' (cf. NM 4:22). Zeraḥyah Ḥen and Anonymous both translate Arab. النار الفارسي as האש הפרסי as well.

אֶשֶׁךְ • מרוח אשך → מְרוֹחַ.

אשק׳ · **scrupel**: Lat. (*e*)*scrupulus* [i.e, the twenty-fourth part of an ounce; cf. DMLBS 3336] (Arab. نصف مثقال; i.e., half a *mithqāl*; i.e, 2.23 grams[21]) · Constantinus Africanus, *Viaticum peregrinantis* · trans. Do'eg ha-Edomi, *Sefer Ya'ir Netiv* V.3.18: ואולם יאות לאמר העזר ונאמר אמת כי כל דבר פותח עוזר אל הקושי הישן מהכבד כמו אבפאטורי אשפיק שרש לבריר מיץ אפי מראטרי אינדוביא ודומיהם. וכן ב׳ אשק׳[22] אשפיק עם מיץ מראטרי יעזור ([Now] I should mention remedies that [open obstructions of the liver]. It is true that any deobstruent is beneficial for a chronic hard liver; [such remedies are] resin spurge, nard, laurel root, celery juice, fennel, chicory/endive, and the like. Two scrupels of nard with fennel juice is also a good remedy). Hebr. אשק׳ is a non-attested abbreviation of אשקרופולוש, Lat. (*e*)*scrupulus*.[23] The term occurs throughout Do'eg's *Sefer Ya'ir Netiv*. Moses ibn Tibbon translates Arab. نصف مثقال as חצי שקל.

אֶתְרוֹג • חמוץ האתרוג → חָמוּץ

---

17 העצמות: العارية add. a.
18 הישנים: emend. ed. היבשים Ms المزمنة a.
19 נאר: emend. ed. נצר Ms.
20 'loss of flesh': Trans. after a.
21 One *mithqāl* equals 4.46 grams; cf. HIM 4–7.
22 אשק׳: אשקרופו Ms Moscow, Russian State Library, Guenzburg 1481, fol. 105[b].
23 Cf. the reading 'ŠQRWPW (*escrupu*[*lus*]) in Ms Moscow, Russian State Library, Guenzburg 1481, fol. 105[b].

ב

נָגַע → הגיע לבגר • בַּגַר/בֶּגֶר.

נָגַע → הגיע לימי הבגרות • בַּגְרוּת.

בַּד • *Plur.* **בדים** · **stems; stalks:** Arab. قضبان · a) Ibn al-Jazzār, *Zād al-musāfir wa-qūt al-ḥādir* · trans. Moses ibn Tibbon, *Sefer Ṣedat ha-Derakhim* IV.15: או יקח בדי לגלגת עם שעור קלוף קלוי רצוץ (Or take common purslane stems with peeled, crushed, and roasted barley). Hebr. *Sing.* בַּד features in NM 5:25 in the sense of 'shoot; twig; branch' (for Arab. غصن) in an attestation from Moses ibn Tibbon, *Sefer Ṣedat ha-Derakhim* III.8.17 (corr.).

b) Maimonides, *Maqāla fī al-rabw* (*On Asthma*) · trans. Samuel Benveniste (*Ma'amar 'al ha-Qaṣeret*) VII.2 (cf. BMA 2:265, ll. 21–23): ואחרי הוסר קצפו יתן בו חצי אוקיה לשון השור ושלשה בדי מנטה ומן התבלין והבשמים לפי השנים והמזג ולפי תכונת האיברים (And when there is no froth left, add to it [i.e., the remedy] half an ounce of borage, three stalks of cultivated mint, and spices according to the age [of the patient], his temperament, and the conditions of his organs). Joshua Shatibi translates Arab. قضبان as קָנֶה (see entry) and Anonymous has קלח (for *Plur.* קלחים ('shoots'), see entry קֶלַח).

בַּהֶרֶת · **deformative disease of the skin; skin sickness involving local patches of lighter or darker color; morphew:** Lat. *morphea* (DMLBS 2398; ND 694) · *Sefer ha-Refu'ot le-Ḥakham Qoṣṭa'ntin*, fol. 227[a]: בבהרת: אמר פלאטיאריש: מורפיאה הוא חולי כשנולדות בהרות בפנים שנשתנה מראה העור בלובן או בשחרות (On morphew: Says Platearius: Morphew is a disease in which morbid eruptions appear on the face whereby the color of the skin changes to white or black). Hebr. בַּהֶרֶת is only attested in the Bible and Rabb. literature in the sense of 'brightness; bright spot; of eruption on the skin' (cf. BDB 97; JD 143; BM 475–476; Low XXXIX). In medieval medical literature it also features in the sense of 'spot or opaque place on the eye; cataract; leucoma' (cf. NM 5:26).

בּוּבְיָא (*Aram.*) · **oven; cooking place; h.l., a pit with hot ashes used for baking bread:** Arab. ملة (NA 567. s.v. *malla*: 'a pit in which bread is baked in hot ashes and stones,' according to Mielck (RMA 50), the term *malla* could refer both to the hot ashes and to the pit in which the bread was baked) · Ibn Zuhr, *K. al-Aghdhiya* · trans. Nathan ha-Me'ati, *Sefer ha-Mezonot*, fol. 2[b]: והמשובח שבכל מיניו מה שישלים אפייתו בתנור ואחריו מה שיאפה בפורני ואיחריו מה שיאפה בבוביא (The best kind [of bread] is that, which is properly baked in a domed clay oven (*tannur*), followed by that which is baked in a brick oven (Aram. *purni*), followed by that which is baked in a pit in hot ashes). Aram. בּוּבְיָא features in SDA 126 in attestations from Talmudic literature in the sense of 'oven; cooking place.'

בּוּלְמוּס · **ravenous hunger (bulimy):** (Gr. βούλιμος; cf. HM 64–65) · Ibn al-Jazzār, *Zād al-musāfir wa-qūt al-ḥādir* · trans. Moses ibn Tibbon, *Sefer Ṣedat ha-Derakhim* IV.3:

השער הג׳ בתאוה הכלבית והוא שאחזו בולמוס (Ch. 3: [When someone suffers from] ravenous hunger [lit., 'canine hunger'], i.e., BWLMWS). The term בּוּלְמוּס is a calque of Gr. βούλιμος and is only attested in Rabb. literature; cf. HM 64–65; JD 146; SDA 127. For the Hebr. synonym חולי רעבון, see entry חֳלִי.

בּוּעָה · **convex side of the liver**: Lat. *gibbus* (cf. *gibbositas*, DMLBS 1347:1: 'protruberance; swelling (on body) *b* (?) part of liver') (Arab. حدبة) · Constantinus Africanus, *Viaticum peregrinantis* · trans. Do'eg ha-Edomi, *Sefer Ya'ir Netiv* V.3: ואם הצמח יהיה בגבהי בועת הכבד נתן דברים שוברים ומטהרים (If the tumor is in the upper parts of the convex side of the liver, we administer [the patient] diuretics and purgatives). Hebr. בּוּעָה only features in the current dictionaries in the sense of 'swelling; abscess' (cf. BM 489; JD 147, s.v. Aram. בועא; SDA 128, s.v. Aram. בּוּעֲתָא), 'bulla or blister on the lung or outside the body' (Low XXXIX), and 'hunchback' (cf. NM 5:27). Moses ibn Tibbon translates Arab. حدبة in the sense of 'hunchback' (Gr. ὗβος) as גַּבְנִינוּת. The latter term is used in the same sense by Nathan ha-Me'ati in his *Pirqei Abuqraṭ* VI.46 (cf. BCD 43 (NM 3:43)).

בּוּרְמָא (*Aram.*) • **בורמא דגללא** · **stone pot**: Arab. إناء حنتم ('glazed, varnished pot,' cf. L 655) · Ibn Zuhr, *K. al-Aghdhiya* · trans. Nathan ha-Me'ati, *Sefer ha-Mezonot*, fol. 6ᵃ: והמשובח שבבצים מה שיעשה מהם כמו שזכר חנין שיקחו ביצים עשרה ותבקעם ותערבם בכלי בורמא[24] דגללא ובער׳ חנתם (The best manner of preparing eggs is the following [recipe] mentioned by Ḥunayn: Take ten eggs, break them, and mix them in a stone pot called ḤNTM in Arab. ...). Aram. בורמא דגללא features in SDA 130. The emended term בורמי might actually be a corruption of *Plur.* בורמ(א)י, cf. SDA 130: בורמ{א}י דגללא.

בזה (*Qal* בָּזָה or *Pi'el* בִּזָּה) · **to neglect**: Lat. *neglego* (Arab. ترك) · Constantinus Africanus, *Viaticum peregrinantis* · trans. Do'eg ha-Edomi, *Sefer Ya'ir Netiv* V.11: ואם תבזה אותו עד שיתקשה בסתימה ובצמח אז יתקשה לעזור ויתארך לרפאת (But if you neglect [an illness of the spleen] until hardness occurs in the obstruction and the tumor, it will be difficult to treat and it will take a long time). In the sense of 'to neglect,' Hebr. בזה is a non-attested semantic bowering from Lat. *neglego*. Moses ibn Tibbon translates Arab. ترك as הונח.

[בחר] • *Part. Nif'al* **נִבְחָר** · **best**: Arab. أجود · Maimonides, *Maqāla fī al-rabw* (*On Asthma*) · trans. Samuel Benveniste, *Ma'amar 'al ha-Qaṣeret* IX.2 (cf. BMA 2:271, ll. 8–9): אבל מי שלחותיו עבות ומדבקות והזקנים וכל שכן בעלי המחלה שחברתי המאמר הזה בגללם הנבחר אצלנו ⟨שירפו⟩ במה שזכר ג׳אלינוס (However, for someone with thick or viscous humors or for old people—and especially for those who suffer from [this] disease [i.e., asthma], for whom I composed this treatise—the best thing to do, in my opinion, is to soften [their stools] with the remedy mentioned by Galen). In the sense of 'best,' Hebr. נִבְחָר

---

24 בורמא דגללא: emend. ed. בורמי וגללא Ms.

is attested in the Bible; cf. BM 508. Joshua Shatibi and Anonymous both render Arab. أجود as טוב.

בִּטּוּל • בטול הרגש · **numbness:** Arab. خدر (Gr. νάρκη; cf. UW 431) · Ibn Sīnā, *K. al-Qānūn fī al-ṭibb*, Hebr. trans. Nathan ha-Me'ati, *Sefer ha-Qanun* II, fol. 116ª: פטר ... יוליד בטול ההרגש הנקר׳ כדר בערבי וההשתקות ובער׳ סכתה (Mushrooms: ... They cause numbness, called *khadar* in Arab., and apoplexy, i.e., *sakta* in Arab.). Hebr. בטול ההרגש is not attested in the current dictionaries. In his *Sefer ha-Peraqim* (*Pirqei Moshe*) XXII.38, 43; XXIII.22, 23, Nathan translates Arab. خدر as תרדמת האברים (cf. BMMN 214, ll. 8, 22; 221, ll. 2–3) and in VII.66 he has תרדמת החוש (cf. BMMN 90, l. 18) (cf. also BMMG no. 1297). Zeraḥyah Ḥen translates Arab. خدر as רִפְיוֹן (see entry).

[בטל] • *Part. Pi'el* • **מְבַטֵּל** · **sedative:** Arab. مخدّر · Ibn Sīnā, *K. al-Qānūn fī al-ṭibb* · trans. Zeraḥyah Ḥen, *Sefer ha-Qanun* II, fol. 175ᵇ: אַפְּוֹן הוא מיץ הפפאורי השחור המצרי מושם לשמש ולא יוסיף בשתייתו על ב׳ דאניקים ויעשה מן החסות המדבריות אפיון גם כן והוא מבטל חלוש ודק (Opium: It is the sun-dried extract of the Egyptian black poppy. Its dose should not exceed two *dāniqs*.[25] It is also prepared from wild lettuce, which itself is a weak, thin sedative). Hebr. *Pi'el* בִּטֵּל features in BCD 32 (NM 1:131) in the sense of 'to benumb [the senses]' in an attestation from Zeraḥyah's *Sefer ha-Peraqim* (*Pirqei Moshe*) VIII.39 (cf. BMMZ 92, l. 17; BMMG no. 1296). Nathan ha-Me'ati translates Arab. مخدّر as מבטל ההרגש.

בֶּטֶן • בשר הבטן → בָּשָׂר.
• **חגרת הבטן** → חֲגֹרָה.
• **חבלי הבטן** → חֵבֶל.
• **החלקים השפלים מהבטן** → חֵלֶק.
• **התיר הבטן** → [נתר].
• **עצר הבטן** → עָצַר¹.
• **הקל הבטן** → [קלל].

בֵּיצָה • *Plur.* **ביצים** • **ביצי בעלי חיים** · **(lit., 'testicles of animals'); castoreum (i.e., medicament often defined as testicles of a water animal; in fact, it is an excretion derived from the scent glands of the Eurasian beaver [*Castor fiber* Linnaeus, 1758]):** Arab. جندبا دستر (cf. DT 2:211 (II.22): 'Bibergeil') · *Shinnui ha-Shemot ha-Niqra'im Synonimi*, fol. 74ª: גנדבי דסדר הוא קשטורו והם ביצי בעלי חיים (GNDBY DSDR (*DSTR); i.e., [Rom.] QŠṬWRW [i.e., castoreum]; that is the testicles of animals). Hebr. ביצי בעלי חיים does not feature in this specific sense in the current dictionaries. A synonym, אשכים, features on fol. 69ª: אשכים ה׳ קסטורו (Testicles, i.e., [Rom.] QSṬWRW [i.e., castoreum]); cf. NM 5:23.

• **ביצי חשועל** · **(lit., 'fox's testicles'); salep (a drug obtained from various species of orchids [Orchidaceae], esp., green-winged orchid [*Orchis morio* L.], early-purple**

25 One *dāniq* varies from 0.52 to 0.74 grams; cf. Ibn Sahl, *Dispensatorium Parvum* (*Al-Aqrābādhīn al-saghīr*), ed. O. Kahl (Leiden 1994), 226.

orchid [*Orchis mascula* (L.) L.], and military orchid [*Orchis militaris* L.]): Arab. خصى الثعلب (cf. MIG no. 1035) · Ibn al-Jazzār, *Zād al-musāfir wa-qūt al-ḥādir* · trans. Abraham ben Isaac, *Sefer Ṣedah la-Oreḥim* VI.1: ואמר דיאסקורידוס כי זה השורש הנק' ביצי אלתעלב ופי' ביצי אלתעלב ביצי השועל והוא שורש אם יתפשט האדם בידו כל זמן שיתפשט אז יעוררהו לתשמיש (Dioscurides said that if one holds the root called [in Arab.] *bayḍā l-thaʿlab*, which means 'fox's testicles,' in one's hand, it will stimulate his lust for coitus as long as he holds it). Hebr. ביצי השועל is a non-attested calque of Arab. *bayḍā l-thaʿlab*, which is a synonym of *khuṣā l-thaʿlab*. The latter term is rendered as אשכי השועל in an anonymous glossary in Ms Oxford, Bodleian Library, Mich. Add. 22, fol. 5[b] (cf. BCD 29 (NM 4:22)).

• **אודם ביצים** → **אֹדֶם**.

בישול → **בִּשּׁוּל**.

בִּלְבּוּל · **turbidity:** Lat. *turbulentia* (Arab. عكر) · Constantinus Africanus, *Viaticum peregrinantis* · trans. Do'eg ha-Edomi, *Sefer Ya'ir Netiv* V.11: וכאשר הטחול ימשוך שמרי הדם ובלבולו הכרח הוא שהדם הוא זך ומזוג (When the spleen attracts the turbid part of the blood and its sediment, the blood necessarily becomes clean ans balanced). Hebr. בִּלְבּוּל does not feature in this sense in the current dictionaries. Moses ibn Tibbon translates Arab. عكر as עכירות.

• **בלבול הגוף** · **indisposition; malaise:** Arab. اضطراب البدن · Maimonides, *Maqāla fī al-rabw* (*On Asthma*) · trans. Samuel Benveniste, *Ma'amar ʿal ha-Qaṣeret* V.6 (cf. BMA 2:261, ll. 14–15): וכאב הקולנג' או כאב הכליות או הטחול או כאב הכבד או כאב הפרקים או בלבול הגוף או פלצות או הסתמר הגוף או קדחת (Pain in the colon, intestines, spleen, liver, or joints; indisposition; shivering fit; shivering; or fever). Hebr. בלבול הגוף is not attested in the current dictionaries. For other combinations in medieval Hebr. medical literature, see BCD 34–35. Joshua Shatibi translates Arab. اضطراب البدن as בלבול הגוף as well and Anonymous renders Arab. اضطراب البدن as שיבוש הגוף (see entry שִׁבּוּשׁ).

בְּלִיטָה · **hernia:** Arab. قرو (cf. UWS 1:552) · al-Rāzī, *K. al-Manṣūrī fī al-ṭibb* · trans. Shem Tov ben Isaac, *Sefer Almansur*, fol. 4[a]: פ"ו: בבליטה והפיתקא ([Chapter] 86: On hernia; [i.e., Aram.] *pitqa*). Hebr. בְּלִיטָה does not feature in this sense in the current dictionaries. For other meanings of this term in medieval medical literature, see BCD 36. Abraham Avigdor translates the parallel Lat. term *eminentia* as בליטה as well. For Aram. פִּיתְקָא, cf. BCD 220 (NM 1:109).

• **בליטת פי הטבעת** · **anal (rectal) prolapse:** Arab. نتوء المقعدة · al-Rāzī, *K. al-Manṣūrī fī al-ṭibb* · trans. Shem Tov ben Isaac, *Sefer Almansur*, fol. 4[a]: ע"ח: בבליטת פי הטבעת והרחם ([Chapter] 78: On anal (rectal) and uterine prolapse). Hebr. בליטת פי הטבעת is not attested in the current dictionaries. Abraham Avigdor translates the parallel Lat. term *exitus ani* as בליטת השת (see entry below).

• **בליטת הרחם** · **uterine prolapse:** Arab. نتوء الرحم · al-Rāzī, *K. al-Manṣūrī fī al-ṭibb* · trans. Shem Tov ben Isaac, *Sefer Almansur*, fol. 4[a]: ע"ח: בבליטת פי הטבעת והרחם

([Chapter] 78: On anal (rectal) and uterine prolapse). In the sense of 'uterine prolapse,' Hebr. בליטת הרחם features in BCD 36 (NM 4:27) in an attestation from Moses ibn Tibbon, *Sefer Ṣedat ha-Derakhim* I.1.4 (IJZ 1–2:441).

• **בליטת חשת** · **anal (rectal) prolapse:** Lat. *exitus ani* · Gerard de Solo, *Practica super nono Almansoris* · trans. Abraham Avigdor, *Ha-Ma'amar ha-Teshi'i le-Sefer ha-Mansuri le-Razi*, fol. 156[a]: שער ברפואת בליטת השת והפתח עורקיו (Chapter on the treatment of anal (rectal) prolapse and of the opening of its vessels). Hebr. בליטת השת is not attested in the current dictionaries. Shem Tov ben Isaac translates the parallel Arab. term نتوء المقعدة as בליטת פי הטבעת (see entry above).

בִּנְיָן · **constitution:** Arab. بِنْية · Maimonides, *Maqāla fī al-rabw* (*On Asthma*) · trans. Samuel Benveniste, *Ma'amar 'al ha-Qaṣeret* IX.16 (cf. BMA 2:276, ll. 16–19): אבל הנהגת הבריאות בהרקה ובהקזה או בשתות המשקים המשלשלים טעות גדולה ואיננו מעצת גדולי הרופאים אך יצטרך להוציא הדם ולשלשול בנפול התחלואים המחייבים לאותו הענין מרוב המלוי והוא שיתקבצו בגופו או שיגבר דמו וירתיח לפי בנין רע או הנהגה רעה נהג עליה (The maintenance of health through evacuation by means of bloodletting or the ingestion of purgatives is a grave mistake and is not part of the advice of the eminent physicians. One should resort to bloodletting and the use of purgatives [only] when diseases occur that require such action, as in the case of someone whose body is full of accumulated [humors] or that his blood cocts and boils because of a bad constitution or a continuously bad regimen). Hebr. בִּנְיָן does not feature in this sense in the current dictionaries. It is mentioned as an antomical term referring to 'the human frame; skeleton,' or 'composition of the body' (JD 177; BM 565; see also PESHAT[26]). Joshua Shatibi and Anonymous both render Arab. بِنْية as בנין as well.

בַּשָּׂם • *Plur.* **בסמים** · **druggists:** Arab. عطّارون · Maimonides, *Maqāla fī al-rabw* (*On Asthma*) · trans. Joshua Shatibi, *Ma'amar 'al ha-Qaṣeret* XII.1 (cf. BMA 2:361, ll. 13–14): אסכרוס[27] וזנגביל שאמי הנקרא רסאן[28] והוא אשר יכירוהו הבסמים במצרים בשם כנף[29] (Lavender and Syrian ginger—i.e., RS'N [read: R'SN, i.e., Arab. *al-rāsan* ('elecampagne')], which the druggists in Cairo know as KNP [i.e., Arab. *janāḥ* ('wing'); cf. IG 316]). Hebr. *Sing.* בַּשָּׂם features in the current dictionaries as a Rabb. term only (cf. BM 567; EM 181). Samuel Benveniste translates Arab. عطّارون as רופאים and Anonymous has רוקחים (see entry רוֹקֵחַ).

בִּסְרִי · **from unripe, sour grapes (*Adj.*):** Arab. حصرمي · Ibn al-Jazzār, *Zād al-musāfir wa-qūt al-ḥādir* · trans. Moses ibn Tibbon, *Sefer Ṣedat ha-Derakhim* IV.11: ותהיה מזונו תרנגולים קטנים מבושלים בתבשיל רמוני או תפוחי או בסרי (He should eat young chickens cooked in a pomegranate dish or an apple dish or a dish of unripe, sour grapes). Hebr. בִּסְרִי features in EM 181 in an attestation from Abraham Isaac Kook, *Orot*.

---

26 https://peshat.org/display/peshat_lemmas_00004724 (accessed March 25, 2022).
27 אסכרוס: أسطوخودس a.
28 רסאן: الراسن a.
29 כנף: الجناح a.

[בעל] • *Nif'al* **נִבְעַל** · **to have sexual intercourse:** Lat. *cohabito* (Arab. أصاب الرجل) · Constantinus Africanus, *Viaticum peregrinantis* · trans. Do'eg ha-Edomi, *Sefer Ya'ir Netiv* VI.11: גם כן יקרה לבתולות בהגיעם לבגר ואינם נבעלות כי הזרע נאסף בהם והיתה הגרישה צריכה כמו לזכרים כי עשיית התולדת ופעולתו דורש זה (This [i.e., hysterical suffocation] can also happen to young women when they have reached sexual maturity, without having sexual intercourse [i.e., virgins]. For when the sperm has collected in them, they need its emission just like men, for this is an act required by nature). Hebr. נִבְעַל features in the sense of 'to have sexual intercourse' in attestations from Rabb. literature only; cf. JD 182; BM 578. Moses ibn Tibbon translates Arab. أصاب الرجل as התחבר לאדם.

בַּעַל • **בעל ארבעים וארבע רגלים** · **centipede:** Arab. ذو الأربعة والأربعين · Ibn Sīnā, *K. al-Qānūn fī al-ṭibb* · trans. Nathan ha-Me'ati, *Sefer ha-Qanun* II, fol. 95[b]: כנתי ... ישקו ממנו שלש דרכמונים לנשיכת השרצים וכשמשקים פרי וציצו ביין יועיל תועלת גדולה מנשיכת עקרב ובעל ארבעים וארבע רגלים וזה שהוא משלשל (Asphodel: ... One should administer three *dirhams* in the cases of insects bites, and if one administers the fruits and flowers with wine, it is particularly useful in scorpion and centipede bites, though it may cause diarrhea). In the sense of 'centipede,' Hebr. בעל ארבעים וארבע רגלים is a non-attested semantic borrowing from Arab. رجل ذو الأربعة والأربعين.

בַּעַל חַיִּים • *Plur.* **בעלי חיים** • ביצי בעלי חיים → בֵּיצָה.

בַּעֲלָה • **בעלת הצד** · **pleurisy:** Arab. ذات الجنب · al-Rāzī, *K. al-Manṣūrī fī al-ṭibb* · trans. Shem Tov ben Isaac, *Sefer Almansur*, fols. 123[b]–124[a]: שער בבעלת הצד הקוראים אותו בני קדר אלגנב כשיתחדש באדם כאב מתחת צלעותיו עוקץ וכל שכן כשישעול עמו שעול יבש ויש לו קדחת (Chapter on pleurisy, which the Arabs call [*dhāt*] *al-janb*: When a person suffers from a biting pain under the ribs, especially at the time that he has a dry cough and he has a fever ...). In the sense of 'pleuritis,' Hebr. בעלת הצד features in BCD 37 (NM 2:32) in a later attestation from Nathan ha-Me'ati, *Sefer ha-Peraqim* (*Pirqei Moshe*) VI.40 (cf. BMMN 71, l. 7; BMMG no. 1999). Abraham Avigdor renders the parallel Lat. term *pleuresis* as בעלת הצד as well.

• **בעלת הריאה** · **pneumonia:** Arab. ذات الرئة · al-Rāzī, *K. al-Manṣūrī fī al-ṭibb* · trans. Shem Tov ben Isaac, *Sefer Almansur*, fol. 124[a]: שער בבעלת הריאה ובלשון הגרי דאת אלראה: כשיתחדש באדם קדחת וצרת הנישום חזקה ואדמימות בלסתות עד שתדמנה צבועות וכאב במוקדם החזה ושיעול ורקיקה (Chapter on pneumonia, [called] in Arab. *dhāt al-ri'a*: When a person suffers from fever, has severe shortness of breath, his jaws are so red as if they have been painted and he feels pain in the front of his chest, and he has to cough and to spit ...). In the sense of 'pneumonia,' Hebr. בעלת הריאה features in BCD 37 (NM 2:32) in a later attestation from Nathan ha-Me'ati, *Sefer ha-Peraqim* (*Pirqei Moshe*) VI.40 (cf. BMMN 71, l. 7; BMMG no. 2000). Abraham Avigdor renders the parallel Lat. term *peripleumonia* as בעלת הריאה as well.

בָּקִי · **experienced:** Arab: دريب · Maimonides, *Maqāla fī al-rabw* (*On Asthma*) · trans. Samuel Benveniste, *Ma'amar 'al ha-Qaṣeret* XIII.30 (cf. BMA 2:308, ll. 4–5): אבל שיהיה

האיש בקי מפני שראה במעשים והביטם והוא אינו יודע זה שקר (But it is impossible for a person to be experienced [in the medical art] because he observed and saw it being practiced, although he has no [theoretical] knowledge [of it]). Hebr. בָּקִי features in JD 185 in the sense of 'expert; versed; familiar' in attestations from Rabb. literature (cf. BM 592–593) and in PESHAT[30] in the sense of 'expert in a field' in attestations from medieval philosophical literature. Joshua Shatibi translates Arab. دريب as *Part. Hofʿal* מֻרְגָּל (see entry [רגל]) and Anonymous has רָגִיל (see entry).

בֶּקִיעַ • *Plur.* **בקיעים** • **cracks:** Arab. شقاق (Gr. ῥαγάς; cf. UW 582) · Ibn Sīnā, *K. al-Qānūn fī al-ṭibb* · trans. Nathan ha-Me'ati, *Sefer ha-Qanun* II, fol. 87b: חבה כצרה ... העדי: ימרוק הפנים והכתם הנק׳ כלף בער׳ והדבק הנק׳ עלך אלאנבאט יועיל לבקיעי הפנים (Terebinth: ... [Its application in] cosmetics: It cleanses the face and removes freckles, called *kalaf* in Arab., while its resin called 'turpentine' is useful in facial cracks). Hebr. בֶּקִיעַ features in the sense of 'fissure' in BM 594 in attestations from the Bible, Rabb. literature, and medieval liturgical literature (cf. NM 5:32). Zeraḥyah Ḥen translates Arab. شقاق as בְּקִיעָה (see entry) and Anonymous has בקיעים just like Nathan.

בְּקִיעָה · **I. hernia; rupture:** Lat. *crepitura* (read: *crepatura*) (Arab. فتوق) · Constantinus Africanus, *Viaticum peregrinantis* · trans. Do'eg ha-Edomi, *Sefer Ya'ir Netiv* VI.8: כל בקיעה אשר בדפים הסובבים הבטן והבצים תקרה מתנועה חזקה כמו במשא כבד אחרי השובע או אשר יגהה[31] מאד בחזקה זהו טושיר או בסיבת צעקה גדולה או שישכב עם אשה אחרי שבעו או אשר ינוע[32] חוץ מתולדת (Every hernia in the membranes around the abdomen and testicles is caused by strenuous activity, such as [the carrying of] a heavy burden on a full stomach, a violent cough, i.e., ṬWoŠYR [i.e., O. Occ. *tossir* (cf. RL 388)], a loud cry, sexual intercourse on a full stomach, an unnatural movement (wrestling) ...). In the sense of 'hernia,' Hebr. בְּקִיעָה features in BCD 38 (NM 2:177) in later attestations, a.o., from Bonfos' trans. of al-Rāzī, *On the Treatment of Small Children* (for Lat. *crepatura*). Moses ibn Tibbon translates Arab. فتوق as בְּקִיעָה as well (see also *Sefer Ṣedat ha-Derakhim* I.1.4 (IJZ 1–2:441); cf. BCD 38 (NM 4:28)) and Abraham ben Isaac translates Arab. فتوق as חולי מרוח אשך.

· **II. crack:** Arab. شقاق (Gr. ῥαγάς; cf. UW 582) · Ibn Sīnā, *K. al-Qānūn fī al-ṭibb* · trans. Zeraḥyah Ḥen, *Sefer ha-Qanun* II, fol. 216b: חַבָּה אלכַּצ׳רָה ... היפוי יטהר הפנים והכלף ועלך אלבטם מועיל לבקיעת הפנים (Terebinth: ... [Its application in] cosmetics: It cleanses the face and removes freckles while its resin (turpentine) is useful in facial cracks). As a medical term in the sense of 'fissure,' Hebr. בקיעה features as בקיעת השפתים ('lip fissures') in BCD 38 (NM 4:28) in an attestation from Moses ibn Tibbon, *Sefer Ṣedat ha-Derakhim* N.4 (cf. IJZ 1–2:440; see also entry בֶּקַע). Nathan ha-Me'ati translates Arab. شقاق as בקיעים (see entry בֶּקִיעַ).

---

30 https://peshat.org/display/peshat_lemmas_00004499 (accessed March 25, 2022).

31 יגהה: *tussiat* L.

32 ינוע חוץ מתולדת: *luctetur* L.

• *Plur.* בקיעות • בקיעות הקורה מן האונגלון · **paronychia; whitlow**: Arab. داحس (Gr. παρωνυχία; cf. MIG no. 587) · Ibn Sīnā, *K. al-Qānūn fī al-ṭibb* · trans. Zeraḥyah Ḥen, *Sefer ha-Qanun* II, fol. 168ᵇ: אֲקָאקִיָא ... ישחיר השערות וייטיב הפנים ויועיל מן הבקיעות הקורה מן האונגלון (Senegal gum: ... It blackens the hair, improves the complexion, and is useful for whitlow (paronychia)). Hebr.-Rom. בקיעות הקורה מן האונגלון is not attested in the current dictionaries. In addition to בקיעות הקורה מן האונגלון, Zeraḥyah renders Arab. داحس also as Rom. פַּנַרִיש (i.e., *panaric*; Lat. *panaricium*). Nathan ha-Me'ati renders Arab. داحس as מורסות האצבע הנקרא דאאס (*דאחס) בערבי, while Anonymous has מורסות ראשי קצות האצבעות; see also entry מֻרְסָה.

בֶּקַע • *Plur.* **בקעים** · **fissures**: Lat. *fissurae* (Arab. شقاق) · Constantinus Africanus, *Viaticum peregrinantis* · trans. Do'eg ha-Edomi, *Sefer Ya'ir Netiv* IV.19: ואם יהיו בעגבות בקעים ומוקד תשים שם מיץ זרע חבושים ומיץ דרגאגן שומן תרנגולת ושומן אניטי שמן ויאולא דונג לבן מוח עגל שמן ורד לובן ביצה (If [the patient suffers from] fissures and burning heat in the anus, one should put on it juice of quince seed and of gum tragacanth, chicken fat and duck fat, violet oil, white wax, brain of a calf, rose oil, and egg white). Hebr. בֶּקַע, *Plur.* בקעים, does not feature in this sense in the current dictionaries, but it features in EM 191 as a modern term in the sense of 'hernia;' cf. the var. בְּקִיעָה with the same meaning featuring above. Moses ibn Tibbon translates Arab. شقاق as סדיקה (see also *Plur.* סדיקות for 'fissures' in *Sefer Ṣedat ha-Derakhim* VII.30.1 (IJZ 7:171, l. 13); cf. BCD 184 (NM 4:118 (corr.))).

בָּקָר • **חמאת בקר** → חֶמְאָה.

• **עין הבקר** → עַיִן.

בַּרְזֶל • **אבק הברזל** → אָבָק.

[ברך] • *Part. Pu'al* **מְבֹרָךְ** • **הרפואה הנקראת מבורך** → רְפוּאָה.

בִּשּׁוּל · **I. stools; excrements**: Lat. *digestio* (cf. DMLBS 860: ... '1c: matter digested or in process of digestion') (Arab. براز) · Constantinus Africanus, *Viaticum peregrinantis* · trans. Do'eg ha-Edomi, *Sefer Ya'ir Netiv* IV.15: כי אנו מבינים זה ממקומות הכאב ומאיכות הדבר המעורב בבישול (For we conclude to this from the sites of pain and from the quality of the matter that is mixed with the excrements). In the sense of 'stools; excrements,' Hebr. בִּשּׁוּל is not attested in the current dictionaries. Note, that Do'eg ha-Edomi explains the term בִּשּׁוּל in this sense in the same chapter when stating: בבשול זהו בתוצאות (cf. BCD 292 (NM 3:240–241)). Moses ibn Tibbon translates the parallel Arab. term براز as יְצִיאָה (see entry).

· **II. diarrhea**: Lat. *egestio* (Arab. إسهال) · Constantinus Africanus, *Viaticum peregrinantis* · trans. Do'eg ha-Edomi, *Sefer Ya'ir Netiv* V.4: ואם הבשול יהיה כמו רחיצת בשר באין עוות ולא כאב ובלא מוקד בקרבים והצבע יתחלף ללבן או לתכלת אז נבין שהקרירות מושל בכבד וכח העושה הדם אפס ועל כן יאות לעזור אליו בדברים מחזקים ובקצת חמום (If the diarrhea looks like meat washed in water [and the patient does not suffer from] colic, nor from burning pain in the intestines, and his face becomes white or livid, we know that cold is dominating his liver, and that the faculty that produces blood has weakened. For this reason he should be treated with ingredients that strengthen the liver and have some heating effect). In the sense of 'diarrhea,' Hebr. בִּשּׁוּל is not attested in the current dictionaries. Moses ibn Tibbon translates Arab. إسهال as שלשול.

· III. *Plur.* **בשולים** · **decoctions:** Lat. *apozemata* (Arab. مطبوخ; Gr. ἀπόζεμα) · Constantinus Africanus, *Viaticum peregrinantis* · trans. Do'eg ha-Edomi, *Sefer Ya'ir Netiv* V.5: ואחרים אפושימש הם בשולים (Other [remedies are called] 'PWŠYMŠ [i.e, Lat. *apozemas*]; i.e., decoctions). Hebr. *Sing.* בִּשּׁוּל is not attested in this sense in the current dictionaries. Moses ibn Tibbon translates the parallel Arab. term مطبوخ as בשולים as well.

• **בשול הדם** · **bloody diarrhea:** Lat. *digestio sanguinis* (Arab. إسهال الدم) · Constantinus Africanus, *Viaticum peregrinantis* · trans. Do'eg ha-Edomi, *Sefer Ya'ir Netiv* IV.15: אבק זה טוב לנגעי המעי מהאדומה והמחודדת ולבשול הדם ולכאב המעים ולעוות (The following powder is beneficial for intestinal ulcers caused by sharp yellow bile, for bloody diarrhea, intestinal pain, and colic). Hebr. בשול הדם does not feature in this sense in the current dictionaries. Moses ibn Tibbon translates the parallel Arab. term إسهال الدم as שלשול הדם.

• **בשול השרשים** · **decoction of roots:** Arab. طبيخ الأصول[33] · Ibn al-Jazzār, *Zād al-musāfir wa-qūt al-ḥādir* · trans. Moses ibn Tibbon, *Sefer Ṣedat ha-Derakhim* VI.9: בשול השרשים מגיר השתן[34] מספר התועלת לבן מאסויה ערובו יקח רוג'ה של צבעים (A prescription for a decoction of roots that makes the urine[35] flow abundantly, taken from the *Book of Success* by Ibn Māsawayh: Take madder ...). Hebr. בשול השרשים is not attested in the current dictionaries. Abraham ben Isaac merely translates the first Arab. term طبيخ as בישול שלאיפוזימא (A decoction of (*i.e.,) 'YPWZYM' [Gr. ἀπόζεμα]). Do'eg ha-Edomi transcribes the parallel Lat. term *rubia* as רוביא. In his *Sefer Ya'ir Netiv* IV.17, Do'eg translates the Lat. synonym *apozima* (read: *apozema*) *de radicibus* (Arab. مطبوخ الأصول) as משקה השרשים (see entry מַשְׁקֶה).

• **האין בשול** → אַיִן.

[בשל] • *Part. Pi'el* **מְבַשֵּׁל** • **חכה המבשל** → פַּחַ.

• *Part. Pu'al* **מְבֻשָּׁל** • **יין מבושל** → יַיִן.

[בשם] *Part. Pu'al* **מְבֻשָּׂם** · **fragrant; aromatic:** Arab. عطري · Ibn al-Jazzār, *Zād al-musāfir wa-qūt al-ḥādir* · trans. Moses ibn Tibbon, *Sefer Ṣedat ha-Derakhim* IV.11: ויחבוש אצטו' בתחבושת קובצת ומבושמת (And one should apply a fragrant, astringent poultice to the stomach). Hebr. מְבֻשָּׂם is not attested in medieval medical literature. Do'eg ha-Edomi translates the parallel Lat. term *odiferus* as אשר ריחו טוב.

---

33 Cf. Ibn al-Tilmīdh, *Aqrābādhīn*, no. 240, in: O. Kahl (ed. and trans.), *The Dispensatory of Ibn at-Tilmīḏ: Arabic Text, English Translation, Study, and Glossaries* (Leiden 2007), 255.

34 השתן: الطنث a.

35 'urine': 'menstrual blood' a.

בֹּשֶׂם • בשם חשם · **(lit., 'fragrance of the Lord'); fruit of the European ash [*Fraxinus excelsior* L.]**: Arab. لسان العصافير (cf. MIG no. 505) · Ibn al-Jazzār, *Zād al-musāfir wa-qūt al-ḥāḍir* · trans. Abraham ben Isaac, *Sefer Ṣedah la-Oreḥim* VI.1: ולשון צפרים הנקרא בלשון ישמעאל לישן אלעצפיר והוא בושם נקרא בושם השם (And fruit of the European ash, called in Arab. LYŠN ʾLʿṢPYR [i.e., *lisān al-ʿaṣāfīr*], is a fragrant ingredient called 'fragrance of the Lord'). Hebr. בשם השם is not attested in the current dictionaries. A Hebr. synonym is לשון עוף (see entry לָשׁוֹן).

• *Plur.* **בשמים • מרקחת בשמים** → מֶרְקַחַת.

בָּשָׂר • בשר הבטן · **the abdominal wall**: Arab. مراقّ البطن (cf. DKT 827) · Ibn al-Jazzār, *Zād al-musāfir wa-qūt al-ḥāḍir* · trans. Moses ibn Tibbon, *Sefer Ṣedat ha-Derakhim* IV.17: וכאשר יתילד הקולון ממורסא האות עליו נראה לעין יושג במשוש כי כשיקרה מורסא בענין הזה תגלה לחוץ בבשר הבטן (When the colic originates from an ulcer, its symptom is evident and can be identified by [the sense of] touch, for the ulcer occurring in this case appears on the outside of the abdominal wall). Hebr. בשר הבטן is not attested in the current dictionaries. Do'eg ha-Edomi translates the parallel Lat. term *inferiores ventris* as החלקים השפלים מהבטן (see entry חֵלֶק).

• **בשר נוסף** · **fleshy excrescence**: Arab. لحم زائد · Ibn al-Jazzār, *Zād al-musāfir wa-qūt al-ḥāḍir* · trans. Moses ibn Tibbon, *Sefer Ṣedat ha-Derakhim* V.20: וצרות המעבר אשר יצא בו השתן יהיה אם מפני סתום בו כמו האבן או דם קרוש או ליחה עבה או מוגלא רבה וכמו דבר יצמח בו כמו יבלת ובשר נוסף (An obstruction in the passage through which the urine passes occurs when it is blocked by something like a stone or by a blood clot or by coarse humor or by much pus or by something that grows there such as a wart or a fleshy excrescence). Hebr. בשר נוסף is not attested in the current dictionaries. Subsequently, the term features in *Sefer ha-Peraqim* (*Pirqei Moshe*) XV.21, 23, and XXII.25 by both, Nathan ha-Me'ati (BMMN 157, ll. 14, 24; 212, l. 20) and Zerahyah Ḥen (BMMZ 156, ll. 3, 12; 210, ll. 5–6) (cf. also BMMG no. 4539). The term also features in the sense of 'nasal polyps; excrescence' (Arab. نواسير) in *Sefer Ṣedat ha-Derakhim* II.13.8 (IJZ 1–2:501; cf. BCD 40 (NM 4:29 (corr.))). Do'eg ha-Edomi translates the parallel Lat. term *caro superflua* as בשר עודף (see next entry).

• **בשר עודף** · **fleshy excrescence**: Lat. *caro superflua* (Arab. لحم زائد) · Constantinus Africanus, *Viaticum peregrinantis* · trans. Do'eg ha-Edomi, *Sefer Ya'ir Netiv* V.20: עצור הדרך מאשר יוצא השתן מהמקוה יקרה בסתימת האבן ואפיסת הדם או הליחות הגסות או הבלוי או מאיזה דבר שנולד שם כמו ורוגא או בשר עודף (An obstruction in the passage through which the urine passes from the bladder occurs when it is blocked by a stone or by a blood clot or by coarse humors or by pus or by whatever grows there such as a wart or fleshy excrescence). Hebr. בשר עודף features in the sense of 'nasal polyps; excrescence' (Arab. نواسير) in *Sefer Ya'ir Netiv* II.13.8 (IJZ 1–2:643). Moses ibn Tibbon translates the parallel Arab. term لحم زائد as בשר נוסף (see previous entry).

• **רחיצת בשר** → רְחִיצָה.

בְּשָׂרִי • השקוי הבשרי → שִׁקּוּי.

ג

גַּב • גב הערוה · **pubic bone; pubes:** Lat. *pecten* (Arab. عانة) · Constantinus Africanus, *Viaticum peregrinantis* · trans. Do'eg ha-Edomi, *Sefer Ya'ir Netiv* v.16: ואם האבן במקוה יהיה הכאב נרגש על גב הערוה והחכוך באמה (If the stone is in the bladder, [the patient] will feel pain in the pubes and itching in the penis). In the sense of 'pubes,' Hebr. גב הערוה features in BCD 42 (NM 2:33; 3:42) in later attestations, a.o., in Nathan ha-Me'ati, *Pirqei Abuqraṭ* IV.80. Moses ibn Tibbon translates Arab. عانة as ערוה.

גְּבוּל • יום הגבול → יום.

גְּבוּלִי · **pertaining to a crisis [of an illness]:** Arab. بحراني · Ibn Sīnā, *K. al-Qānūn fī al-ṭibb*[36] · trans. Nathan ha-Me'ati, *Sefer ha-Qanun*, Ms Oxford, Bodleian Library, Poc. 353, Uri Heb. 314 (Neubauer 2111), fol. 246[b]: לפעמים יהיה מחולשה שלא יסבול מה שיגיע אליו מן המזון ויוזקו בו לפיפותיו וגם יתחדש בתנועות הליחות הגבוליות ויחדשו כובד וכאב בצדדי הכבד (Sometimes [pain in the liver] occurs when it cannot endure the food that reaches it and that harms its membrane (capsule). Pain can also be caused by the movements of the humors that bring the illness to a crisis and that cause heaviness and pain in parts of the liver).[37] Hebr. גְּבוּלִי features in BM 676 in attestations from the *Sefer ha-Qanun* and is explained by Ben Yehuda as 'pertaining to the *gevul* of an illness.' The noun גְּבוּל is explained by him as 'an absolute change in a disease for better or for worse, for health or for death' (cf. BM 676; see also Hebr. גְּבוּל in the sense of 'crisis' in Nathan's *Sefer ha-Peraqim* (*Pirqei Moshe*) N (cf. BCD 42 (NM 2:33); BMMN 20, l. 20; BMMG no. 186)).

גִּבּוּן · **cheese-like substance:** Arab. جبنية (Gr. τυρώδης; cf. UWS 2:510) · Ibn Sīnā, *K. al-Qānūn fī al-ṭibb* · trans. Nathan ha-Me'ati, *Sefer ha-Qanun* II, fol. 99[b]: לבן ... החלב מורכב משלשה עצמים ממימיות וגבון ודשנות (Milk: ... Milk consists of three substances: a watery substance, a cheese-like substance, and a fatty substance).[38] Hebr. גִּבּוּן features in BM 676 in an attestation from the *Sefer ha-Qanun* and is explained by Ben Yehuda as הפוך החלב לגבינה ('milk turning into cheese'). Zeraḥyah Ḥen and Anonymous both translate Arab. جبنية as גַּבְנִיּוּת (see entry).

גַּבְנִיּוּת · **cheese-like substance:** Arab. جبنية (Gr. τυρώδης; cf. UWS 2:510) · Ibn Sīnā, *K. al-Qānūn fī al-ṭibb* · trans. Zeraḥyah Ḥen, *Sefer ha-Qanun* II, fol. 232[b]: לבן חלב ... החלב מורכב מעצמים שלשה ממימיות וגבניות ודשניות (Milk: ... Milk consists of three substances:

36 Cf. ed. Bulaq 1877, 2:367.

37 The same text is quoted by the copyist of Moses ibn Tibbon, *Sefer Ṣedat ha-Derakhim*, in the same manuscript (Ms Oxford, Bodleian Library, Poc. 353, Uri Heb. 314 (Neubauer 2111), fol. 43[b]).

38 Cf. Galen, *De simplicium medicamentorum temperamentis ac facultatibus* X.2.7, ed. Kühn, 12:266, ll. 2–3: σύγκειται δ' ἐκ τριῶν οὐσιῶν ἅπαν γάλα, τυρώδους, ὀρρώδους, λιπαρᾶς.

a watery substance, a cheese-like substance, and a fatty substance).[39] Hebr. גַּבְנִיּוֹת is not attested in the current dictionaries. Nathan ha-Me'ati translates Arab. جبنية as גְּבוּן (see entry).

גֵּד • *Plur.* **גידים** • **[pulp of] colocynth**: Arab. شحم الحنظل · Ibn al-Jazzār, *Zād al-musāfir wa-qūt al-ḥāḍir* · trans. Moses ibn Tibbon, *Sefer Ṣedat ha-Derakhim* IV.19: וזה כשנעיין ואם היה חזק נשלשלהו בסמים אשר ישלשלו בקביצות כמו מיראבולנוש סיטרינוש ואינדיאוש וקיבוליש ואימבליקוש ובליריקוש ומה שדומה להם ונרחיק משלשל אותו בסמים חמים כאלואי ואשקמוניא וגידים (We should pay attention: If [the patient suffering from hemorrhoids] is strong we purge him with astringent purgatives, such as citrine, Indian, chebulic, emblic, and belleric myrobalans, and the like. We should avoid purging him with hot remedies, such as aloe, scammony, and [pulp of] colocynth). Hebr. גֵּד, *Plur.* גידים, features in BM 691 in the sense of 'wormwood' and in the sense of 'colocynth' in ibid., n. 3; referring to, a.o., Jonah ibn Janah.[40] For the parallel Aram. term גִּידָא, *Plur.* גידין, in *Sefer Ṣedat ha-Derakhim* IV.17, see entry below. Do'eg ha-Edomi transcribes the parallel Lat. term *coloquintida* as קולוקונטידא.

גִּדּוּל • **nutritive quality**: Lat. *nutrimentum* (Arab. غذاء) · Constantinus Africanus, *Viaticum peregrinantis* · trans. Do'eg ha-Edomi, *Sefer Ya'ir Netiv* VI.1: וכן רָאבַש והפולים מולידים רוח ומגדלים מאד אך גדולם נוטה לקרירות (Likewise, turnips and beans: They produce flatulence and are very nutritious but their nutritive quality tends to be cold). Hebr. גִּדּוּל does not feature in this sense in the current dictionaries. Moses ibn Tibbon translates Arab. غذاء as מזג and Abraham ben Isaac has כח.

[גדל] • *Part. Pi'el* **מְגַדֵּל** • **nourishing; nutritious**: Lat. *nutritivus* (Arab. مغذّ) · Constantinus Africanus, *Viaticum peregrinantis* · trans. Do'eg ha-Edomi, *Sefer Ya'ir Netiv* VI.1: וכן רָאבַש והפולים מולידים רוח ומגדלים מאד אך גדולם נוטה לקרירות (Likewise, turnips and beans: They produce flatulence and are very nutritious but their nutritive quality tends to be cold). Hebr. *Pi'el* גִּדֵּל, *Part.* מְגַדֵּל, does not feature in this sense in the current dictionaries. Moses ibn Tibbon translates the parallel Arab. term مغذّ as זן.

גִּהוּק • **belching; eructation**: Arab. جشاء · Ibn al-Jazzār, *Zād al-musāfir wa-qūt al-ḥāḍir* · trans. Moses ibn Tibbon, *Sefer Ṣedat ha-Derakhim* IV.9: כי המזונות אם נשתנו אל ליחה לבנה יהיה הגיהוק חמוץ (When the foods change into phlegm there will be sour belching). Hebr. גִּהוּק features in BM 712 in later attestations from the *Sefer ha-Qanun*. Do'eg ha-Edomi transcribes the parallel Lat. term *oxiregimina* as אוקשירימיא. Synonyms featuring in medieval medical literature are גְּעוּשׁ (cf. BCD 48 (NM 2:35, corr. 4:229)); גַּעַשׁ (BCD 48 (NM 4:33–34)); פִּהוּק (cf. BCD 219 (NM 3:187)); and Aram. קַבְסָא (cf. BCD 236 (NM 3:198)).

---

39 Cf. Galen, *De simplicium medicamentorum temperamentis ac facultatibus* X.2.7, ed. Kühn, 12:266, ll. 2–3: σύγκειται δ' ἐκ τριῶν οὐσιῶν ἅπαν γάλα, τυρώδους, ὀρρώδους, λιπαρᾶς.

40 Cf. Marwān ibn Janāḥ, *The Book of Hebrew Roots* (*K. al-Uṣūl*), ed. A. Neubauer (Oxford 1875), 123, n. 43.

גּוֹדָל • המקור שהוא בין הגודל והאצבע → מָקוֹר.

גווייש ‣ **dyspnea; shortness of breath; asthma**: Lat. *asma* · Gerard de Solo, *Practica super nono Almansoris* · trans. Abraham Avigdor, *Ha-Ma'amar ha-Teshi'i le-Sefer ha-Mansuri le-Razi*, fol. 102[a]: שער נ״ו: בהתיצבות הנשימה הנקרא גווייש (Chapter 56: On breathing difficulty called GWYYŠ). The term גווייש, a non-attested loan word from O. Occ. **gois*, features in NM 5:36 in an attestation from Moses ibn Tibbon, *Sefer Ṣedat ha-Derakhim* III.11. Shem Tov ben Isaac translates the parallel Arab. term ربو as צרות הנשום (see entry צָרוּת).

גּוּף • בלבול הגוף → בִּלְבּוּל.
 • שיבוש הגוף → שִׁבּוּשׁ.

גָּזַר • גזר דין ‣ **to define**: Lat. *diffinio* (Arab. حدّ)· Constantinus Africanus, *Viaticum peregrinantis* · trans. Do'eg ha-Edomi, *Sefer Ya'ir Netiv* IV.14: וגליאנוס גזר דין תחולי הזה בקצרה מאד ואמר: ליאנטריא הוא כאשר המאכל בשום ענין אינו מתחלף באסטומכא לא בהזלה ולא בצבע ולא בריח בהעדרת הבשול (Galen gave a very short definition of this illness [i.e., lientery] saying: lientery [occurs] when the food in the stomach does not undergo any change, not in a fluid substance, in smell, nor in color, because of a lack of concoction). Hebr. גזר דין does not feature in this sense in the current dictionaries. Moses ibn Tibbon translates the parallel Arab. term حدّ as גדר.

גִּיד • גיד הערוה ‣ **penis**: Arab. ذَكَر · Ibn al-Jazzār, *Zād al-musāfir wa-qūt al-ḥāḍir* · trans. Abraham ben Isaac, *Sefer Ṣedah la-Oreḥim* VI.1: וימשח בו גיד הערוה ואז יעמוד בחוזק ויתחזק (And rub the penis with it, for then he will have a strong erection). Hebr. גיד הערוה features in medieval medical literature in the sense of 'urethra' in Do'eg ha-Edomi, *Sefer Agur* IV.82 (cf. BCD 45 (NM 3:44)). For גִּיד alone in the sense of 'penis,' see BM 752 and BCD 44 (NM 1:18, 81, 133). Moses ibn Tibbon translates Arab. ذَكَر as זַכְרוּת (see entry).
 • כשזב הזרע מן הגיד בלא רצון → [זוב].
 • עמד הגיד → עָמַד.
 • כשיעמוד גיד הערוה תדיר → עָמַד.
 • עמידת הגיד → עֲמִידָה.

גִּידָא (*Aram.*) **•** *Plur.* גידין ‣ **[pulp of] colocynth**: Arab. شحم الحنظل · Ibn al-Jazzār, *Zād al-musāfir wa-qūt al-ḥāḍir* · trans. Moses ibn Tibbon, *Sefer Ṣedat ha-Derakhim* IV.17: תאר תחבושת מועיל לקולון: יקח סחיטת קשואים מרים ואשקמוניאה ומררת שור וגידין מ״א חלק (Recipe of a plaster (salve) that is good for colon: Take one part each of extract of squirting cucumber, scammony, ox bile and colocynth pulp …). As a botanical term, Aram. גִּידָא, *Plur.* גידין, is only attested in Rabb. literature in the sense of 'wormwood' (cf. SDA 221). For the Hebr. counterpart גֵּד, *Plur.* גידים, in *Sefer Ṣedat ha-Derakhim* IV.19, cf. entry above. Do'eg ha-Edomi transcribes the parallel Lat. term *colocontida* as קולוקונטידא.

גיעול → גְּעוּל.

גִּירְסָא (*Aram.*) ‣ **memorizing**: Arab. حفظ · Maimonides, *Maqāla fī al-rabw* (*On Asthma*)

· Anonymous, *Sefer ha-Qaṣeret* XIII.19 (cf. BMA 2:442, ll. 21–24): וכשיהיה גאלינוס עם טוב שכלו ואורך שניו במעשה הרפואות והפרדו לזו המלאכה וחוזק השתדלותו עליה יסתפק במעשיו וחוזר[41] בהם היאך יהיה העניין באלו המקומות שכבר קצרו הרופאים בהתעסקות הרבה עם עוצם מה שצריך אליו מהגירסא ואורך חלקיה (And if Galen—with his excellent intellect and long experience in the practice of medicine, his devotion to this art, and his strong aspirations [to excel] in it—casts doubts on his own practice and is tentative about it, how much more should this be the case in our generations, in which physicians have only very little experience, while [at the same time] much memorizing is needed, since the different parts of medicine have become so lengthy!). Aram. גִּירְסָא is attested for in Rabb. literature in the sense of '1. learning; study; 2. reciting; recitation; 3. textual tradition' (SDA 227; cf. NM 5:39). For the Hebrew counterpart גִּירְסָה; cf. BM 846; s.v. גרסה: 'text; variant.' Samuel Benveniste translates Arab. حفظ as זכרנות and Joshua Shatibi has שמירה.

גֶּלֶד • *Plur.* גלדים • גלדי האצטומכה · **the layers (coats) of the stomach**: Arab. طبقات المعدة · Ibn al-Jazzār, *Zād al-musāfir wa-qūt al-ḥādir* · trans. Moses ibn Tibbon, *Sefer Ṣedat ha-Derakhim* IV.6: ואם היה הצמא בסבת מרה כרכומית עצורה בגלדי האצטומ׳ ראוי להריק אותה בקיא או בשלשול (If thirst is caused by yellow bile that is retained in the layers of the stomach, it should be evacuated through vomiting or provoking diarrhea). Hebr. *Sing.* גֶּלֶד features in the Bible in the sense of 'skin' (KB 1:191); in Rabb. literature as 'coating; skin; thickness' (JD 1:245), and in medieval literature as 'peel' (e.g., of an onion) (BM 770). In the sense of 'membrane [of the eye]' it is attested in Shem Tov ben Isaac, *Sefer ha-Shimmush* XXX.2.21 (cf. BCD 46 (NM 1:82)).

גְּלָלָא (*Aram.*) • בורמא דגללא → בּוּרְמָא.

גְּמִיעָה · **linctus**: Arab. لعوق · Maimonides, *Maqāla fī al-rabw* (*On Asthma*) · trans. Joshua Shatibi, *Ma'amar 'al ha-Qaṣeret* XII.3 (cf. BMA 2:362, ll. 15–16): וכבר זכרו האחרונים אחריו הרכבה אחרת והוא תלתן ותאנים יבושלו ויסונן המים ויצרף דבש דבורים ויעבהו והיא גמיעה (Later physicians mention another compound drug: Cook fenugreek and figs, strain the water, add bee honey to it, and thicken this until it becomes a linctus). Hebr. גְּמִיעָה features in the current dictionaries in the sense of 'quaffing; a full draught' (JD 252 (s.v. גמיאה); BM 799). Samuel Benveniste translates Arab. لعوق as לְחִיכָה (see entry) and Anonymous has לְעִיטָה (see entry). For a var. reading גְּמִיאָה for Arab. مضمضة ('mouthwash'), cf. NM 5:40.

גָּמַר · **to become fixed, settled**: Arab. تمكّن (Gr. στηρίζω; cf. UW 638) · Ibn al-Jazzār, *Zād al-musāfir wa-qūt al-ḥādir* · trans. Moses ibn Tibbon, *Sefer Ṣedat ha-Derakhim* V.5: ואמ׳ דיאשקורידש כי שתני התישים כשישתם בכל יום והם חמים עם אשפיקא נרדי ויתמיד זה יתיך השקוי הבשרי קודם שיגמור[42] ויגירהו בשתן והשלשול (Dioscurides said if one contin-

41 וחוזר: ويتردّد a.

42 שיגמור: Ms London, British Library, Add. 27542, fol. 87b.

ues to drink every day the urine of a he-goat with Indian spikenard while it is still hot, it dissolves anasarca before it becomes fixed (settled). It expels the [fluid] with the urine and diarrhea).[43] Hebr. גָּמַר does not feature in this sense in the current dictionaries.

• *Nif'al* **נִגְמַר** · **to be fully developed, reach its climax:** Arab. انتهى · Ibn al-Jazzār, *Zād al-musāfir wa-qūt al-ḥādir* · trans. Moses ibn Tibbon, *Sefer Ṣedat ha-Derakhim* v.3: ואם נגמרה המורסא הנה ראוי שיעורב עם הרפואות האלו אשר זכרנו דברים מתיכים משקיטים (When the tumor is fully developed, the remedies I mentioned should be mixed with ingredients that have a dissolving and alleviating effect). Hebr. *Nif'al* נִגְמַר does not feature in this sense in the current dictionaries. Do'eg ha-Edomi translates the parallel Lat. term *status* as עֹמֶד in his *Sefer Ya'ir Netiv* II.18.11 (corr.) (cf. NM 5:150; IJZ 1–2:648) and also as הַעֲמָדָה in v.13 (see entry).

גַּס • **המעי הגס** → מְעִי.

גִּעוּל · **(nocturnal) pollution:** Lat. *pollutio* (Arab. احتلام) · Constantinus Africanus, *Viaticum peregrinantis* · trans. Do'eg ha-Edomi, *Sefer Ya'ir Netiv* VI.4: ולפעמים יראה אשה ויחשוק אותה והנפש בתוך שנתו מציירת אותה אצלו כאלו היה שם ומשם יחול הגיעול ההוא כי ציור הנפש אינו כי אם חבור הגוף (Sometimes a man sees a woman and longs for her. When he is asleep the soul imagines her near to him as if he was (had intercourse) with her and this causes the nocturnal pollution, for the imagination of the soul is nothing else but a temperament of the body). Hebr. גִּעוּל features in BM 820 in the sense of 'loathing; abhorrence.' Moses ibn Tibbon and Abraham ben Isaac both translate Arab. احتلام as קרי. In Do'eg's *Sefer Ya'ir Nativ*, Hebr. גִּעוּל also features as 'sordes (earwax)' (II.7) and 'blemish; fault; defect' (II.17); cf. NM 5:40–41. A synonym for גִּעוּל featuring in *Sefer Ya'ir Netiv* VI.4 is גרישת הזרע בתוך השינה (see entry גְּרִישָׁה).

גָּרָב • **הגרב המנוגע** · **ulcerating scabies:** Arab. الجرب المتقرّح · Ibn Sīnā, *K. al-Qānūn fī al-ṭibb* · trans. Nathan ha-Me'ati, *Sefer ha-Qanun* II, fol. 68[a]: באן ... כשמערבין אותו באספלנית הנקרא מרהם בערבי עם חומץ יועיל מהקלוף והגרב המנוגע ויועיל מהסמנים[44] הרפים והמספחת הנקרא סעפה[45] בערבי (B'N [i.e., fruit of the ben oil tree [*Moringa oleifera* Lam.]]: When it is mixed with vinegar in an ointment, called *marham* in Arab., it is useful for exfoliating and ulcerating scabies, 'milk-like'[46] pimples, and favus, called *sa'fah* in Arab.). Hebr. הגרב המנוגע is not attested in the current dictionaries. For גָּרָב in the sense of 'scabies,' cf. BM 830; see also BCD 48 (NM 2:177). Hebr. נָגַע, *Part. Pu'al* מְנֻגָּע, features in the sense of 'ulcerous' (Lat. *vulneratus*) in BCD 170 (NM 3:132). Zer-

---

43 Cf. Dioscurides, *De materia medica* II.81, ed. by M. Wellmann (Repr. Berlin, 1958), 165; trans. by L.Y. Beck (Hildesheim 2005), 126.

44 מהסמנים הרפים (= البثور اللينة): البثور اللبنية a.

45 סעפה: emend. ed. סחפה Ms سعفة a.

46 "'milk-like' pimples': Trans. after a.

aḥyah Ḥen translates Arab. الجرب المتقرّح as הגרב כשיתנגע and Anonymous has הגרב המשתחן.

גַּרְגִּיר • גרגיר הקרא · **tapeworms**: Arab. حبّ القرع · Ibn al-Jazzār, *Zād al-musāfir wa-qūt al-ḥādir* · trans. Moses ibn Tibbon, *Sefer Ṣedat ha-Derakhim* IV.18: ומהם מה שיתילד במעים הדקים העליונים ואלו נקראים נחשים בעבור שהם ארוכים ומהם מה שיתילד במעים העבים אשר למטה מן הטבור ויקראו גרגיר הקרא (Of the [intestinal worms] there are those that originate in the upper small intestine and they are called *neḥashim* [lit., 'snakes;' h.l., roundworms] because they are long; others originate in the large intestine below the navel and are called *gargir ha-qara'* [lit., 'pumpkin seeds;' i.e., tapeworms]). Hebr. גרגיר הקרא does not feature in the current dictionaries. For the Hebr. synonyms גרגרי הדלעת and גרגרי הדלועים, replacing the Arab. term for 'pumpkin' (قرع), with the Hebr. one (*Sing.* דלעת and *Plur.* דלועים); cf. BCD 49 for attestations from Nathan ha-Me'ati, *Sefer ha Peraqim* (*Pirqei Moshe*) VII.31 (cf. NM 2:35; BMMN 85, l. 15; BMMG no. 769) and Shem Tov ben Isaac, *Sefer ha-Shimmush* XXVII (cf. NM 4:34). Do'eg ha-Edomi transcribes the parallel Lat. term *ascarides et cucurbini* as אישקרידיש גם קוקורביטין.

גַּרְגְּרָנוּת · **gluttony**: Arab. نهم · Maimonides, *Maqāla fī al-rabw* (*On Asthma*) · Anonymous (*Sefer ha-Qaṣeret* V.3 (cf. BMA 2:403, ll. 20–21): וכבר ראיתי מקצת אנשי הגרגרנות לפעמים מלא[47] בטנו עד שיצא המאכל לפיו כמו הבהמות המעלות גרה (I have sometimes seen certain gluttons belching[48] and [thereby] returning the food [from their stomachs] to their mouths, just like ruminating animals). Hebr. גַּרְגְּרָנוּת is attested in Rabb. and halakhic literature (cf. JD 265; BM 833). Samuel Benveniste translates Arab. أهل النهم ('gluttons') as גרגרנים and Joshua Shatibi as זוללים.

גֶּרֶד · **shreds [of intestinal tissue]**: Lat. *rasura* (Arab. خراطة) · Constantinus Africanus, *Viaticum peregrinantis* · trans. Do'eg ha-Edomi, *Sefer Ya'ir Netiv* IV.15: ואם הוא במעי האמצעי הכאב עשוי בגבהי הטבור והתוצאות מעורבים עם הדבר שהוא סבה מהדיסנטיריא. ואם הוא במעי השפל יצא דם או דבר נקי וזך כמו גרד יוצא משם (If the dysentery is in the middle intestines, the pain is in the region above the navel and the stools are mixed with the matter that causes the dysentery. If it is in the lower intestines, blood or matter is discharged that is clean like intestinal shreds). Hebr. גֶּרֶד features in JD 265 and BM 834 in the sense of 'erasure.' Moses ibn Tibbon translates the parallel Arab. term خراطة as גְּרִידָה (see entry).

גָּרוֹן • נחור הגרון → נְחוֹר.

• ערלת הגרון → עָרְלָה.

• הרוח הנדחה דרך הגרון → רוּחַ.

גְּרִידָה · **shreds [of intestinal tissue]**: Arab. خراطة · Ibn al-Jazzār, *Zād al-musāfir wa-qūt al-ḥādir* · trans. Moses ibn Tibbon, *Sefer Ṣedat ha-Derakhim* IV.15: ואם יהיה החולי

---

47 מלא בטנו: تجشّأ a.

48 'belching': Trans. after a.

באמצעיים יהיה מה שיצא מעורב עם הדבר העושה החולי מן הגרידה ויהיה הכאב בטבור לא למעלה ממנו ולא למטה ממנו (If the illness [i.e., dysentery] is in the middle [intestines], the stools are mixed with the matter, i.e., shreds [of intestinal tissue] that causes the illness and the pain is [in the region of] the navel, not higher and not lower). In the sense of 'shred,' Hebr. גְּרִידָה features in BCD 50 (NM 2:35–36) in a later attestation from Nathan ha-Me'ati, *Sefer ha-Peraqim* (*Pirqei Moshe*) VI.82 (cf. BMMN 77, l. 6; BMMG no. 1339). For גְּרִידָה in the sense of 'abrasion' (for Arab. سحج), see BCD 50 (NM 3:48); 'scarification' (for Lat. *scarificatio*), see BCD 50 (NM 1:19); and 'peel' (for Arab. جرادة), see NM 5:42. Do'eg ha-Edomi translates the parallel Lat. term *rasura* as גֶּרֶד (see entry).

גְּרִישָׁה • גרישה לחוץ · extracting; extraction: Lat. *eiectio* (Arab. إخراج) · Constantinus Africanus, *Viaticum peregrinantis* · trans. Do'eg ha-Edomi, *Sefer Ya'ir Netiv* V.16: ואם היא גדולה שלא תוכל לצאת בשתן נמהר להסירה מצואר המקוה ולא ירפא כי אם בכריתות ובגרישת האבן לחוץ (If [the bladder stone] is so large that it cannot come out with the urine, we should hurry to remove it from the neck of the bladder; it can only be cured by surgery and by extracting the stone). Hebr. גְּרִישָׁה features in NM 5:43 in the sense of 'vomiting; spitting' (for Lat. *reiectio*) in an attestation from Do'eg ha-Edomi, *Sefer Ya'ir Netiv* III.8. Moses ibn Tibbon translates the parallel Arab. term إخراج as הוציא.

• גרישת חזרע בתוך השינה · nocturnal pollution: Lat. *effusio spermatis in somno* (Arab. احتلام)· Constantinus Africanus, *Viaticum peregrinantis* · trans. Do'eg ha-Edomi, *Sefer Ya'ir Netiv* VI.4: בגרישת הזרע בתוך השינה הוא קרי (On nocturnal pollution; i.e., *qeri*). Hebr. גרישת הזרע בתוך השינה does not feature in the current dictionaries. Hebr. קרי (*qeri*) is the standard Hebr. synonym, cf. BM 6180–6182 and entry גִּעוּל, a synonym used by Do'eg for Lat. *pollutio*. Moses ibn Tibbon translates the parallel Arab. term احتلام as מקרה לילה (see entry מִקְרֶה) and Abraham ben Isaac has קרי הנקר' בחלום.

[גרען] *Pi'el* **גִּרְעֵן · to make pills:** Arab. حبّب · Maimonides, *Maqāla fī al-rabw* (*On Asthma*) · Anonymous, *Sefer ha-Qaṣeret* XII.8 (cf. BMA 2:434, ll. 20–23): אחר יותר חזק ממנו זרע אנגורה ובסביאג מכל אחד דרהם מי קשואים של חמור חצי דרהם שחם חנטל רביע דרהם כתירא ומקל תכלתי מכל אחד רביע דרהם תוך פסתק ג' גרעינים יולש במי כרפס ומגרענין אותו בשמן שקדים וזה יוציא לחויות עבות מתדבקות רעות (Another [purgative] stronger than this one: [Take] one *dirham*[49] each of Roman nettle seed and common polypody, half a *dirham* of the juice of squirting cucumber, one quarter of a *dirham* of pulp of colocynth, one quarter of a *dirham* each of gum tragacanth and blue bdellium and three grains of shelled pistachio nuts; knead [these ingredients] with celery juice and make pills from them, using almond oil. This [purgative] expels the bad, thick, and viscous humors). Hebr. גִּרְעֵן, a denominal verb coined from גַּרְעִין, is not attested

49 The standard *dirham* is 3.125 grams; cf. HIM 3.

in the current dictionaries. Samuel Benveniste and Anonymous both render Arab. حبّب as עשה גרגרים.

[גרש] • *Pi'el* גֵּרֵשׁ ‣ **to emit, eject**: Lat. *emitto* (Arab. إلقاء) · Constantinus Africanus, *Viaticum peregrinantis* · trans. Do'eg ha-Edomi, *Sefer Ya'ir Netiv* VI.1: והכין להם התולדת אברים בענין לגרש זרע אחד לקבל זרע אחר (Nature prepared organs for them [i.e., man and woman]; for the one to emit the sperm and for the other to receive it). Hebr. גֵּרֵשׁ does not feature in this sense in the current dictionaries. Moses ibn Tibbon translates Arab. إلقاء as השליך. See also NM 5:43 for Do'eg's use of *Pi'el* גֵּרֵשׁ in the sense of 'to insufflate' (for Lat. *insufflo*) in *Sefer Ya'ir Netiv* II.15.4 (cf. IJZ 1–2:644).

גֶּשֶׁם • *Plur.* **גשמים** ‣ **winter**: Arab. شتاء · Maimonides, *Maqāla fī al-rabw* (*On Asthma*) · trans. Samuel Benveniste, *Ma'amar 'al ha-Qaṣeret* VI.5 (cf. BMA 2:264, ll. 14–15): ואני איעץ למעלתך בכל זה ובמקום כוסות יין בגשמים תשתה כמו משליש ליטרא[50] למחצית ליטרא מהדבש המתוקן (I advise my Master to do all this, but to take—instead of a glass of wine—in winter between one third of a liter and half a liter[51] of refined hydromel). Hebr. גשמים stands for ימות הגשמים, which features in Rabb. literature in the sense of 'the rainy season' (i.e., autumn and winter); cf. JD 274; BM 855. For 'the sunny season' (i.e., summer), see also entry חַמָּה (for ימות החמה). Joshua Shatibi translates Arab. شتاء as סתיו and Anonymous has קור (cf. BCD 248 (NM 3:207)).

---

50 ליטרא: رطل a.

51 'liter': Arab. *raṭl*. The weight of the *raṭl* is varying according to region and period; from the twelfth century on, its general weight in Egypt is 450 grams; cf. HIM 28–33, esp. 29.

ד

דִּבּוּק · **I. stickiness; viscosity**: Arab. لزوجة · Maimonides, *Maqāla fī al-rabw* (*On Asthma*) · trans. Samuel Benveniste, *Ma'amar 'al ha-Qaṣeret* IV.6 (cf. BMA 2:256, ll. 19–20): וזה עוזר לעכל מאד ויתיך הבלגם וימרק האסטומכה[52] ויחתך דבוק הליחות ולא יחמם חמום יותר (This [mustard preparation] is very good for the digestion; it dissolves the phlegm, cleans the[53] lining of the stomach, dissolves the stickiness of the humors, and does not heat excessively). Hebr. דִּבּוּק is not attested in medieval medical literature in the current dictionaries. Joshua Shabiti translates Arab. لزوجة as דבקות (cf. BCD 54 (NM 3:50), s.v. *Plur.* דבקויות (for Arab. لزوجات) in the sense of 'viscous matters') and Anonymous renders Arab. لزوجة as התדבקות.

· **II. firmness**: Arab. تلزز · Maimonides, *Maqāla fī al-rabw* (*On Asthma*) · trans. Samuel Benveniste, *Ma'amar 'al ha-Qaṣeret* X.4 (cf. BMA 2:278, ll. 16–19): וראוי להרגיל בו המים החמים ביותר עד שיקרב עור הראש להאדים כי זה מחמם המוח חמימות יתישרו בו פעולותיו ויחסרו הנוספים ממנו ויקנה לעור הראש דבוק וכח עד שלא ירגיש למעט סבה שימצאהו (One should accustom oneself to water that is so hot that the skin of the head almost turns red, because this warms the brain with a balanced heat so that its activities improve and its superfluities are reduced. It also makes the skin of the head firmer and stronger so that it is not affected [anymore] by the slightest cause). Joshua Shatibi translates Arab. تلزز as קביצה and Anonymous has קִבּוּץ (see entry).

· **III. agglutination**: Arab. تغرية · Ibn Sīnā, *K. al-Qānūn fī al-ṭibb* · trans. Nathan ha-Me'ati, *Sefer ha-Qanun* II, fol. 70ª: ביץ ביצים ... יש בו קבוץ וקל וחומר באודם הצלוי ממנו והלובן שלו ישקיט כל הכאבים הנושנים וזה בדבוק אשר בו (Eggs: ... They are constipative, especially the fried yolk. The egg white relieves all chronic pains due to its agglutination). Zeraḥyah Ḥen translates Arab. تغرية as דִּבּוּק as well and Anonymous has דבקות (cf. NM 5:45).

• **הפרד הדבוק** → **[פרד]**.

דביד · **electuary**: Arab. دبيد (cf. FAQ 182) · Ibn al-Jazzār, *Zād al-musāfir wa-qūt al-ḥāḍir* · trans. Moses ibn Tibbon, *Sefer Ṣedat ha-Derakhim* V.2: או ישתה דביד ורדים העשוי במשקה סוכר או עוגות ברבריס עם אוקשימל (He [i.e., a person suffering from a liver obstruction] may also take an electuary of roses prepared with julep or barberry pastilles with oxymel). Hebr. דביד, often faultily spelled as דביר, is a non-attested calque of Arab. دبيد. Subsequently, the term features in Samuel Benveniste, *Ma'amar 'al ha-Qaṣeret* XIII.41 (cf. BMA 2:313, l. 19); while Joshua Shabiti renders Arab. دبيد in the same paragraph as יין (cf. BMA 2:382, l. 16). The term דביד also features in Ms Munich,

---

52 האסטומכה: خمل المعدة a.

53 'the lining of the stomach': Trans. after a.

Bayerische Staatsbibliothek, Cod. hebr. 8, in an anonymous list of parallel medical terms entitled *Sha'ar Shinnui ha-Shemot ha-Niqra'im Synonimis* (*Chapter on Different [Medical] Terms Called 'Synonyms'*),[54] fol. 197b: דביר (*דביד) הוא שם רפואה בלשון ארמית ועל כן יאמר דביר (*דביד) וורד דביר (*דביד) לאקא (DBYD is the name of a [kind of] remedy in Aram.; accordingly it is said: 'a rose electuary; a lac electuary'). The Arab. term دبيد does not come from Syriac, but from Pers.; cf. VL 1:810, s.v. *dabīd*: 'term. techn. med. medicamentum; 2. sec. al. electuarium.'

[דבק] • *Pi'el* **דִּבֵּק** · **to cause to heal**: Arab. ألزق (Gr. κολλάω; cf. UW 354–355) · Ibn Sīnā, *K. al-Qānūn fī al-ṭibb* · trans. Nathan ha-Me'ati, *Sefer ha-Qanun* II, fol. 72a: בלוט ... ועלי הבלוט ידבק המכות כששוחקים אותו וזורים אותו עליהם (Oak: ... Oak leaves cause wounds to heal when they are pulverized and sprinkled over them). In a medical context, Hebr. *Pi'el* דִּבֵּק features in the sense of 'to seal' (for Arab. ألحم (corr.)) in Nathan's *Sefer ha-Peraqim* (*Pirqei Moshe*) III.13 (cf. BCD 53 (NM 2:36); BMMN 41, l. 8; BMMG no. 4515), and in the sense of 'to set [broken bones]' (for Arab. جبر) in Zeraḥyah Ḥen, *Sefer ha-Peraqim* (*Pirqei Moshe*) XV.64 (cf. BCD 53 (NM 1:135); BMMZ 162, l. 21; BMMG no. 552). Zeraḥyah translates Arab. ألزق *in his Sefer ha-Qanun* as דִּבֵּק as well. In comparison, Anonymous has *Hif'il* הִדְבִּיק (cf. Nathan's use of הִדְבִּיק (for Arab. ألحم) in his *Sefer ha-Peraqim* XV.17 (cf. BMMN 156, l. 23; BCD 53 (NM 2:36); BMMG no. 4516) in the same sense ('to allow to heal up') as he uses *Pi'el* דִּבֵּק in the *Sefer ha-Qanun*, and Abraham ben Isaac uses *Hif'il* הִדְבִּיק in the sense of 'to apply' (for Arab. ألزق) in his *Sefer Ṣedah la-Oreḥim* I.6.5 (NM 5:44; IJZ 1–2:547)).

• *Hitpa'el* **הִתְדַּבֵּק** · **to close, heal**: Arab. التئم (cf. WKAS 2.1:58) · Ibn al-Jazzār, *Zād al-musāfir wa-qūt al-ḥāḍir* · trans. Moses ibn Tibbon, *Sefer Ṣedat ha-Derakhim* V.13: ואם נפתחה המורסא וראינו המוגלא נגרה הנה ראוי שנמהר לרפאת הנגע ההוא בכל ענין עד שיתדבק (When the ulcer bursts and we see pus streaming out, we should hurry to treat the wound in every possible way until it closes). Hebr. הִתְדַּבֵּק features in a similar sense of 'to grow [together again]' (for Arab. نمى) in a later attestation in BCD 53 (NM 3:50). Do'eg ha-Edomi translates the parallel Lat. term *solidatio* as הדביק וחיזק (see next entry). The Lat. verb *solido* is translated by him in the same paragraph as חזק והדביק (see entry [חזק]).

• *Hif'il* **הִדְבִּיק** • **הדביק וחיזק** · **to close**: Lat. *solidatio* (Arab. التئم) · Constantinus Africanus, *Viaticum peregrinantis* · trans. Do'eg ha-Edomi, *Sefer Ya'ir Netiv* V.13: ואם הצמח נבקע והבלוי יזל משם יאות שנמהר להדביק ולחזק הנגע עם חלב חמורה (If the wound bursts and the pus streams out, one should hurry to close the wound with donkey's milk). Moses ibn Tibbon translates the parallel Arab. term التئم as *Hitpa'el* הִתְדַּבֵּק (see previous entry). In the same paragraph, Do'eg translates the Lat. verb *solido* as חזק והדביק (see entry [חזק]).

54 For this list, cf. G. Bos, S. Lauschus, and F. Savelsberg, 'Substitute Drugs in the Hebrew Tradition' (forthcoming).

• חזק והדביק → [חזק].

• *Part. Hifʿil* מַדְבִּיק • הרפואות המדביקות → רְפוּאָה.

דֶּבֶק · **resin**: Arab. علك · Ibn Sīnā, *K. al-Qānūn fī al-ṭibb* · trans. Nathan ha-Me'ati, *Sefer ha-Qanun* II, fol. 87b: חבה כצרה ... העדי: ימרוק הפנים והכתם הנקר' כלף בער' והדבק הנק' עלך אלאנבאט יועיל לבקיעי הפנים (Terebinth: ... [The application of its resin in] cosmetics: It cleanses the face and removes freckles, called *kalaf* in Arab., while its resin called 'turpentine' is useful in facial cracks). Hebr. דֶּבֶק does not feature in this sense in the current dictionaries. Zeraḥyah Ḥen transcribes Arab. علك as עלך.

• **דבק הזהב** · **chrysocolla**: Arab. لزاق الذهب (from Gr. χρῡσοκόλλα 'gold-solder; malachite; basic copper carbonate;' cf. LS 2010; WKAS 2:544) · Ibn Sīnā, *K. al-Qānūn fī al-ṭibb* · trans. Zeraḥyah Ḥen, *Sefer ha-Qanun* II, fol. 229b: לַאזֻוֵרְד אֶזוּר: המהות כחו ככח דבק הזהב וחלוש ממנו מעט (Le'ZeWaRəD 'eZWuR [i.e., lapis lazuli]: What is it (*ha-mahut*)?:[55] Its potency is similar to that of chrysocolla, but it is slightly weaker in action). Hebr. דבק הזהב is a non-attested calque of Arab. لزاق الذهب. A var. reading used by Zeraḥyah in his *Sefer ha-Peraqim* (*Pirqei Moshe*) XXIII.101 is דבקות הזהב (cf. BCD 54 (NM 1:136); BMMZ 231, l. 4), while Nathan ha-Me'ati translates Arab. لزاق الذهب as מדביק הזהב (cf. BMMN 232, l. 1) (cf. also BMMG no. 4604). Shem Tov ben Isaac has מדביק הזהב as well in his *Sefer ha-Shimmush* XXIX, list 1 (cf. SHS 1:332–333 (Mem 63)).

דֶּבֶק • הפרדת הדבקים → הַפְרָדָה.

דְּבֵקוּת · **connection**: Arab. إتّصال · Ibn al-Jazzār, *Zād al-musāfir wa-qūt al-ḥāḍir* · trans. Moses ibn Tibbon, *Sefer Ṣedat ha-Derakhim* VI.15: ואם יהיו ליחות מתעוררות בגוף המעוברת ראוי להשקותן רפואה משלשלת כאשר יעברו על העובר ד' חדשים וזה הזמן הממוצע בין זמני ההריון אשר יהיה בו דבקות העובר ברחם טוב וחזק (If the humors are stirred up in the body of a pregnant woman, one should administer her a laxative once the fetus is four months old, because the time between four and seven months is the middle period of the pregnancy in which the connection of the fetus with the uterus is sound and strong). For Hebr. דְּבֵקוּת in a medical context, cf. entry דִּבּוּק. The term features in PESHAT[56] in the sense of a.o., 'contiguity; adhesion; physical attachment.'

דָּבָר • **דברים מחליקים** · **laxatives**: Arab. الأشياء المزلقة · Maimonides, *Maqāla fī al-rabw* (*On Asthma*) · trans. Samuel Benveniste, *Ma'amar 'al ha-Qaṣeret* IX.6 (cf. BMA 2:272, ll. 20–22): ולא יצטרך לרפות במשקים ולא בדומיהם מפני שהם מחלישים עור האסטומכה ויעוררו הקיא כמשפט רוב הדברים המחליקים בשעת האכילה (But one should not resort to taking decoctions and the like for softening [the stools] because they loosen the lining of the stomach and cause nausea, as most laxatives do when taken). Hebr. דברים מחליקים features in BCD 55 (NM 2:26) in the sense of 'mollifacients' (for Lat. *leni-*

55 See entry מָהוּת.

56 https://peshat.org/display/peshat_lemmas_00000620 (accessed January 9, 2022).

ficantia) in an attestation from Hillel ben Samuel, *Sefer Keritut*. Joshua Shatibi and Anonymous render Arab. الأشياء المزلقة as דברים מחליקים as well.

• **דברים שוברים** ‣ **diuretics:** Lat. *diuretica* (Arab. الأدوية المدرّة) · Constantinus Africanus, *Viaticum peregrinantis* · trans. Do'eg ha-Edomi, *Sefer Ya'ir Netiv* v.2: ואם הוא מחתוך אחד מן האברים נצוה להקיזו ונתן לו דברים שוברים כאשר הזכרנו (If [the obstruction of the liver] is caused by an amputation of a limb, we order [the patient] to be bled and to give him diuretics as we mentioned [before]). Hebr. דברים שוברים is not attested in the current dictionaries. For *Part.* שׁוֹבֵר on its own (for Lat. *diureticus*), cf. entry [שבר] below. Moses ibn Tibbon translates Arab. الأدوية المدرّة as הרפואות המגירות השתן. A synonym similar to the term used by Moses ibn Tibbon and also featuring in medieval medical literature (for Arab. الدواء المدرّ للبول, in Anonymous, *Sammim Libbiyim*) is הסם המגיר השתן (cf. BCD 187 (NM 4:125)).

דִּבְשִׁי • **המורסות הדבשיות** → מֻרְסָה.

דוחק → דֹּחַק.

[דחה] • *Part. Nif'al* נִדְחֶה • **הרוח הנדחה דרך הגרון** → רוּחַ.

דֹּחַק • **דוחק בחזה** ‣ **angina pectoris:** Arab. ضيق الصدر · Ibn al-Jazzār, *Zād al-musāfir wa-qūt al-ḥāḍir* · trans. Abraham ben Isaac, *Sefer Ṣedah la-Oreḥim* vi.12: וכאשר יתגדל יקרה בגידולו כאב באשטומכה וניפוח במקום[57] ודוחק בחזה גם רפיון וחלשות (If [the tumor in the uterus] gets worse (grows) it will be followed by pain in the stomach, swelling under the epigastrium,[58] angina pectoris, languor, and weakness). Hebr. דוחק בחזה is not attested in the current dictionaries. Moses ibn Tibbon translates Arab. ضيق الصدر as צרות החזה (see entry צָרוּת).

דִּין ‣ **crisis [of an illness]:** Lat. *crisis* (Arab. بحران) · Constantinus Africanus, *Viaticum peregrinantis* · trans. Do'eg ha-Edomi, *Sefer Ya'ir Netiv* iv.11: דבר טוב אל הגוף אם הקיא נעשה אליו בטרם הצורך ואם הוא צריך יעשה אותו כפי הדין הוא קרישיס (It is good for the body when a person vomits before it is necessary, but if that is the case he should vomit in accordance with the crisis; i.e., QRYŠYS [i.e., Lat. *crisis*]). Hebr. דִּין does not feature in this sense in the current dictionaries. Moses ibn Tibbon translates the parallel Arab. term بحران as נקיון הוא בחראן בערבי (cf. BCD 180 (NM 1:62–63) for Hebr. נִקָּיוֹן in his *Sefer Ṣedat ha-Derakhim* vii.7.1 (cf. IJZ 7:135, l. 5)).

• **גזר דין** → גְּזַר.

דְּלִיפָה ‣ **flowing; streaming:** Arab. هطل · Maimonides, *Maqāla fī al-rabw* (*On Asthma*) · trans. Samuel Benveniste, *Ma'amar 'al ha-Qaṣeret* xi.2 (cf. BMA 2:284, ll. 1–2): ופעמים ⟨יהיה⟩ הדבר היורד חד דק יצטרך למה שידקקהו ויחתכהו וזה מוסיף להוריד מה שידלוף ואע"פ שהדליפה נשארת (Sometimes the descending secretion is sharp and fine and [nevertheless] needs something to thin and cut it [even more]. This increases the des-

---

57 במקום: في ما دون الشراسيف a.

58 'epigastrium': Trans. after a.

cending flow, when there is still [something] left [of it to stream down]). Hebr. דְּלִיפָה features in BM 945 in the sense of 'dripping.' Joshua Shatibi and Anonymous both render Arab. هطل as נזילה.

דָּלַף · to flow, stream: Arab. هطل · *Maqāla fī al-rabw* (*On Asthma*) · trans. Samuel Benveniste, *Ma'amar 'al ha-Qaṣeret* XI.2 (cf. BMA 2:283, l. 22–284, l. 1): פעמים יהיה הדבר המצער המונע מהשינה הוא הדבר שידלוף מהמוח בעת רדתו ופעמים יהיה הדבר הדוחק הוא מהם מה שכבר הגיע בריאה (Sometimes that which causes agitation and sleeplessness is that which streams and descends from the brain, while that which causes [a feeling of] pressure is that which is [already] there in the lungs). Hebr. דָּלַף features in the current dictionaries in the sense of 'to drop, drip' (cf. BM 947). Joshua Shatibi translates Arab. هطل as נזל and Anonymous has ירד.

דָּם • דם קרוש · blood clot: Arab. علق · Ibn al-Jazzār, *Zād al-musāfir wa-qūt al-ḥādir* · trans. Moses ibn Tibbon, *Sefer Ṣedat ha-Derakhim* V.20: וצרות המעבר אשר יצא בו השתן יהיה אם מפני סתום בו כמו האבן או דם קרוש או ליחה עבה או מוגלא רבה וכמו דבר יצמח בו כמו יבלת ובשר נוסף (An obstruction in the passage through which the urine passes occurs when it is blocked as, e.g., by a stone or by a blood clot or by coarse humor or by much pus or by something that grows there such as a wart and a fleshy excrescence). In the sense of 'blood clot,' Hebr. דם קרוש features (for Arab. عبيط) in BCD 57 (NM 3:52–53) in a later attestation from Nathan ha-Me'ati, *Pirqei Abuqraṭ* IV.69. Arab. عبيط is translated by Ibn Tibbon on the other hand as דם קפוי in his *Perush Aphorismi shel Apuqraṭ* (*Pirqei Abuqraṭ*) IV.69 (206) (cf. BMCH 1:372, l. 18). Do'eg ha-Edomi translates the parallel Lat. term *sanguis coagulata* as אפיסת הדם (see entry אֲפִיסָה).

- **אפיסת הדם** → **אֲפִיסָה**.
- **אפיסת דם נידות** → **אֲפִיסָה**.
- **בשול הדם** → **בִּשּׁוּל**.
- **השתנת הדם** → **הַשְׁתָּנָה**.
- **עכוב דם הנדות** → **עִכּוּב**.
- **העיצר דם הנדות** → **עֶצֶר**.
- **שלשל דם הוסת** → **שִׁלְשֵׁל**.
- **שפע הדם** → **שֶׁפַע**.
- **שפעת הדם** → **שִׁפְעָה**.

דַּף • *Plur.* דפים • דפי האסטומכא · the layers of the stomach: Lat. *pelliculae stomachi* (Arab. أغشية) · Constantinus Africanus, *Viaticum peregrinantis* · trans. Do'eg ha-Edomi, *Sefer Ya'ir Netiv* IV.1: ואחרי שהליחות יגורשו מדפי האסטומכא והוא נטהר מהליחות הרעות טוב לתת לו גירא פיגרא מאשר השני חלקים מאלואין והשלישי מסמנין (Once the [coarse, viscous] humors have been removed from the layers of the stomach so that it is clean from bad humors, it is good to administer *hiera picra*, two thirds of which consist of aloe and one third of [the other] ingredients). Hebr. דַּף, *Plur.* דפים, features also in the sense of 'membranes' in BCD 5:52 in an attestation from *Sefer Ya'ir Netiv* I.18.1 (cf. IJZ 1–2:619). Moses ibn Tibbon translates the parallel Arab. term أغشية as קרומות.

דְּפוּס • *Plur.* **דפוסים** • **דפוסי הזרע** · **seminal vesicles**: Arab. أوعية المني · Ibn al-Jazzār, *Zād al-musāfir wa-qūt al-ḥādir* · trans. Abraham ben Isaac, *Sefer Ṣedah la-Oreḥim* VI.3: דע כי יציאת הזרע וזיבתו תדיר בלא רצון ולא תאוה ולא עינוג יהיה מחמת כחישות כח התופס לדפוסי[59] הזרע (A constant involuntary flow and excretion of sperm, without enjoyment, is caused by weakness of the retentive faculty in the seminal vesicles). Hebr. דפוסי הזרע is not attested in the current dictionaries. Moses ibn Tibbon translates Arab. أوعية المني as כיסי הזרע (see entry כִּיס). Do'eg ha-Edomi translates the parallel Lat. term *vasa spermatis* as כלי הזרע (see entry כְּלִי).

דְּפִיקָה · **I. stretching; tension (tetanus)**: Lat. *techinatio*[60] (Arab. امتداد) · Constantinus Africanus, *Viaticum peregrinantis* · trans. Do'eg ha-Edomi, *Sefer Ya'ir Netiv* V.2: ואם העשן נאסף בכבד ואינו יכול לצאת אז לא ירגיש הכובד לבדו אך השתטחות גם דפיקה זה טיטנוס וכאב רב בין צמידי הראש והכבד (If the vapor collects in the liver but does not have a way out, [the patient] will not only feel heaviness but also stretching and tension (tetanus), and severe pain in the region between the collarbones and the liver). Hebr. דְּפִיקָה features in the sense of 'tension' (for Lat. *tensio*; Arab. تمدّد) in NM 5:52 in an attestation from *Sefer Ya'ir Netiv* II.1.2 (cf. IJZ 1–2:632). In his *Sefer Agur* IV.57, Do'eg uses the synonym דפק הגידים (cf. BCD 49 (NM 3:54)).

· **II. throbbing**: Arab. ضربان · Ibn Sīnā, *K. al-Qānūn fī al-ṭibb* · trans. Nathan ha-Me'ati, *Sefer ha-Qanun* II, fol. 70a: ביץ ביצים ... הלובן שלו ישקיט כאב העין והאודם שלו עם הזעפראן ושמן ורדים יועיל מאד מדפיקת העין (Eggs: ... The white of an egg relieves ophthalgia and its yolk mixed with saffron and rose oil is very useful in the throbbing of the eye). Hebr. דְּפִיקָה features in the sense of 'pulsation' in BM 977. It also features as 'throbbing pain; tension' in Moses ibn Tibbon, *Sefer Ṣedat ha-Derakhim* II.1.9 (cf. BCD 58 (NM 4:39); IJZ 1–2:487) and in Do'eg ha-Edomi, *Sefer Ya'ir Netiv* II.1.2 (cf. NM 5:52; IJZ 1–2:632). Zeraḥyah Ḥen translates Arab. ضربان as חֲבָטָה (see entry). See also entry דֶּקֶר.

דַּק · **skillful; skilled; accomplished**: Arab. لطيف (cf. WKAS 2.2:730) Ibn al-Jazzār, *Zād al-musāfir wa-qūt al-ḥādir* · trans. Moses ibn Tibbon, *Sefer Ṣedat ha-Derakhim* IV.19: והנה אמר גלי' כי הנאצור דומה לצנור של קנה אשר לו מכסה מבפנים ומחוץ והוא חלול ושהוא לא יתרפא כי אם במעשה היד בעקור ושרפואתו ובריאותו בעקור כשיהיה במקום חכם דק במעשה הברזל (Galen said that a fistula is similar to a hollow reed that is covered inside and outside and that can only be cured by being removed through surgery. [He further said that] its removal through surgery can only be successful in a place where a skill-

59 לדפוסי: emend. ed. דפסי Ms.

60 Lat. *techinatio*, i.e., 'stretching; tension; tetanus' does not feature in any Lat. dictionary; a var. reading *techinositas* features in the *Viaticum peregrinantis* II.2, where it stands for Arab. تمدّد ('tension; stretching (tetanus)'); Do'eg renders Lat. here also as דפיקה. The same Arab. term is rendered as *tethinositas* in the *Viaticum peregrinantis* I.12, which is again rendered by Do'eg as דפיקה in his *Sefer Ya'ir Netiv*.

ful surgeon is present). In the sense of 'skilled,' Hebr. דַּק is as non-attested semantic borrowing from Arab. لطيف.

• *Plur.* **דקים** · **intestines**: Arab. أمعاء · Ibn al-Jazzār, *Zād al-musāfir wa-qūt al-ḥādir* · trans. Moses ibn Tibbon, *Sefer Ṣedat ha-Derakhim* IV.13: העוות יקרה לדקים הם בני מעים כשיסתבך בם כימוס עב או ליחה מררית בה עובי כמו המתילד מאכילת כרתי ומה שדומה לזה (The intestines are affected by a colic when thick chyme or bilious thick phlegm gets stuck in them, such as that which originates from the consumption of leek and the like). In the sense of 'intestines,' Hebr. דקים (an abbr. of מעים דקים) features in NM 5:54–55 in an attestation from R. Isaiah's trans. of Guillaume de Congenis, *Chirurgia* (*Treatise on Surgery*). Ben Yehuda (BM 981) mentions דקים in the sense of 'intestines; bowels' in an attestation from Maimonides, *Mishneh Torah: Ma'akhalot Asurot*.

• **השחין הדק** → שְׁחִין.

דֶּקֶר · **throbbing [of pain]**: Arab. ضربان · Ibn al-Jazzār, *Zād al-musāfir wa-qūt al-ḥādir* · trans. Abraham ben Isaac, *Sefer Ṣedah la-Oreḥim* VI.6: אם יהיה אותו רפש מיסוד קר אז יהיה דמות הפלגמוני כדמות מראה הגוף ולא יהיה עמו לא כאב ולא דקר (If that residu [that reaches the testicles] consists of a cold humor, then the color of the tumor [on the testicles] will be the same as that of the body and there will be no throbbing pain). Hebr. דֶּקֶר features in BM 989 in an attestation from the *Sefer Asaph ha-Rofe* and is explained by Ben Yehuda as 'a kind of pain resulting from stabbing' (כעין כאב מדקירה). Moses ibn Tibbon translates Arab. ضربان as דפק. Do'eg ha-Edomi uses the same Hebr. term to render the parallel Lat. term *pulsatio*. See also entry דְּפִיקָה.

דַּרְגָּה • דרגה דרגה · **gradually**: Arab. على تدريج · Maimonides, *Maqāla fī al-rabw* (*On Asthma*) · trans. Samuel Benveniste, *Ma'amar 'al ha-Qaṣeret* IX.16 (cf. BMA 2:276, ll. 19–22): ומי שנהג להקיז או לשתות משקה בעתים הידועים ילך על פי מנהגו וירחיק בין אותן הזמנים מעט מעט ויחסר שעור ההרקה דרגה דרגה עד שיגיע לשנות הזקנה וכבר פסק מנהג ההקזה והשלשול (If someone is accustomed to bloodletting or to the ingestion of [purgatives] at fixed times, he should watch his habits [and see] if he can gradually increase the intervals between the fixed times and gradually decrease the evacuated amounts, so that when he reaches old age, his habit of bloodletting and using purgatives has ceased). Hebr. דרגה דרגה is not attested in the current dictionaries. Joshua Shatibi renders Arab. على تدريج as בהדרגה (see entry הַדְרָגָה) and Anonymous has במדרגות (see entry מַדְרֵגָה).

דרדני · **gums**: Arab. لثة · al-Rāzī, *K. al-Manṣūrī fī al-ṭibb* · trans. Shem Tov ben Isaac, *Sefer Almansur*, fol. 3[b]: מ"ג: בדרדני אשר יגר מהם דם ([Chapter] 43: On bleeding gums). The unidentified Hebr. term דרדני features in BCD 60 (NM 1:85–86, corr. 4:229; 4:40) in attestations from Shem Tov's *Sefer ha-Shimmush* XXVII; XXX.2.95. Moses ibn Tibbon, *Sefer Ṣedat ha-Derakhim* II.18.1 (cf. BCD 127 (NM 4:81); IJZ 1–2:508) and subsequently Abraham Avigdor translate Arab. لثة as ככים (see entry כַּךְ).

דֶּרֶךְ • בדרך רחוק · **rarely**: Arab. في الندرة · Ibn al-Jazzār, *Zād al-musāfir wa-qūt al-ḥādir* · trans. Moses ibn Tibbon, *Sefer Ṣedat ha-Derakhim* IV.6: ומן הפיהוק מה שהוא נקל להרפא

וממנו מה שהוא קשה לרפאתו כפיהוק אשר מהרקה ואי אפשר שיהיה כי אם בדרך רחוק (Hiccups can be easy but also difficult to cure, like the hiccups caused by emptying [the body through vomiting], although this only occurs rarely). In the sense of 'rarely,' Hebr. בדרך רחוק is not attested in the current dictionaries. Do'eg ha-Edomi translates the parallel Lat. term *rarus* as ברחוק (see entry רָחוֹק).

• **רוּחַ → הרוח הנדחה דרך הגרון.**

• *Plur.* **דרכים · rules; instructions:** Arab. قوانين · Maimonides, *Maqāla fī al-rabw* (*On Asthma*) · trans. Samuel Benveniste, *Ma'amar 'al ha-Qaṣeret* X.1 (cf. BMA 2:277, ll. 11–13): אבל בעת רפואת החוליים אל יתן אל לבו לשנות המנהג בשום פנים ולא בשום ענין אבל יזהר בו זהירות שלם כמו שבאר ג׳אלינוס לנו בדרכיו המועילים (But in the case of the healing of diseases, one should not consider changing the habit in any manner or for any reason. Instead, it should be observed with utmost attention, as Galen explained to us in his helpful instructions). In the sense of 'rules,' Hebr. דרכים features in BCD 60 (NM 3:55) in an earlier attestation from Moses ibn Tibbon, *Perush Aphorismi shel Apuqraṭ* (*Pirqei Abuqraṭ*) N (16) (BMCH 1:322, l. 1). Joshua Shatibi renders Arab. قوانين as סדרים (see entry סֵדֶר) and Anonymous has עקרים (see entry עִקָּר).

דרמך · bran-free fine white flour: Arab. درمك (cf. NA 559; NTT 469) · Ibn Zuhr, *K. al-Aghdhiya* · trans. Nathan ha-Me'ati, *Sefer ha-Mezonot*, fol. 2b: לחם שעורים ... קר ויבש בשווי מזונו פחות ממזון לחם החטה ויחסר מזונו ממזון לחם החטה בשעור מה שיחסר מזון לחם החטה ממזון לחם הדרמך[61] כי הדרמך יותר זו שבהם (Barley bread ... is moderately cold and dry; it is less nutritious than wheat bread in the same degree that wheat bread is less nutritious than DRMK bread [i.e., bread made from fine bran-free flour]. Actually DRMK bread is the most nutritious bread). Hebr. דרמך is a non-attested calque of Arab. درمك. It is rendered as Hebr. סלת נקיה ('pure fine flour') in a marginal gloss. The term דרמך also features in Shem Tov ben Isaac, *Sefer ha-Shimmush* XXVII (cf. BCD 225, s.v. פַּת (NM 4:41–42)).

דִּשּׁוּן · fatness: Arab. دسومة · Maimonides, *Maqāla fī al-rabw* (*On Asthma*) · trans. Samuel Benveniste, *Ma'amar 'al ha-Qaṣeret* IV.7 (cf. BMA 2:256, ll. 21–22): ודע שהדברים החמים היבשים מזיקים ביותר לחולי זה כל שכן למזג זה הנזכר מפני שהם מדבקות הלחות שיש בהן דשון ויקשרו ויקפיאו מה שאין בו דשון (Know that the hot and dry ingredients are extremely harmful for this disease [i.e., asthma], especially for the temperament that we mentioned because they make the fatty humors sticky and thicken and coagulate those humors that have no fatness). Hebr. דִּשּׁוּן is attested in Rabb. literature in the sense of 'removal of ashes; cleaning' (cf JD 306; BM 1009) and for medieval halakhic literature (Yehudai Gaon, *Halakhot Qetsuvot*) in the sense of 'fattening' (cf. BM, ibid.). Joshua Shatibi translates Arab. دسومة as דשנות and Anonymous has הִתְדַּשְּׁנוּת (see entry).

---

61 הדרמך: סלת נקיה Ms1.

ה

הֲבָרָה · **intestinal rumblings (borborygmus)**: Lat. *gurgulatio* (Arab. قرقرة) · Constantinus Africanus, *Viaticum peregrinantis* · trans. Do'eg ha-Edomi, *Sefer Ya'ir Netiv* IV.17: ובהיות זה החולי מרוח גס נתבונן בו בנסוע הכאב ממקום למקום ומההברה ומנפח הבטן ומאותות אחרות הנראות לסובלי הלבנה (When this illness [i.e., colic] is caused by coarse flatulence, it is indicated by pain traveling from spot to spot, intestinal rumblings, swelling of the stomach, and other symptoms that one can observe in those suffering from phlegm). In the sense of 'intestinal rumblings,' Hebr. הֲבָרָה features in BCD 61 (NM 4:40) in a later attestation from Shem Tov ben Isaac, *Sefer ha-Shimmush* XXVII. In addition to הֲבָרָה, Do'eg translates Lat. *gurgulatio* as רַעַם (see entry) in *Sefer Ya'ir Netiv* IV.13. Moses ibn Tibbon translates the parallel Arab. term قرقرة as רַעַם as well.

הַגָּרָה · **I. flow; discharge; secretion**: Arab. سيلان · Ibn Sīnā, *K. al-Qānūn fī al-ṭibb* · trans. Nathan ha-Me'ati, *Sefer ha-Qanun* II, fol. 71b: בקלה אלחמקה ... יש בו קבוץ ימנע יציאת הדם וההגרות הישנות והזנתו מעט (Common purslane: ... It is astringent, stops chronic bleeding and [other] discharges, has little nutritive value ...). Hebr. הַגָּרָה features in BM 1041 as a noun derived from the verb [נגר], *Hif'il* הִגִּיר, 'to pour.' In his *Sefer ha-Peraqim* (*Pirqei Moshe*) IX.102, Nathan uses the term הַגָּרָה to render Arab. قيلة ('hernia,' cf. BCD 61 (NM 2:38); BMMN 117, l. 26; BMMG no. 4307). For compound nouns with הַגָּרָה, see below and BCD 62. Zeraḥyah Ḥen translates Arab. سيلان as הַגָּרָה as well and Anonymous has ההגרה וההזלה.

· **II. purging**: Arab. إحدار · Ibn al-Jazzār, *Zād al-musāfir wa-qūt al-ḥādir* · trans. Moses ibn Tibbon, *Sefer Ṣedat ha-Derakhim* IV.9: ואם ימנע הגרתו בקיא יעשה קלוחים רכים ורפים ורפואות משלשלות (If it is impossible to purge [the spoiled food] through vomiting, one should apply light clysters and purgatives). Hebr. הַגָּרָה does not feature in this sense in the current dictionaries.

• **הגרת הבטן** · **cholera**: Arab.: هيضة (Gr. χολέρα; cf. UWS 2:691) · Ibn al-Jazzār, *Zād al-musāfir wa-qūt al-ḥādir* · trans. Moses ibn Tibbon, *Sefer Ṣedat ha-Derakhim* IV.8: וכשישתה מי רמונים ממוצעים וחמיצות אתרוג יועיל מהפיהוק אשר ממרה אדומה וישקיט הקבסא והגרת הבטן (If one drinks sweet and sour pomegranate juice and citron pulp, it is beneficial for hiccups caused by yellow bile, it alleviates eructation and cholera). Hebr. הגרת הבטן features in BCD 62 (NM 3:55–56) in the sense of 'diarrhea.' A wide variety of synonymous terms for 'cholera,' showing the lack of standardization, can be found in medieval Hebrew medical literature; in different trans. of Hippocrates' *Aphorisms*, we find: הרקת הירוקה מלמעלה ומלמטה (Joseph Delmedigo, III.30; cf. BCD 73 (NM 3:70)); כאב הקיבה (Anonymous, *Perush Aphorismi shel Apuqraṭ* (*Pirqei Abuqraṭ*) I.12 (39); cf. BCD 123 (NM 3:113); BMCH 1:523, l. 10); or שפיכה (Moses ibn Tibbon, *Perush Aphorismi shel Apuqraṭ* (*Pirqei Abuqraṭ*) III.30 (136); cf. BCD 282 (NM 3:233–234); BMCH 1:356, l. 20). In his *Sefer ha-Peraqim* (*Pirqei Moshe*), Nathan ha-Me'ati renders Arab. هيضة as ליאנטריא הנק' היצא (III.60; cf. BMMN 48, l. 15) or

חולי הנקרא היצא הנקרא ליאנטריא (VII.42; cf. BMMN 87, l. 10) or חולי היצא הוא ליאנטריא (XXIII.83, cf. BMMN 229, l. 18), and Zeraḥyah Ḥen has אנשטיאון בער׳ היצה (III.60; cf. BMMZ 42, l. 2) or שלשול הנק׳ איניישטיאון (VII.42, cf. BMMZ 81, l. 18) or אינגישטיאון הנקרא בערבי היצה (XXIII.83, cf. BMMZ 228, l. 13) (cf. also BMMG no. 5419). Cf. BCD 277 (NM 4:206).

• **הגרת הזרע מבלי רצון** · **involuntary flow of sperm (nocturnal emission)**: Lat. *gonorrhoea* · *Sefer ha-Refu'ot le-Ḥakham Qosṭa'ntin*, fol. 207[a]: בהגרת הזרע מבלי רצון: אמר פלוטיאריש: גונוריאה הוא חולי שמוציא זרע כל היום ומטפטף בלא תאות אשה ובלו קושי (On involuntary flow of sperm: Says Platearius: GWNWRY'H [i.e., Lat. *gonorrhoea*] is the illness in which a person emits and drips sperm every day without desiring a woman (sexual lust) and without an erection). Hebr. הגרת הזרע מבלי רצון is not attested in the current dictionaries.

• **הגרת השתן מבלי חפץ** · **urinary incontinence (unvoluntary urination, polyuria)**: Arab.: سلس البول (cf. FL 2:340, s.v. سَلَس: 'profluvium urinae; diabetes;' SN 1:112 (266): 'Krampfhafte Harnruhr (*Diabetes spasticus*)') · al-Rāzī, *K. al-Manṣūrī fī al-ṭibb* · trans. Shem Tov ben Isaac, *Sefer Almansur*, fol. 134[a]: שער בהגרת השתן מבלי חפץ: כשתרבה השתנת החולה בלי חריפות או ישתין והוא ישן ולא יהיה עם זה צמא ולא כחשות הגוף צריך להשקותו סם מחזיק השתן (On urinary incontinence (unvoluntary urination, polyuria): When the patient urinates frequently but has no burning sensation, or he urinates while he is asleep but he is not thirsty and his body is not meager, one should administer him a [medicinal potion] that holds the urine [in the body]). Hebr. הגרת השתן מבלי חפץ is not attested in the current dictionaries. In addition, Shem Tov translates Arab. سلس البول also as **יציאת השתן מבלי הרגש** (*Sefer Almansur*, fol. 4[a]) and Do'eg ha-Edomi translates the parallel Lat. term *lubrica urina* ('polyuria; diabetes') in his *Sefer Ya'ir Netiv* V.18 as **יציאת השתן** (for both terms, see entry יְצִיאָה).

הַדְרָגָה • **בהדרגה** · **gradually**: Arab. على تدريج · Maimonides, *Maqāla fī al-rabw* (*On Asthma*) · trans. Joshua Shatibi, *Ma'amar 'al ha-Qaṣeret* IX.16 (cf. BMA 2:352, ll. 3–5): ומי שירגיל ההקזה או שתיית הסם המשלשל בעתות ידועות יעיין במנהגו וירחיק בין אלו העתים מעט מעט וימעיט בשעורי ההרקה בהדרגה עד שלא יבואו שני הזקנה כי אם כבר נכרת מנהג ההקזה או השלשול (If someone is accustomed to bloodletting or to the ingestion of [purgatives] at fixed times, he should watch his habits [and see] if he can gradually increase the intervals between the fixed times and gradually decrease the evacuated amounts, so that when he reaches old age his habit of bloodletting and using purgatives has ceased). Hebr. בהדרגה is attested in medieval philosophical literature; cf. KTP 1:159; HCD 12. Samuel Benveniste renders Arab. على تدريج as דרגה דרגה (see entry דַּרְגָּה) and Anonymous has במדרגות (see entry מַדְרֵגָה).

הִדְרָקוֹן (read: יְרָקוֹן) · **jaundice**: Lat. *ictericia* (Arab. يرقان 'jaundice') · Constantinus Africanus, *Viaticum peregrinantis* · trans. Do'eg ha-Edomi, *Sefer Ya'ir Netiv* V.10: מהדרוקן זהו איקטיריסיא שם איקטיריסיא נתפס מעוף אחד שיש לו צבע מכורכם כזהב (On jaundice, i.e, 'YQṬYRYSY' [i.e., Lat. *ictericia*]. The term *ictericia* hails from a bird with a saffron color like gold …). Hebr. הִדְרָקוֹן (from Gr. ὑδερικόν [πάθος]) only features in the current dictionaries in the sense of 'dropsy;' cf. JD 335; Low XLVII; s.v. הִידְרוֹקָן. Do'eg consistently translates Lat. *ictericia* ('jaundice') as הִדְרָקוֹן ('dropsy'), probably confusing it with the regular Hebr. term יֵרָקוֹן for 'jaundice,' which features in Moses ibn Tibbon, *Sefer Ṣedat ha-Derakhim* I.0.4 (cf. IJZ 1–2:441).

הוֹרָאָה • *Plur.* **הוראות** › **symptoms**: Arab: دلائل · Maimonides, *Maqāla fī al-rabw* (*On Asthma*) · trans. Samuel Benveniste, *Ma'amar 'al ha-Qaṣeret* XIII.19 (cf. BMA 2:303, l. 18–304, l. 1): אך אם יראה שאם היה הדבר בהפך מה שחשב שיזיקהו הזק גדול לא יעשה כפי סברתו וכפי שהורו ההוראות (But if he concluded that, if the case was the opposite of what he thought, [the purgative] would cause serious harm, [then] he would not act according to his reason nor according to the symptoms). In the sense of 'symptom,' Hebr. *Sing.* הוֹרָאָה features in BCD 63–64 (NM 4:42) in an attestation from Jacob ibn Tibbon, *Hanhagat ha-Beri'ut le-Abu 'Ali ben Zuhr* (cf. RSA 162). Joshua Shatibi translates Arab. دلائل as הוראות as well, and Anonymous has ראיות (see entry רְאָיָה).

הַזָּלָה › **flow; flux**: Lat. *fluxus* · Constantinus Africanus, *Viaticum peregrinantis* · trans. Do'eg ha-Edomi, *Sefer Ya'ir Netiv* V.15: גם יועילו אל הדם שהורק בתוך האסטומכא היורדת מהזלת דם הנחירים ([These pastilles] are also beneficial for the blood that flows down to the stomach because of a nosebleed). Hebr. הַזָּלָה features in BM 1065 in the sense of 'flowing (of menstrual blood)' in an attestation from Meir Aldabi, *Shevilei Emunah*. It features in a later attestation in BCD 64 (NM 3:60–61) in the sense of 'diarrhea' or 'flux.' Synonymous terms featuring in medieval medical texts are יְרִידָה (cf. BCD 120 (NM 3:110–111)), נְזִילָה (cf. BCD 172 (NM 3:152–153)), and אֲרֻבָּה (cf. NM 5:23).

• **הזלת השתן** › **strangury**: Arab: تقطير البول (Gr. δυσουρία/στραγγουρία; cf. UW 212–213; 642) · Ibn Sīnā, *K. al-Qānūn fī al-ṭibb* · trans. Nathan ha-Me'ati, *Sefer ha-Qanun* II, fol. 74ᵃ: גואשיר … ירכך קשי הרחם ויועיל להזלת השתן וישתה ממנו שיעור לוז[62] במים חמים לשלשול השתן[63] ודם הוסת והרחם הקר ופריו כמו כן ישלשל דם הוסת ויותר עם האפסנתין (Opopanax: … It softens the hardness of the uterus and is useful for strangury. A dose of one hazelnut[64] is taken orally with warm water for diuresis, menstruation, and a cold uterus. Its fruit, especially when taken with absinth wormwood, stimulates menstruation). In the sense of 'strangury,' Hebr. הזלת השתן is not attested in the current dictionaries. It features in BCD 65 (NM 3:63) in the sense of 'micturiction' (for Arab. إدرار البول) in an attestation from Anonymous, *Perush Aphorismi shel Apuqraṭ* (*Pirqei Abuqraṭ*) I.2 (29) (cf. BMCH 1:520, l. 19). Zeraḥyah Ḥen and Anonymous both

62 לוז: بندقة a.

63 השתן (= Ms Paris, BnF, héb. 1136, fol. 71ᵇ): emend. ed. השעור Ms.

64 'hazelnut' (Arab. *bunduqa*): I.e., 3.4 grams, cf. IG 164.

translate Arab. تقطير البول as הטפת השתן (cf. BCD 66 for attestations from Do'eg ha-Edomi, *Sefer Agur* v.58 (cf. NM 3:64) and Shem Tov ben Isaac, *Sefer ha-Shimmush* XXVII (cf. NM 4:44)).

• *Plur.* **הזלות** · **defluxions; catarrhs**: Arab. نزلات · Maimonides, *Maqāla fī al-rabw* (*On Asthma*) · trans. Samuel Benveniste, *Ma'amar 'al ha-Qaṣeret* VIII.1 (cf. BMA 2:269, ll. 6–7): וראוי לך שתזהר מן ההזלות הקרות והחמות כל מה שתוכל (You should be extremely careful to avoid cold and hot defluxions). Joshua Shatibi translates Arab. نزلات as נזלות and Anonymous has ירידות. For the synonomous *Sing.* terms נְזִילָה and יְרִידָה, see entry הַזָּלָה above.

הַטְמָנָה · **dark grey color**: Arab: كهبة · Ibn Sīnā, *K. al-Qānūn fī al-ṭibb* · trans. Nathan ha-Me'ati, *Sefer ha-Qanun* II, fol. 115b: פודנג ... הסימנים:[65] כשיבושל עם יין וקל וחומר הלח ממנו ועושים ממנו תחבושת יסיר הסמנים השחורים מהגוף וההטמנה שנולדת אחר[66] העין (Mint: ... [Its use in] cosmetics:[67] When it is boiled with wine, especially fresh mint, and used as a plaster, it removes black spots from the body and the dark grey color (circles) under[68] the eyes). Hebr. הַטְמָנָה does not feature in this sense in the current dictionaries. Zeraḥyah Ḥen translates Arab. كهبة as הַסְתָּרָה (see entry) and Anonymous has כמינת הדם.

הַכְאָבָה · **causing pain**: Arab: تصديع · Ibn Sīnā, *K. al-Qānūn fī al-ṭibb* · trans. Zeraḥyah Ḥen, *Sefer ha-Qanun* II, fol. 260b: מֶנְטְרַשְׁטְרֵי[69] ... מיצו ימית התולעים באוזן ויש בו הכאבת ראש (Mint: ... The extract kills earworms but may cause headache). Hebr. הַכְאָבָה is not attested in medieval medical literature. Nathan ha-Me'ati translates Arab. تصديع as מכאיב.

הַכָּאָה · **blow**: Arab: ضربة · Ibn al-Jazzār, *Zād al-musāfir wa-qūt al-ḥāḍir* · trans. Moses ibn Tibbon, *Sefer Ṣedat ha-Derakhim* v.3: ואם תהיה המורסא המתילדת בכבד מפני הכאה או נפילה שקרה בכבד מחוץ נשקה החולה הברברי ציני חצי שקל ביין (If the tumor that arises in the liver is caused by a fall or blow affecting the liver from the outside, we give the patient a potion consisting of half a *sheqel*[70] of Chinese rhubarb with wine). Hebr. הַכָּאָה is not attested in a medical context in the current dictionaries (cf. BM 1082–1083). For הַכָּאָה in the sense of 'beat [of the pulse],' see BCD 67 (NM 3:64) for an attestation from *Sefer Ṣedat ha-Derakhim* I.20.2 (cf. IJZ 1–2:472); and for הַכָּאָה in the sense of 'throbbing,' see also BCD 67 (NM 4:44) for an attestation from Anonymous, *Perush Aphorismi shel Apuqraṭ* (*Pirqei Abuqraṭ*) VII.21 (373) (cf. BMCH 1:600, l. 1).

---

65 הסימנים: الزينة a.
66 אחר: تحت a.
67 'cosmetics': Trans. after a.
68 'under': Trans. after a.
69 מֶנְטְרַשְׁטְרֵי: פּוּדַנְגּ' Ms1.
70 Hebr. *sheqel* stands for Arab. *mithqāl*; one *mithqāl* is 4.46 grams; cf. HIM 4–7.

הַמְלָטָה · **labor pains:** Arab. طلق · Ibn al-Jazzār, *Zād al-musāfir wa-qūt al-ḥādir* · trans. Moses ibn Tibbon, *Sefer Ṣedat ha-Derakhim* VI.14: ופעמים שיסור הרחם ממקומו ויצא לחוץ בסבת המלטה חזקה (Sometimes, the uterus suffers from a displacement and prolapse because of severe labor pains). Hebr. הַמְלָטָה features in BM 1115 in the sense of 'parturition' in an attestation from the *Sefer ha-Qanun*. A synonym used by Moses ibn Tibbon to render Arab. طلق is הַתָּרָה (see entry). Abraham ben Isaac translates Arab. طلق as הלידה בקושי and as צירים וחבלים (cf. also entry הַתָּרָה). Do'eg ha-Edomi translates the parallel Lat. term *expressio* as עִשּׂוּי (see entry).

הסת · **nightmare:** Arab: كابوس · al-Rāzī, *K. al-Manṣūrī fī al-ṭibb* · trans. Shem Tov ben Isaac, *Sefer Almansur*, fol. 114b: שער בהסת: כשיהיה האדם בעת השינה כמו דבר כבד נופל עליו כי זה הוא ההסת ואין ראוי להתרשל מרפואתו כי זה מקדמת הכפיון (Chapter on nightmare: When a person is asleep and feels as if something heavy falls upon him, it is a nightmare. One should not be lazy (negligent) to treat it, because it precedes epilepsy). Hebr. הסת (from the root סות ('to incite, instigate, entice')) is a non-attested var. reading of הסתה, which is featuring in Rabb. literature in the sense of 'seduction; enticement' (JD 359) and in medieval medical literature, e.g., in Nathan ben Jo'el Falaquera, *Ṣori ha-Guf* for Arab. كابوس ('nightmare'); cf. BM 4018, n. 1: בחולי הנקרא כאבוס ובלשון התלמוד הסתה ובלע״ז פריקמא האלכאבוס הוא חלי ירגיש בו האדם בעת השינה כאלו דבר יפול עליו ויקרר נשימתו ויפסק קולו ותנועתו ויכבד עליו ראשו כאלו רוצה להחנק לסתום הנקבים וכשיכלה זה יעור משנתו פתאום כמבוהל (On the illness called K'BWS [i.e., Arab. *kābūs*, 'nightmare'], in the Talmud *hassatah*, and in o.l. PRYQM'. The *al-kābūs* is an illness during which a person feels when he is asleep as if something falls upon him; his breathing becomes cold; he loses his voice and possibility to move, his head becomes heavy as if he is being strangled because his [respiratory] passages are closed. When this stops, he wakes from his sleep all of a sudden, frightened). Gerard de Cremona translates Arab. كابوس as *incubus*.

הִסְתַּעֲרוּת · **disturbance:** Arab. قلق (Gr. ταραχή; '[physiological] disturbance; upheaval;' cf. UWS 2:429–430) · Ibn al-Jazzār, *Zād al-musāfir wa-qūt al-ḥādir* · trans. Moses ibn Tibbon, *Sefer Ṣedat ha-Derakhim* VI.12: ואם היתה המורסא מתילדת ממותר חם כרכומית או דמי יהיה עם מה שהקדמנו קדחת חמה ושרפה ברחם עם כח הכאב וימשך אחר זה צמא והסתערות בצד אשר תהיה בו המורסא (If the tumor originates from a hot superfluity of yellow bile or of blood, there is—besides what we have mentioned before—high fever and a burning sensation in the uterus with severe pain in the side where the tumor is and it is followed by thirst and disturbance). Hebr. הִסְתַּעֲרוּת features in the sense of 'disturbance' (for Arab. اضطراب) in BCD 69 (NM 3:65–66).

הַסְתָּרָה · **dark grey color:** Arab: كهبة · Ibn Sīnā, *K. al-Qānūn fī al-ṭibb* · trans. Zeraḥyah Ḥen, *Sefer ha-Qanun* II, fol. 260b: מֻנְטְרַשְׁטְרֵי[71] ... היפוי: כשיבושל וכל שכן החדש עם יין

71 מֻנְטְרַשְׁטְרֵי: פֿנדנג׳ Ms[1].

ויחבוש בו יעביר הרשמים השחורים מן הגוף וההסתרה שמתחת לעין (Mint: ... [Its use in] cosmetics: When it is boiled with wine, especially fresh mint, and used as a plaster it removes black spots from the body and dark grey color (circles) under the eyes). Hebr. הַסְתָּרָה does not feature in this sense in the current dictionaries. Nathan ha-Me'ati translates Arab. كهبة as הַטְמָנָה (see entry).

הַעֲדָרָה ‧ **withholding; retention**: Lat. *ablatio* (Arab. احتباس) · Constantinus Africanus, *Viaticum peregrinantis* · trans. Do'eg ha-Edomi, *Sefer Ya'ir Netiv* VI.12: וצמח אחר עשוי מרוח גס או מהכאה או מהעדרת הפרחים (Other tumors [in the uterus] are caused by a coarse wind or by an injury or by retention of the menstruation). Hebr. הַעֲדָרָה features in the sense of 'absence; lack; want' (for Lat. *carentia*) in NM 5:59–60 in an attestation from Do'eg ha-Edomi, *Sefer Ya'ir Netiv* III.11. Moses ibn Tibbon translates Arab. احتباس as עצירה and Abraham ben Isaac has אפיסות והפסקה (see entry אֲפִיסוּת).

הַעֲמָדָה ‧ I. **retention [of food] (constipation)**: Arab. احتباس (Gr. ἐπίσχεσις/ἐποχή (UW 1:390, 395)) · Maimonides, *Maqāla fī al-rabw* (*On Asthma*) · trans. Samuel Benveniste, *Ma'amar 'al ha-Qaṣeret* N.4 (cf. BMA 2:243, l. 17): הפרק התשיעי: בהנהגת ההרקה וההעמדה (Chapter nine: On the [proper] regimen for evacuation and retention). Hebr. הַעֲמָדָה does not feature in this sense in the current dictionaries. Joshua Shatibi translates Arab. احتباس as העצר and Anonymous has אִמּוּץ (see entry).

‧ II. **culmination; climax**: Lat. *status* (Arab. منتهى) · Constantinus Africanus, *Viaticum peregrinantis* · trans. Do'eg ha-Edomi, *Sefer Ya'ir Netiv* V.13: ונתן לו טרוסישקש עוזרים להעמדת הצמחים (And we give [the patient] pastilles when the ulcers culminate (reach their final stage)). In the sense of 'culmination,' Hebr. הַעֲמָדָה features (for Arab. منتهى) in BCD 69 (NM 2:40) in a later attestation from Nathan ha-Me'ati, *Sefer ha-Peraqim* (*Pirqei Moshe*) VIII.6 (cf. BMMN 92, l. 20; BMMG no. 5308). Do'eg also translates Lat. *status* as עֲמֹד (in *Sefer Ya'ir Netiv* II.18.11 (corr.); cf. NM 5:150; IJZ 1–2:648). Moses ibn Tibbon translates the parallel Arab. term منتهى as הגמר (for *Nif'al* נִגְמַר, see entry גָּמַר).

הָפוּךְ (*Part. Pass.*) → **[הפך]**.

[הפך] • *Part. Pass.* **הָפוּךְ** ‧ **on one's back**: Lat. *supinus* (Arab. على ظهره) · Constantinus Africanus, *Viaticum peregrinantis* · trans. Do'eg ha-Edomi, *Sefer Ya'ir Netiv* VI.2: ונצוה אליו שישכב כל פעם מן הצד ולא הפוך (And we tell him [i.e., someone suffering from priapism] to always lay down (sleep) on his side, but not on his back). Hebr. הָפוּךְ does not feature in this sense in the current dictionaries. Moses ibn Tibbon and Abraham ben Isaac both translate Arab. على ظهره as על גבו.

• *Hitpa'el* **הִתְהַפֵּךְ** • **השער המתהפך בעפעפים** → **שֵׂעָר**.

הֶפְסֵד ‧ **loss [of life]; perdition; death**: Arab. تلف · Ibn al-Jazzār, *Zād al-musāfir wa-qūt al-ḥāḍir* · trans. Moses ibn Tibbon, *Sefer Ṣedat ha-Derakhim* IV.17: ונזכור עתה רפואתו ונאמר כי הוא ראוי ברפואת כל חולי שתהיה הכונה בה אל גשם חומרו ולהסירו אם לא שיהיו מקריו קשים יהיה ראוי להתפחד עמהם מההפסד (Now I will mention its cure [i.e., of a colic] and say that to heal any disease one should pay attention to the substance of the matter [that causes the illness] and its removal. [One should do so] unless the symptoms of the disease are so severe that one has to fear [that the patient might die]). Hebr. הֶפְסֵד does not feature in this sense in the current dictionaries.

הֶפְסֵק · **rupture; cut:** Arab. انقطاع · Ibn al-Jazzār, *Zād al-musāfir wa-qūt al-ḥādir* · trans. Moses ibn Tibbon, *Sefer Ṣedat ha-Derakhim* v.15: ואם תהיה השתנת הדם מפני הפסק עורק בכליות ובמעבר אשר בין הכליות והמקוה או מפני הפתח פי העורק נצוה אליו תמיד מנוחה ומרגוע (If the urination of blood is caused by a rupture (cut) in an vessel of the kidneys or in a passage between the kidneys and the urinary bladder or because of a burst in the opening of a vessel, we tell the patient to frequently rest and relax). Hebr. הֶפְסֵק features in the current dictionaries in the sense of 'interruption; suspension' only (cf. JD 362; BM 1158). Do'eg ha-Edomi translates the parallel Lat. term *incisus* as נתק.

הַפְסָקָה • **אפיסות והפסקה** → **אֲפִיסוּת**.

הַפְרָדָה • **הפרדת הדבקים** · **dissolution of continuity; separation of connected parts:** Lat. *separatio iuncture* (Arab. انحلال الفرد) · Constantinus Africanus, *Viaticum peregrinantis* · trans. Do'eg ha-Edomi, *Sefer Ya'ir Netiv* v.5: ועוד כי התחלואים הקרובים לכבד אינם יוצאים מכלל שלשה ומהם אמרו הרופאים כי כל איברי הגוף סובלים והם חבור רע תחלואי המשרתים הם הנקראים אופציאלש והפרדת הדבקים ([You should also know that] according to the physicians there are three [kinds] of diseases that affect all the organs but especially the liver. [These three kinds are]: a bad temperament, functional illnesses called ʾWPṢYʾLŠ [i.e., Lat. *officiales*] and dissolution of continuity). Hebr. הפרדת הדבקים is not attested in the current dictionaries. Lat. *separatio iuncture* is also translated by Do'eg as הפרדת החבור (see next entry). Moses ibn Tibbon translates the parallel Arab. term انحلال الفرد as פרוד החבור (see entry פֵּרוּד). For Hebr. synonyms, see ibid.

• **הפרדת החבור** · **dissolution of continuity; separation of connected parts:** Lat. *separatio iuncture* (Arab. انحلال الفرد) · Constantinus Africanus, *Viaticum peregrinantis* · trans. Do'eg ha-Edomi, *Sefer Ya'ir Netiv* v.4: הזלת דם מהכבד נעשית מענינים רבים והדם יוצא מתמונות משתנות כי הוא יהיה או מהפרדת החבור כמו כאשר עצומו נגוע (There are many causes for the streaming of blood from the liver, while the [kinds] of blood that is evacuated vary, because it hails either from the dissolution of continuity, as is the case when the substance of the liver is affected). Hebr. הפרדת החבור is not attested in the current dictionaries. Lat. *separatio iuncture* is also translated by Do'eg as הפרדת הדבקים (see previous entry). Moses ibn Tibbon translates the parallel Arab. term انحلال الفرد as פרוד החבור (see entry פֵּרוּד).

הַפְּרָדוּת • **הפרדות החיבור** · **dissolution of continuity; separation of connected parts:** Arab. تفرّق الاتّصال · Maimonides, *Maqāla fī al-rabw* (*On Asthma*) · Anonymous, *Sefer ha-Qaṣeret* v.1 (cf. BMA 2:403, ll. 9–11): וכלל הדבר בזה כולו ההזהרות מהשובע המביא להתמשך האצטומכא שכל אבר שיתמשך תפסדנה פעולותיו בהכרח שההתמשכות ממיני הפרדות החיבור (The main principle in this entire matter is to avoid satiation, which causes distension of the stomach, because when any organ is distended, its functions are necessarily impaired. For distension is a kind of separation of connected parts (dissolution of continuity)). Hebr. הפרדות החיבור is not attested in the current dictionaries. Samuel Benveniste translates Arab. تفرّق الاتّصال as הפרד הדבוק (see entry [פרד]) and Joshua Shatibi has פרוק החבור (see entry פֵּרוּק).

הֶפְשֵׁט • הפשט המעיים · abrasion of the intestines: Arab. سَحْج · Ibn Zuhr, *K. al-Aghdhiya* · trans. Nathan ha-Me'ati, *Sefer ha-Mezonot*, fol. 5[b]: ואם תגמעה שלוקה בלתי קשה תועיל מהפשט המעיים (If you drink [an egg] that has been boiled but is not yet hard, it is good for intestinal abrasion). Hebr. הפשט המעיים features as הפשט במעיים in BCD 71 (NM 2:40–41) in an attestation from Nathan's *Sefer ha-Peraqim* (*Pirqei Moshe*) XXI.27 (cf. BMMN 199, l. 6) and as הפשט המיעים in his glossary to the *Sefer ha-Qanun*: סחג הוא הפשט המיעים הנקרא דסינטריא (SḤG (abrasion). This is HPŠṬ HMYʿYM (abrasion of the intestines) called DSYNṬRY') (cf. NM 2:117, 152 (Samekh 8)).

הַפְשָׁטָה · abrasion (excoriation): Lat. *excoriatio* (Arab. سحوج) · Constantinus Africanus, *Viaticum peregrinantis* · trans. Do'eg ha-Edomi, *Sefer Ya'ir Netiv* IV.15: ואם הנגעים והפשטה יהיו במעי השפל יאות לעיין מאין הם (If the ulcers and abrasion (excoriation) are in the lower intestines, one should investigate their origin). Hebr. הַפְשָׁטָה features in BM 1163 as a synonym of הֶפְשֵׁט (cf. BCD 71 (NM 2:40–41)) in the sense of 'dysentery; stripping (of the skin)' in attestations from the *Sefer ha-Qanun*. As 'abrasion (excoriation),' it features in NM 5:61 in a later attestation from R. Isaiah's trans. of Guillaume de Congenis, *Chirurgia* (*Treatise on Surgery*). Hebr. הַפְשָׁטָה features in the sense of 'ulceration' in Hillel ben Samuel, *Sefer Keritut* (cf. BCD 71 (NM 1:22)). Moses ibn Tibbon translates the parallel Arab. term سحوج as חמרמרות (cf. BCD 104 (NM 1:56) for an attestation from *Sefer Ṣedat ha-Derakhim* VII.29.1 (cf. IJZ 7:171, l. 3)) and Shem Tov ben Isaac has עִצּוּם in his *Sefer ha-Shimmush* XXVII (cf. BCD 207 (NM 4:152), s.v. העיצום וההפשטה).

הַצָּבָה • הצבת הניפוש · orthopnea:[72] Arab. انتصاب النفس (cf. UW 471, s.v. ὀρθόπνοια: نفس الانتصاب) · Ibn Sīnā, *K. al-Qānūn fī al-ṭibb* · trans. Zeraḥyah Ḥen, *Sefer ha-Qanun* II, fol. 260[b]: מֶנְטְרַשְׁטְרֵי[73] ... בישולו יועיל מהצבת הניפוש (Mint: ... Its decoction is beneficial for orthopnea). Hebr. הצבת הניפוש is not attested in the current dictionaries. A var. reading from the same root יצב used by Zeraḥyah in his *Sefer ha-Peraqim* (*Pirqei Moshe*) XXIV.38 is מַצָּב (cf. BCD 156 (NM 1:165); BMMZ 238, l. 22; BMMG no. 5143). Nathan ha-Me'ati translates Arab. انتصاب النفس as הצבת הנשימה (see next entry).

• הצבת הנשימה · orthopnea:[74] Arab. انتصاب النفس · Ibn Sīnā, *K. al-Qānūn fī al-ṭibb* · trans. Nathan ha-Me'ati, *Sefer ha-Qanun* II, fol. 115[b]: פודנג ... תבשילו יועיל מהצבת הנשימה (Mint: ... Its decoction is beneficial for orthopnea). Hebr. הצבת הנשימה is

---

72 I.e., discomfort in breathing that is brought on or aggravated by lying flat (cf. BMA 1:2, n. 5).

73 פֻּנדַּנְג׳: מֶנְטְרַשְׁטְרֵי Ms[1].

74 I.e., discomfort in breathing that is brought on or aggravated by lying flat (cf. BMA 1:2, n. 5).

not attested in the current dictionaries. A var. reading from the same root יצב used by Nathan in his *Sefer ha-Peraqim* (*Pirqei Moshe*) XXIV.38 is הִתְיַצְּבוּת (cf. BCD 75 (NM 2:42); BMMN 239, l. 1; BMMG no. 5143). Zeraḥyah Ḥen translates Arab. انتصاب النفس as הצבת הניפוש (see previous entry) and Anonymous has a combination of both terms by Nathan: התיצבות הנשימה.

הֲקָאָה · **vomiting**: Arab. قيء · Ibn al-Jazzār, *Zād al-musāfir wa-qūt al-ḥādir* · trans. Moses ibn Tibbon, *Sefer Ṣedat ha-Derakhim* IV.11: ופעמים תהיה הקאת הדם מהדחותו אל האצטו׳ מאברים אחרים והוא אות רע (Sometimes, vomiting of blood occurs when it is pushed to the stomach from other organs. This is a bad symptom). Hebr. הֲקָאָה features in the current dictionaries in an attestation from David Kimhi, *Sefer ha-Shorashim* only (cf. BM 1168).

הַקְטָרָה • *Plur.* **הקטרות** · **fomentations**: Lat. *suffumigationes* (Arab. تنطيل) · Constantinus Africanus, *Viaticum peregrinantis* · trans. Do'eg ha-Edomi, *Sefer Ya'ir Netiv* V.5: ועם הרפואה השנית נטהר המים המכורכמים ונגרש אותם בזיעה ובהתרה וזה נעשה במרחץ ועם הקטרות (With the second [kind] of remedies, we cleanse and expel the yellowish fluid [of dropsy] through sweating and dissolution. This should be done by bathing and fomentations [with these remedies]). Hebrew הַקְטָרָה features in the current dictionaries only in the sense of 'letting rise in smoke; burning on the altar; burning incense' (cf. JD 364; BM 1172; EM 402). Moses ibn Tibbon translates Arab. تنطيل as נְטִילָה (see entry).

הַקָּרָה · **cooling**: Arab. تبريد · Ibn al-Jazzār, *Zād al-musāfir wa-qūt al-ḥādir* · trans. Moses ibn Tibbon, *Sefer Ṣedat ha-Derakhim* V.1: או ישתה מן העוגות המורכבות המועילות לחום הכבד לפי מה שנזכור במה שאחר זה מזה המאמר מן המשקים הקרים אשר להם מן ההקרה כח ינגב ויפתח ויחזק הכבד (He may also take one of the compound pastilles that are good for the heat of the liver and that I will mention later on in the section on cold potions that have a cooling force that dries, opens, and strengthens the liver). Hebr. הַקָּרָה does not feature in the current dictionaries.

הֶרְגֵּל · **experience**: Arab. دربة · Maimonides, *Maqāla fī al-rabw* (*On Asthma*) · trans. Joshua Shatibi, *Ma'amar 'al ha-Qaṣeret* XIII.30 (cf. BMA 2:377, ll. 22–23): ומן הטעות גם כן הדמיון בשהאיש יהיה לו הרגל אמיתי במעשה הרפואה גם שלא יהיה לו בה ידיעה (Another mistake is to imagine that one can have experience in the practice of medicine without knowledge). Hebr. הֶרְגֵּל features in the current dictionaries in the sense of 'habit; training' (BM 1182–1183; KT 1:211) only. Samuel Benveniste translates Arab. دربة as בקיאות and Anonymous has זְרִיזוּת (see entry).

הֶרְגֵּשׁ • בטול ההרגש → **בִּטּוּל**.

הַרְגָּשָׁה • *Plur.* **הרגשות** · **senses**: Arab. حواسّ · Ibn Sīnā, *K. al-Qānūn fī al-ṭibb* · trans. Nathan ha-Me'ati, *Sefer ha-Qanun* II, fol. 112ᵇ: ענבר ... יועיל אל המוח וההרגשות (Ambergris: ... It is beneficial for the brain and the senses). Hebr. הַרְגָּשָׁה features in PESHAT[75]

75 https://peshat.org/display/peshat_lemmas_00001161 (accessed February 6, 2022).

in attestations from medieval philosophical literature in the sense of 'sense perception; sensory faculty.' In medieval medical literature, it features as 'conjecture' in Zeraḥyah Ḥen, *Sefer ha-Peraqim* (*Pirqei Moshe*) XI.1 (cf. BCD 72 (NM 1:140–141); BMMZ 131, l. 7; BMMG no. 851). Here, Zeraḥyah Ḥen and Anonymous both translate Arab. حواسّ as חושים.

הַרְחָבָה · **rejoicing**: Arab. انبساط · Maimonides, *Maqāla fī al-rabw* (*On Asthma*) · trans. Samuel Benveniste, *Ma'amar 'al ha-Qaṣeret* VIII.2 (cf. BMA 2:269, ll. 14–15): והגילה והשמחה יעשו הפכם להרחבת הנפש ותנועת הדם והרוח היוצא מהגוף ויראו פעולות האברים בכל שלמות שיתכן (But joy and pleasure have an effect opposite to all these things because of the rejoicing of the soul and the movement of the blood and pneuma to the outside of the body so that the functions of the organs seem to be at their very best). In the sense of 'rejoicing,' Hebr. הַרְחָבָה is a non-attested semantic borrowing from Arab. انبساط. Joshua Shatibi translates Arab. انبساط as *Inf. Hitpa'el* הִתְפַּשֵּׁט (see entry פָּשַׁט) and Anonymous has הִתְפַּשְּׁטוּת (see entry).

הֶרְיוֹן • עוצר ההריון → עֹצֶר.

הַשְׁוָיָה · **equilibrium**: Arab. اعتدال · Maimonides, *Maqāla fī al-rabw* (*On Asthma*) · Anonymous, *Sefer ha-Qaṣeret* II.3 (cf. BMA 2:394, ll. 3–4): ואין ראוי לצאת בה עד[76] התכלית מפני מה שזכרנוהו מהשוית הגוף בדקות ובבריאות (But one should not pursue it [i.e., a thinning regimen] to the extreme—[and this is] according to what we mentioned about the equilibrium of the body in leanness and fatness[77]). Hebr. הַשְׁוָיָה, a var. reading of הַשְׁוָאָה, does not feature in this sense in the current dictionaries. In PESHAT[78] it features in the sense of 'comparison.' Samuel Benveniste translates Arab. اعتدال as מצוע and Joshua Shatibi has שווי.

הַשְׁמָטָה · **sliding; slip**: a) Lat. *lubricatio* (Arab. زلق) · Constantinus Africanus, *Viaticum peregrinantis* · trans. Do'eg ha-Edomi, *Sefer Ya'ir Netiv* VI.15: וכן העובר ברחם כי בנפול הזרע ברחם יהיה הקשר חלש ועל כן הוא סובל היזק מפני דלוג או השמטה או נפילה (The same is the case with the fetus in the uterus, for [in the beginning], when the sperm falls into the uterus, its connection [with it] is weak; therefore it will suffer harm [when the pregnant woman] jumps, slips, or falls]). Hebr. הַשְׁמָטָה does not feature in this sense in the current dictionaries. In medieval medical literature, it features in BCD 73 (NM 1:14) in the sense of 'dislocation' for Arab. خلع in an attestation from Zeraḥyah Ḥen, *Sefer ha-Peraqim* (*Pirqei Moshe*) XV.46 (cf. BMMZ 159, l. 24; BMMG no. 1539). Moses ibn Tibbon translates the parallel Arab. term زلق also as הַשְׁמָטָה (see next entry) and Abraham ben Isaac has חלקה רגליה.

b) Arab. زلق · Ibn al-Jazzār, *Zād al-musāfir wa-qūt al-ḥāḍir* · trans. Moses ibn Tibbon, *Sefer Ṣedat ha-Derakhim* VI.15: ואם יקרה לאשה דלוג או השמטה או נפילה או

---

76 ובבריאות: والضخامة a.

77 'fatness': Trans. after a.

78 https://peshat.org/display/peshat_lemmas_00049701 (accessed March 27, 2022).

שתשתה רפואה משלשלת ... יהיה נתר דבקות העובר ברחם מהר (When it occurs to a woman that she jumps or slips or falls or that she takes a laxative ... the connection between the fetus and uterus is quickly severed). Abraham ben Isaac translates Arab. زلق as חלקה רגליה and Do'eg ha-Edomi has also הַשְׁמָטָה for the parallel Lat. term *lubricatio* (see previous entry).

הִשְׁתַּטְּחוּת · **spasm; cramp; convulsion**: Arab. امتداد (Gr. σπασμός; cf. UW 626–627) · Ibn Sīnā, *K. al-Qānūn fī al-ṭibb* · trans. Nathan ha-Me'ati, *Sefer ha-Qanun* II, fol. 73[a] (Ms Paris, BnF, héb. 1136, fol. 70[b]): בול ... יועיל מהכאבים העצביים וקל וחומר שתן העזים הגדלים בבתים ושתן הסוסים ויותר אל הקווץ וההשתטחות[79] וכן יועיל אם עושים ממנו סעוט אל ההשתטחות (Urine: ... especially of domestic goats and horses is useful for neural pains. It is also useful for convulsions and spasms. It is useful for spasms when it is dripped into the nose). Hebr. הִשְׁתַּטְּחוּת is not attested in this sense in the current dictionaries. In his *Sefer ha-Peraqim* (*Pirqei Moshe*) IX.91, Nathan translates Arab. امتداد as מְתִיחָה (cf. BMMN 116, l. 9; BMMG no. 4732) and uses the same term for the Arab. synonym تمدّد ('tetanus') in his *Pirqei Abuqraṭ* IV.57 (cf. BCD 167 (NM 3:148)). Anonymous also translates Arab. امتداد as מְתִיחָה, while Zeraḥyah Ḥen has טוּמוֹר.

הַשְׁתָּנָה • השתנת הדם · **urinating blood (hematuria)**: Lat. *mictus sanguinis* (Arab. بول الدم) · i. Constantinus Africanus, *Viaticum peregrinantis* · trans. Do'eg ha-Edomi, *Sefer Ya'ir Netiv* V.15: מהשתנת הדם (On urinating blood). Hebr. השתנת הדם features also in BCD 74 (NM 4:49) in a later attestation for the parallel Arab. term بول الدم in Moses ibn Tibbon, *Sefer Ṣedat ha-Derakhim* I.0.4 (IJZ 1–2:441).

· ii. *Sefer ha-Refu'ot le-Ḥakham Qosṭa'ntin*, fol. 204[a]: בהשתנת הדם: אמר פלאטיאריש: לפעמים בא החולי לאדם שישתין דם או בפני עצמו או בשתן מעורב (On urinating blood: Says Platearius: Sometimes a person is affected by the illness that he urinates blood either on its own or mixed with urine).

הִתְאַבְּנוּת • התאבנות הפרקים · **stiffness of the joints (ankylosis)**: Arab. حجر المفاصل · Ibn Sīnā, *K. al-Qānūn fī al-ṭib* · Anonymous, *Sefer ha-Qanun* II, fols. 75[a]–76[a]: גבן הוא גבנה ... תשחק הישנה ממנו בשמן או במי כרעי החזיר מלוחים וירטה בו התאבנות הפרקים (Cheese: ... old cheese, pounded with olive oil or saltish water of pig's trotters, is used as a plaster for stiffness of the joints). Hebr. התאבנות הפרקים is not attested in the current dictionaries. Nathan ha-Me'ati translates Arab. حجر المفاصل as אבון הפרקים (see entry אִבּוּן) and Zeraḥyah Ḥen has קושי הפרקים.

הִתְדַּשְּׁנוּת · **fattening; fatness**: Arab. دسومة · Maimonides, *Maqāla fī al-rabw* (*On Asthma*) · trans. Anonymous, *Sefer ha-Qaṣeret* IV.7 (cf. BMA 2:400, ll. 20–22): ודע שהדברים החמים היבשים ביותר מזיקים בזה החלי ובלבד לזה המזג הנזכר מפני שהן מדבקין מהלחות מה שיש בהן התדשנות ומעמידין ומקפיאין מה שאין בו התדשנות (Know that the hot and dry

79 וההשתטחות: Ms Paris, BnF, héb. 1136, fol. 70[b] וההשטטחות Ms Oxford, Bodleian Library, Can. Or. 88, fol. 73[a].

ingredients are extremely harmful for this disease [i.e., asthma], especially for the temperament that we mentioned because they make the fatty humors sticky and thicken and coagulate those humors that have no fatness). Hebr. הִתְדַּשְּׁנוּת does not feature in the current dictionaries. Samuel Benveniste translates Arab. دسومة as דִּשּׁוּן (see entry) and Joshua Shatibi has דשנות.

הִתְחוֹלְלוּת · **dissolution:** Arab. تحلّل · Maimonides, *Maqāla fī al-rabw* (*On Asthma*) · trans. Anonymous, *Sefer ha-Qaṣeret* X.3 (cf. BMA 2:421, ll. 24–26): אמר גאלינוס דברים אלו לשונם אמר: ראוי שתדע שהוא אין דבר מועיל כתועלת השינה אחר הרחיצה בבישול מה שיתכונן בישולו והתחוללות הלחויות הרעות עצמן (Galen said the following, and these are his very words: You should know that nothing compares to sleeping immediately after a bath for cocting what can be cocted and dissolving the bad humors themselves). Hebr. הִתְחוֹלְלוּת only features in BM 1225 in an attestation from Simeon ben Zemah Duran, *Tiferet Yisra'el*. Samuel Benveniste translates Arab. تحلّل as להמס and Joshua Shatibi has להתיך.

הִתְיַצְּבוּת · **orthopnea:**[80] Arab. انتصاب (cf. UW 471, s.v. ὀρθόπνοια: نفس الانتصاب) · Maimonides, *Maqāla fī al-rabw* (*On Asthma*) · trans. Anonymous, *Sefer ha-Qaṣeret* N.2 (cf. BMA 2:388, l. 1–4): וכבר ידעתי מהראות ובמה שזכרתו ההדרה לי שסבת זה הרבו ירידה יורדת ממוח הראש בעתות רובן בחורף ושההתיצבות והילילה לא יסורו ימים בלילותם כפי אורך המשמרה או קצרותה עד שתקל ויתבשל מה שבא בריאה עד שתתנקה (I know—from what I have witnessed [with my own eyes] and from what [my Master] has described to me—that the cause of this asthma is a defluxion that descends from the brain at certain times [of the year], but mostly in winter. [And I know] that the orthopnea and distress do not cease through the night for days on end, according to the length or brevity of the attack, until the defluxion decreases and until that [fluid], which has reached the lungs, has been cocted so that the latter have become clean). In the sense of 'orthopnea,' Hebr. הִתְיַצְּבוּת features in BCD 75 (NM 2:42) in an attestation from Nathan ha-Me'ati, *Sefer ha-Peraqim* (*Pirqei Moshe*) XXIV.38 (cf. BMMN 239, l. 1; BMMG no. 5143). Samuel Benveniste translates Arab. انتصاب as זְקִיפָה (see entry) and Joshua Shatibi has קִימָה (see entry). Other synonyms featuring in Moses ibn Tibbon's trans. are עֲמִידָה (in his *Hanhagat ha-Beri'ut* IV.22, see entry) and נשימת הזקיפה (in his *Sefer Ṣedat ha-Derakhim* III.11, cf. NM 5:136).

הִתְכּוֹנְנוּת · **preparation; disposition:** Arab. استعداد · Maimonides, *Maqāla fī al-rabw* (*On Asthma*) · trans. Samuel Benveniste, *Ma'amar 'al ha-Qaṣeret* V.6 (cf. BMA 2:261, ll. 6–10): וכבר מנה גאלינוס מספר מקרים ואמר בנוסח זה שכל אחד מאלו נראה הוא לעין יקרה למי שלא יתעכל מאכלו ובאר לנו שהוא אינו רוצה בזה שכל מי שלא יתעכל מאכלו יתחדשו בו אותם המקרים כלם כי פעמים יתחדש לאחד מבני אדם אחד מאותם המקרים או רבים מהם לפי השתנות הטבעים והשנים והתכוננות הגוף והשתנות מיני המסעדים שנפסדו (Galen has enumerated a

80 I.e., discomfort in breathing that is brought on or aggravated by lying flat (cf. BMA 1:2, n. 5).

number of symptoms and these are his very words: In all such cases, we observed with our own eyes that it occurred to him whose food is not digested. It is clear to us that Galen does not mean by this that all these symptoms happen to everyone whose food is not digested, for one or more of these symptoms [may] occur to every individual person according to the different temperaments [of people], their age, their bodily dispositions, and the different kinds of foods that are corrupted). In the sense of 'preparation,' Hebr. הִתְכּוֹנְנוּת features in EM 430 as a modern term only. Joshua Shatibi translates Arab. استعداد as הכנה and Anonymous has הכנות.

הִתְפַּשְּׁטוּת · **rejoicing**: Arab. انبساط · Maimonides, *Maqāla fī al-rabw* (*On Asthma*) · trans. Anonymous, *Sefer ha-Qaṣeret* VIII.2 (cf. BMA 2:413, ll. 14–15): והשמחה והגילה עושין הפך אלו כולן להתפשטות הנפש ותנועת הדם והנפש[81] למחוץ לגוף ויראו פעולות האיברים על יותר שלמות מה שיהיה (But joy and pleasure have an effect opposite to all these things because of the rejoicing of the soul and the movement of the blood and pneuma[82] to the outside of the body so that the functions of the organs seem to be at their very best). In the sense of 'rejoicing,' Hebr. הִתְפַּשְּׁטוּת is a non-attested semantic borrowing from Arab. انبساط. Samuel Benveniste translates Arab. انبساط as הַרְחָבָה (see entry) and Joshua Shatibi has *Inf. Hitpa'el* הִתְפַּשֵּׁט (see entry פָּשַׁט).

• **ההתפשטות המתחדש בעין** · **dilation of the pupil (mydriasis)**: Arab. انتشار (HLA 178) · al-Rāzī, *K. al-Manṣūrī fī al-ṭibb* · trans. Shem Tov ben Isaac, *Sefer Almansur*, fol. 3^b: כח' בהתפשטות המתחדש בעין ([Bk. 9], ch. 28: On dilation of the pupil). Hebrew ההתפשטות המתחדש בעין does not feature in the current dictionaries. The term הִתְפַּשְּׁטוּת on its own features in the sense of 'dilatation (of the palpebral membrane)' in NM 5:63–64 in a later attestation from Nathan ha-Me'ati, *Sefer ha-Peraqim* (*Pirqei Moshe*) XXIII.69 (cf. BMMN 227, l. 19; BMMG no. 5129). Abraham Avigdor translates the parallel Lat. term *dilatio pupile* as ההתפשטות המתחדש בעין as well.

הַתָּרָה · I. **relaxation; looseness [of the bowels]**: Lat. *solutio* (Arab. إسهال) · Constantinus Africanus, *Viaticum peregrinantis* · trans. Do'eg ha-Edomi, *Sefer Ya'ir Netiv* IV.14: ונזכיר כאן העזר המורכב לכל מיני התרת המעים ומן החלקות ומן האפיסה ומהאסטומכא שאינו יכול להחזיק המאכל (I will now mention compound remedies for all kinds of looseness of the bowels [and soft stools], for weakness of the stomach that cannot hold the food). Hebr. הַתָּרָה features in BCD 77–78 as Hebr. התרת הבטן in the sense of 'diarrhea' or 'looseness of the bowels' in later attestations from Zeraḥyah Ḥen, *Sefer ha-Peraqim* (*Pirqei Moshe*) VII.42 (cf. NM 1:143; BMMZ 81, l. 18; BMMG no. 3185) and Moses ibn Tibbon, *Perush Aphorismi shel Apuqraṭ* (*Pirqei Abuqraṭ*) II.14 (66) (cf. NM 3:74; BMCH 1:338, l. 1). Moses ibn Tibbon translates the parallel Arab. term إسهال as שלשול.

81 והנפש: والروح a.
82 'pneuma': Trans. after a.

• **11. labor pains:** Arab. طلق · Ibn al-Jazzār, *Zād al-musāfir wa-qūt al-ḥādir* · trans. Moses ibn Tibbon, *Sefer Ṣedat ha-Derakhim* v.16: כשתגיע עת הלידה הטבעית אשר שער אותה ה׳ ית׳ וית׳ יקרה לאשה ההתרה ויתנועע האבר תנועה יותר חזקה שבתנועות לסבת מעוט מזונו ויתרחב הרחם בעבור ההתרה ההיא (When a woman reaches the time that God—blessed be He—has ordained for natural childbirth, she develops labor pains, whereby [the fetus] makes very strong movements because of the little amount of food left for it and the uterus widens because of those labor pains). Hebr. הַתָּרָה does not feature in this sense in the current dictionaries. A synonym used by Moses ibn Tibbon is הַמְלָטָה (see entry). Abraham ben Isaac translates Arab. طلق as צירים וחבלים and as הכאב והצירים.

שִׁלְשֵׁל → **שלשל דם הוסת • וֶסֶת**.

וֶרֶד · **blossom; flower**: Arab. ورد (cf. FL 4:454, s.v. وَرْد: 'In genere Flos arboris') · i. Ibn al-Jazzār, *Zād al-musāfir wa-qūt al-ḥādir* · trans. Moses ibn Tibbon, *Sefer Ṣedat ha-Derakhim* IV.14: ויועיל לשלשול הנושן אשר מחלקות המעים שישלוק אותה במים שנתבשל בהם איפוקישטידוש הוא טראתית בע׳ וגלנש וקשטנייאש ומעט מורד הרמונים וקלפותיהם (For chronic diarrhea caused by lientery it is beneficial to boil [the mentioned ingredients] in water in which hypocist, i.e., *ṭarāthīth* in Arab. [cf. IG 416], acorns, chestnuts, and some blossom and peels of the pomegranate have been cooked). In the sense of 'blossom; flower,' Hebr. וֶרֶד is a non-attested calque of Arab. ورد.

· ii. Ibn Sīnā, *K. al-Qānūn fī al-ṭibb* · trans. Zeraḥyah Ḥen, *Sefer ha-Qanun* II, fol. 248ᵃ: סוּרַנְגֶ׳אן אַרְמוֹדַקְטִילִי שורש צמח שיש לו ורד לבן וישוב[83] ציטרינו (SWuR-aNəĞe'N [i.e., Arab. *sūranjān*; 'autumn crocus' [*Colchicum autumnale* L.]; cf. IG 654]; 'aRəMWoDaQəṬiYLiY [i.e., Rom. *ermodactili*]: The root of a plant that has white and yellow flowers). Nathan ha-Me'ati translates Arab. ورد as *Plur.* ורדים and Anonymous has *Sing.* וֶרֶד, just like Zeraḥyah.

83 וישוב ציטרינו: وأصفر a.

זָב (*Part.*) → [זוב].

זָבַח · **to slaughter**: Arab. ذبح · Ibn Zuhr, *K. al-Aghdhiya* · trans. Nathan ha-Me'ati, *Sefer ha-Mezonot*, fol. 4b: והנהיגו הרופאים הקדמונים לזבוח אלו העופות קשי הבשר קודם התבשלם בשעות הרבה ויעזבו תלויים בנוצתם (The ancient physicians used to slaughter these birds with firm meat many hours before cooking them and to let them hang from their feathers). Hebr. זָבַח features in the current dictionaries in attestations from the Bible and Rabb. literature only; cf. BM 1283–1284; JD 378. In their *Sefer ha-Peraqim* (*Pirqei Moshe*) XVII.34, XX.9, and XXIV.43, Zeraḥyah Ḥen is the one who translates Arab. ذبح as זָבַח (cf. BMMZ 173, l. 6; 182, l. 8; 239, l. 17), while Nathan has שָׁחַט there (cf. BMMN 175, l. 7; 185, l. 3; 239, l. 20) (cf. also BMMG no. 1956).

זָהָב • דבק הזהב → דֶּבֶק.

זְהָבִי • מרקחת יקרא הזהבי → מֶרְקַחַת.

[זוב] • *Part.* זָב • כשזב הזרע מן הגיד בלא רצון · **spermatorrhea (gonorrhea)**: Arab. سيلان المني من غير إرادة · Ibn al-Jazzār, *Zād al-musāfir wa-qūt al-ḥādir* · trans. Abraham ben Isaac, *Sefer Ṣedah la-Oreḥim* VI.3: השער השלישי יזכיר כשזב הזרע מן הגיד בלא רצון (Ch. 3: On spermatorrhea (gonorrhea)). Hebr. כשזב הזרע מן הגיד בלא רצון is not attested in the current dictionaries. A more concise term used by Abraham ben Isaac for 'spermatorrhea' is זיבות הזרע (see entry זִיבוּת). Moses ibn Tibbon translates the Arab. term as הגרת הזרע מבלי רצון (cf. BCD 62 (NM 4:41)) and Do'eg ha-Edomi simply transcribes the parallel Lat. term *gonorrhea* as גּוֹנוֹרֵיאָה.

זוּז · ***zuz*** **(measure of weight equivalent to one *dirham* (= 3.125 grams))**: Arab. درهم (Gr. δραχμή); cf. HIM 3[84] · Ibn Sīnā, *K. al-Qānūn fī al-ṭibb* · trans. Nathan ha-Me'ati, *Sefer ha-Qanun* II, fol. 69b: בזר קטונא ... אם יקלו ממנו משקל שני זוזים בלול בשמן ורדים יעצר הבטן ויועיל מנגעי המעיים הנקרא סחג׳ בערבי ויותר אל הנערים (Fleawort seed: ... If one roasts the weight of two *zuzim* of fleawort seed and mixes it with rose oil, it causes constipation. It is useful for intestinal abrasions called *saḥaj* in Arab., particularly of infants). As a measure of weight, Hebr. *Sing.* זוז occurs in Rabb. literature where it is used interchangeably with the דינר (Lat. *denarius*), which in turn is parallel to Gr. δραχμή. Zeraḥyah Ḥen renders Arab. درهم as *Plur.* דראהם and Anonymous has זוזים, just like Nathan.

זחיר (*Arab.* زحير) • חולי הזחיר → חֳלִי.

זִיבָה · **flow of sperm; spermatorrhea (gonorrhea)**: Arab. سيلان المني · Ibn al-Jazzār, *Zād al-musāfir wa-qūt al-ḥādir* · trans. Moses ibn Tibbon, *Sefer Ṣedat ha-Derakhim* VI.3: או יקח רודא וזרע קנילאדא מ״א חלק ויודק וישתה ממנו שקל במשקה הדס וחומץ כי הוא יועיל מרבוי הזיבה (Or take rue and henbane seed, of each one part; pulverize [these ingredients]

84 Cf. also M. Ullmann, *Die Medizin im Islam* (Leiden 1970), 318.

and take one *sheqel*[85] with myrtle juice and vinegar, for it is good for frequent flow of sperm (gonorrhea)). Hebr. זִיבָה is only attested in Rabb. literature in the sense of 'gonorrhea' (cf. JD 390; BM 1318).

זִיבוּת • **זיבות הזרע** · **flow of sperm; spermatorrhea (gonorrhea)**: Arab. سيلان المني · Ibn al-Jazzār, *Zād al-musāfir wa-qūt al-ḥādir* · trans. Abraham ben Isaac, *Sefer Ṣedah la-Oreḥim* VI.3: ואם תרצה להסיר זיבות הזרע גם תאות התשמיש קח גלנר וזרע פורקקלי וזרע לטוקא וזרע קנבי מכל א׳ ב׳ שקלים (If you want to stop the flow of sperm (gonorrhea) and extinguish the lust for sexual intercourse, take flower of the pomegranate, common purslane seed, lettuce seed, and hemp seed, two *sheqels*[86] of each ...). Hebr. זִיבוּת is only attested in Rabb. literature in the sense of 'gonorrhea' (cf. JD 391; BM 1319). For the expression כשזב הזרע מן הגיד בלא רצון, also used by Abraham ben Isaac for 'spermatorrhea (gonorrhea)' in the same paragraph, see entry [זוב]. Moses ibn Tibbon translates Arab. سيلان المني as הגרת הזרע.

זילוף → זִלּוּף.

[זיף] • *Part. Puʿal* מְזוּיָּף · **adulterated**: Arab. مغشوش · Ibn Sīnā, *K. al-Qānūn fī al-ṭibb* · trans. Nathan ha-Me'ati, *Sefer ha-Qanun* II, fol. 74ᵃ: גואשיר ... והשחור הרך הוא מזוייף ומזייפין אותו באשק (Opopanax: ... The black and soft variety is [often] adulterated, namely with gum ammoniac). Hebr. *Part. Puʿal* מְזוּיָּף is not attested in medieval medical literature in the current dictionaries (cf. BM 1325). Zeraḥyah Ḥen and Anonymous translate Arab. مغشوش as מְזוּיָּף as well.

זְכוּכִי · **vitreous**: Lat. *vitreus* (Arab. زجاجي) · Constantinus Africanus, *Viaticum peregrinantis* · trans. Do'eg ha-Edomi, *Sefer Ya'ir Netiv* IV.15: או מהלבנה המלוחה או מחודדת ובמליחותה עושה זה הדבר עצמו למעי כמו שנראה במלאכת הניטרי או בלבנה הזכוכית (It [i.e., excoriation (abrasion) of the intestines] may also be caused by sharp salty phlegm, by the very effect of its saltiness on the intestines, as we can see from the effect of borax (sodium borate). It may also be caused by vitreous phlegm). In the sense of 'vitreous,' Hebr. זְכוּכִי features in BM 1332 in later attestations, a.o., from the *Sefer ha-Qanun*. Moses ibn Tibbon translates the parallel Arab. term زجاجي as זְכוּכִי as well.

זְכוּכִית • **זכוכית לבנה** · **white vitriol**: Arab. قلقطار (Gr. χαλκῖτις) ('a variety of vitriol,' cf. MIG no. 817) · [*Synonima*], Ms Vatican, Biblioteca Apostolica, ebr. 550, fol. 128ᵃ: קלקטאר הוא זכוכית לבנה (QLQṬ'R [Arab. *qulquṭār*]; i.e., [Hebr.] *zekhukhit levanah* [lit., 'white glass']). Hebr. זכוכית לבנה is not attested in the current dictionaries. Shem Tov ben Isaac remarks about this type of vitriol in his glossary to the *Sefer Almansur*: קלקטאר: לבן ינגב שכבת הזרע ויסיר התאוה (QLQṬ'R (a type of vitriol): It is white; it dries the sperm and takes the sexual lust away) (cf. BMZ 70–71 (Qof 10)).

[זכך] • *Piʿel* זִכֵּךְ · **to filter, strain**: Arab. صفّى · Maimonides, *Maqāla fī al-rabw* (*On

---

85 Hebr. *sheqel* stands forn Arab. *mithqāl*; one *mithqāl* is 4.46 grams; cf. HIM 4–7.

86 See fn. above.

Asthma) · trans. Joshua Shatibi, *Ma'amar 'al ha-Qaṣeret* IX.1 (cf. BMA 2:347, ll. 4–6): וכבר שבח אבו מרואן בן זהר לרככו בזה אמר: ימרס מן התמר הנדי י״ דרהם במה שישקעהו ממים חמים וישרה בו מן אלראונד צני רצוץ שלשה רבעיות דרהם כ״ד שעות ויזכך על[יו] אוקיא משקה קליפת אתרוג (Abu Marwan ibn Zuhr has recommended softening them [i.e., the stools] with the following [drug]: Macerate ten *dirhams* of Indian tamarind in sufficient warm water to cover them, and then soak three-quarters of a *dirham* of ground Chinese rhubarb for twenty-four hours and strain this into one ounce of lemon peel juice). In the sense of 'to strain, filter,' Hebr. *Pi'el* זִיכֵּךְ is a non-attested semantic borrowing from Arab. صفّى. Samuel Benveniste translates the Arab. term as *Pi'el* צִלֵּל (see entry [צלל]) and Anonymous has סִינֵן.

זַכְרוּת · **penis**: Arab. ذَكَر · Ibn al-Jazzār, *Zād al-musāfir wa-qūt al-ḥāḍir* · trans. Abraham ben Isaac, *Sefer Ṣedah la-Oreḥim* VI.1: וימשח בשמן ההוא הבטן והזכרות כי הוא יקשה (And rub with that oil the abdomen and penis, for it produces an erection). In the sense of 'penis,' Hebr. זַכְרוּת is not attested in medieval Hebr. medical literature. Abraham ben Isaac translates Arab. ذَكَر as גיד הערוה (see entry גִּיד).

זִלּוּף · **massage**: Arab. دلك · Maimonides, *Maqāla fī al-rabw* (*On Asthma*) · trans. Anonymous, *Sefer ha-Qaṣeret* X.6 (cf. BMA 2:422, ll. 21–22): אמר גאלינוס דברים אלו לשונם אמר: אמנם זילוף האברים החלושים ראוי להשמר מעשיתו בעתים שיתעוררו בהן החליים שלהם (Galen has said the following, and these are his very words: One should beware of applying massage to weak limbs at times when their diseases are stirred up in them). Hebr. זִלּוּף only features in the current dictionaries in the sense of 'sprinkling' in attestations from Rabb. literature (cf. JD 394; BM 1345). Samuel Benveniste translates Arab. دلك as מִשּׁוּשׁ (see entry) and Joshua Shatibi as חֲפִיפָה (cf. BCD 105–106 (NM 1:57, 151; 2:48; 3:95–96)).

[זלף] • *Pi'el* זִלֵּף · **I. to massage**: Arab. دلك · Maimonides, *Maqāla fī al-rabw* (*On Asthma*) · trans. Anonymous, *Sefer ha-Qaṣeret* XIII.14 (cf. BMA 2:441, ll. 7–8): אמר גאלינוס: ולפיכך היה הדבור שהישר למשוח הזקן בבקר בשמן ויזלף יהיה פועל הזילוף כמו שראוי מהקשה שבדברים (Galen said: Therefore, it is easy to say that it is correct to rub the elderly in the morning with oil and to massage them, but to massage them properly is a most difficult thing). Hebr. *Pi'el* זִלֵּף features in the current dictionaries in the sense of 'to pour, drip, sprinkle' (cf. JD 402; BM 1348). Joshua Shatibi translates Arab. دلك as *Pi'el* חִפֵּף (cf. BCD 106 (NM 2:49)).

· **II. to foment, bathe, apply as a douche**: Arab. نطل (Gr. καταντλέω; cf. UW 331) · Ibn Sīnā, *K. al-Qānūn fī al-ṭibb* · trans. Nathan ha-Me'ati, *Sefer ha-Qanun* II, fol. 92[b]: כשכש ... ואם עושים ממנו תחבשת על מצח בעל התעורה וכן אם יזלפו בתבשילו (Poppy: ... [It is beneficial] if it is applied as a plaster on the forehead of patients of insomnia. Likewise, when [the forehead] is fomented with its decoction). In his *Sefer ha-Peraqim* (*Pirqei Moshe*) IX.6 and XV.17, Nathan translates Arab. نطل as יצק (cf. BMMN 103, l. 24; 156, l. 24; BMMG no. 5171).

זַעַף · **foam**: Arab. رغوة · Ibn Sīnā, *K. al-Qānūn fī al-ṭibb* · trans. Nathan ha-Me'ati, *Sefer* *ha-Qanun* II, fol. 69[a]: בורק ... איברי הראש: יועיל מהילפת הנקרא חזאז בערבי ומהזעף הנקרא רעונה[87] בערבי עם דבש וכשמטיפים ממנו באזן ינקה ויועיל מהחרשות (Borax (sodium borate): ... The parts of the head: It is useful for dandruff called *ḥazāz* in Arab. Ear drops made from its foam, called R'WNH (*R'WH) [in Arab.] mixed with honey cleanses the ears and is good for deafness). Hebr. זַעַף only features in the current dictionaries in the sense of 'anger; rage;' cf. BM 1376. Ben Yehuda (ibid., n. 1) remarks that the Arab. verb زعف, which is a parallel to the Hebr. verb זָעַף, has the meaning of 'to kill instantly,' but in some places also that of קָצַף ('to be angry'). Zeraḥyah Ḥen translates Arab. رغوة as standard קֶצֶף and Anonymous has קֶצֶף as well. Shem Tov ben Isaac translates it as חֶלְאָה in his *Sefer ha-Shimmush* XXVII (cf. BCD 94 (NM 4:66)).

זְקִיפָה · **I. orthopnea:**[88] Arab. انتصاب (cf. UW 471, s.v. ὀρθόπνοια: نفس الانتصاب) · Maimonides, *Maqāla fī al-rabw* (*On Asthma*) · trans. Samuel Benveniste, *Ma'amar 'al ha-Qaṣeret* N.2 (cf. BMA 2:242, l. 6–8): וכבר ידעתי בעדות ובמה שספרת לנו שסבת החולי הזה הזלה מן המוח בזמנים שרובם בסתו והזקיפה והכאב לא יסורו ימים בלילותם לפי ארך המשמרה וקצורה עד שתעמד ההזלה ויתבשל מה שהגיע בריאה עד שתנקה (I know from what I have witnessed [with my own eyes] and from what [my Master] has described to me that the cause of this illness is a defluxion that descends from the brain at certain times [of the year], but mostly in winter. [And I know] that the orthopnea and distress do not cease through the night for days on end, according to the length or brevity of the attack, until the defluxion decreases and until that [fluid] which has reached the lungs has been cocted so that the latter have become clean). Hebr. זְקִיפָה does not feature in this sense in the current dictionaries. Joshua Shatibi translates Arab. انتصاب as קִימָה (see entry), and Anonymous has הִתְיַצְּבוּת (see entry). Other synonyms featuring in Moses ibn Tibbon's trans. are עֲמִידָה (in his *Hanhagat ha-Beri'ut* IV.22, see entry) and נשימת הזקיפה (in his *Sefer Ṣedat ha-Derakhim* III.11, cf. NM 5:136).

· **II. (penile) erection:** Lat. *erigo* (Arab. إنعاظ) · Constantinus Africanus, *Viaticum peregrinantis* · trans. Do'eg ha-Edomi, *Sefer Ya'ir Netiv* VI.1: ואותה הזקיפה באה מן הלב כי הלב שולח לכל הגוף הרוח הרוחני (And that [power of] erection comes from the heart because the heart sends the spiritual[89] pneuma [i.e., animal pneuma] to the whole body). Hebr. זְקִיפָה features in MD 265, s.v. 'erection; *erectio*.' Moses ibn Tibbon translates Arab. إنعاظ as קֹשִׁי (cf. the use of the same Hebr. term, also for Arab. إنعاظ, in his *Perush Aphorismi shel Apuqraṭ* (*Pirqei Abuqraṭ*) VI.30 (322) (cf. BCD 251–252 (NM 3:211); BMCH 1:399, l. 3)), and Abraham ben Isaac has עמידת הגיד (see entry עֲמִידָה).

• **זקיפת האמה ברוב** · **priapism:** Lat. *nimia erectio virgae* (Arab. الإنعاظ الدائم) · Constantinus Africanus, *Viaticum peregrinantis* · trans. Do'eg ha-Edomi, *Sefer Ya'ir Netiv*

87 רעונה (*רעוה): رغوة a.

88 I.e., discomfort in breathing that is brought on or aggravated by lying flat (cf. BMA 1:2, n. 5).

89 'spiritual pneuma [i.e., animal pneuma]': الروح الحيوانية a.

vi.2: זקיפת האמה ברוב ([On] priapism). Hebr. זקיפת האמה ברוב is not attested in the current dictionaries. Moses ibn Tibbon translates Arab. الإنعاظ الدائم as קושי מתמיד (see entry קֹשִׁי) and Abraham ben Isaac has כשיעמוד גיד הערוה תדיר (see entry עָמַד).

זָקַף • *Part.* זוֹקֵף • **having an erection**: Lat. *erigor* (Arab. نعظ) · Constantinus Africanus, *Viaticum peregrinantis* · trans. Do'eg ha-Edomi, *Sefer Ya'ir Netiv* vi.1: גם נמצאו רבים אחרים שיש להם תאוה רבה ואינם זוקפים גם זרע אינו יכול לצאת מהם (Many others have sexual lust but have no erection and ejaculate no sperm). Hebr. זָקַף, *Part.* זוֹקֵף, is not attested in this sense in the current dictionaries. Do'eg also uses *Pass. Part.* זָקוּף (see next entry) to render Lat. *erigens*. Moses ibn Tibbon translates the parallel Arab. term نعظ as *Hitpa'el* הִתְקַשָּׁה (see entry [קשה]), and Abraham ben Isaac has עמד הגיד (see entry עָמַד).

• *Pass. Part.* זָקוּף • **having an erection**: Lat. *erigens* (Arab. إنعاظ)· Constantinus Africanus, *Viaticum peregrinantis* · trans. Do'eg ha-Edomi, *Sefer Ya'ir Netiv* vi.4: ואלה הרואים קרי תמיד ראויים להעזר עם רפואות קרות או עם מאכלים או עם משיחות כמו שהזכרנו על הזקופים תמיד (Those who suffer from frequent nocturnal emissions should be treated with cold remedies, foodstuff, or unguents, as we have mentioned for someone who has a permanent erection). Hebr. *Pass. Part.* זָקוּף does not feature in this sense in the current dictionaries. Do'eg also uses *Part.* זוֹקֵף (see previous entry) to render Lat. *erigor*. Moses ibn Tibbon translates the parallel Arab. term إنعاظ ('erection') as קושי.

זְרִיזוּת · **experience**: Arab. دربة · Maimonides, *Maqāla fī al-rabw* (*On Asthma*) · trans. Anonymous, *Sefer ha-Qaṣeret* xiii.30 (cf. bma 2:446, ll. 3–4): ומהטעיה גם כן הדמיון שהאיש יהיה אצלו זריזות במעשי הרפואה ואף על פי שאין לו הבנה (Another mistake is to imagine that one can have experience in the practice of medicine without knowledge). Hebr. זְרִיזוּת does not feature in this sense in the current dictionaries. Samuel Benveniste translates Arab. دربة as בקיאות and Joshua Shatibi has הֶרְגֵּל (see entry).

זֶרַע • גרישת הזרע בתוך השינה → גְּרִישָׁה.

• דפוסי הזרע → דְּפוּס.

• הגרת הזרע מבלי רצון → הַגָּרָה.

• כשזב הזרע מן הגיד בלא רצון → [זוב].

• כיסי הזרע → כִּיס.

• כלי הזרע → כְּלִי.

ח

חִבּוּר · **composition [of a remedy]**: Arab. تأليف · Ibn al-Jazzār, *Zād al-musāfir wa-qūt al-ḥādir* · trans. Moses ibn Tibbon, *Sefer Ṣedat ha-Derakhim* v.7: תאר עוגות ריברברי מועילות מסיתומי הכבד והטחול ומחזקות האצטו׳ חבור יצחק וכבר נסיתים (A recipe for rhubarb pastilles that are good for obstructions in the liver and spleen and that strengthen the stomach and that were composed by Isḥāq [ibn ʿImrān] and that I tried). Hebr. חִבּוּר does not feature in a medical context in the current dictionaries. Do'eg ha-Edomi translates the parallel Lat. term *Rx* ('recipe') as מַעֲשֶׂה (see entry).

- **הפרדת החבור** → **הַפְרָדָה**.
- **הפרדות החיבור** → **הַפְרָדוֹת**.
- **פרוד החבור** → **פֵּרוּד**.
- **פרוק החבור** → **פֵּרוּק**.

חֲבָטָה · **I. torpor; shock**: Arab. وهن (cf. D 2:846: 'faiblesse du corps; torpeur des membres;' FL 512: 'debilitas in agendo') · Ibn al-Jazzār, *Zād al-musāfir wa-qūt al-ḥādir* · trans. Moses ibn Tibbon, *Sefer Ṣedat ha-Derakhim* v.3: ואם יקרה לחולה עם המורסא חום בכבד נשקהו בלבשטיאש ובול ארמיני במיץ פלנטאגי או במיץ מורילא. וכל מיני בול יועילו למורסות אשר מדם יקרו בתוך הגוף והרצוץ והחבטה והכתישה ויחבוש בתחבושת צנדל ומה שדומה לזה (If in addition to the tumor the patient suffers from heat in the liver, we should give him rose or blossom of the wild pomegranate, and Armenian earth with juice of plantain or of black nightshade. All kinds of earth are good for bodily tumors that originate from blood; [they are also good for] a bruise, shock, and contusion. [The patient] should apply a poultice of sandalwood and the like). Hebr. חֲבָטָה features in the current dictionaries in the sense of 'blow; stroke; shock' in attestations from Rabb. literature (cf. JD 417–418; BM 1420). In his *Sefer Ṣedat ha-Derakhim* VII.25, Ibn Tibbon translates the same Arab. term وهن as רסוס (cf. IJZ 7:166, l. 15).

· **II. throbbing**: Arab. ضربان · Ibn Sīnā, *K. al-Qānūn fī al-ṭibb* · trans. Zeraḥyah Ḥen, *Sefer ha-Qanun* II, fol. 184b: ביצות ... הלובן שבו משכך כאב העין והאודם שבו עם הזעפראן ושמן מורדים מועיל מאד מחבטת העין (Eggs: ... The white of an egg relieves ophthalgia and its yolk, mixed with saffron and rose oil, is very useful for the throbbing of the eye). Nathan ha-Me'ati translates Arab. ضربان as דְּפִיקָה (see entry).

חֲבִישָׁה · **astringency**: Arab. قبض · Maimonides, *Maqāla fī al-rabw* (*On Asthma*) · trans. Samuel Benveniste, *Ma'amar 'al ha-Qaṣeret* v.4 (cf. BMA 2:260, ll. 10–11): וכמו כן יקדם מה שיש בו רפיון ויאחר מה שיש בו חבישה לפי קצת הסברות (Similarly, one should first [eat] that which has a diluting effect and then [eat] that which is astringent, according to the opinion of some [physicians]). In the sense of 'astringency,' Hebr. חֲבִישָׁה is a non-attested semantic borrowing from Arab. قبض. A synonymous term used by Samuel Benveniste is חֲבִישׁוּת (see next entry). Joshua Shatibi renders Arab. قبض as קביצות (cf. 236 (NM 2:78)) and Anonymous has אִמּוּץ (see entry).

חֲבִישׁוּת · **astringency**: Arab. قبض · Maimonides, *Maqāla fī al-rabw* (*On Asthma*) · trans.

Samuel Benveniste, *Ma'amar 'al ha-Qaṣeret* XI.1 (cf. BMA 2:283, ll. 7–8): ועל כל פנים בחזקנו כל אבר ואבר עד שנשיבהו אל מזגו הטבעי צריך שנשים ברפואותיו מה שיש בו חבישות לכל אבר כפי הראוי לו (To strengthen any organ and to restore its natural temperament, it is unavoidable that we use astringent drugs in accordance with what is appropriate to each organ). Hebr. חֲבִישׁוּת, a synonym of חֲבִישָׁה (see previous entry), does not feature in the current dictionaries. Joshua Shatibi renders Arab. قبض as קביצות (cf. 236 (NM 2:78)) and Anonymous has עִפּוּץ (see entry).

חֶבֶל • *Plur.* **חבלים** • **חבלי הבטן** · **gripes; colic**: Arab. مغص (Gr. στρόφος; cf. UW 644) · Ibn Sīnā, *K. al-Qānūn fī al-ṭibb* · Anonymous, *Sefer ha-Qanun* II, fols. 51[a]–51[b]: ... בורק משלשל אם יונח למטה ואם יאכל עם רודא וכמון או בשול רודא ושבת ישקיט חבלי הבטן (Borax (sodium borate): ... When one applies it in a suppository, or eats it with rue and cumin or takes a decoction with rue and dill, it alleviates gripes (colic)). Hebr. חבלי הבטן is not attested in the current dictionaries. Nathan ha-Me'ati translates Arab. مغص as עקיצת המעיים (see entry עֲקִיצָה), and in his *Pirqei Abuqraṭ* V.41 as חבלים (cf. BCD 88 (NM 3:78)). Zeraḥyah Ḥen translates the Arab. term as פונטורא (cf. Lat. *punctura*). For other synonyms, see entries חִיל, חִתּוּךְ, and מַשְׁבֵּר.

[חבר] • *Part. Pi'el* **מְחַבֵּר** • **המחיצה המחברת** → מְחִיצָה.

• *Part. Hitpa'el f.* **מִתְחַבֶּרֶת** · **conjunctiva**: Lat. *coniunctiva* · Gerard de Solo, *Practica super nono Almansoris* · trans. Abraham Avigdor, *Ha-Ma'amar ha-Teshi'i le-Sefer ha-Mansuri le-Razi*, fol. 74[a]: ראוי שתדע שזאת הנקודה האדומה המתחדשת בעין מהותה דם נקפא מתדבק ביריעה הנקראת המתחברת (Know that this red spot (*macula rubea*) that occurs in the eye is essentially coagulated blood that adheres to the membrane called 'conjunctiva'). Hebr. *Part. Hitpa'el f.* מִתְחַבֶּרֶת does not feature in this sense in the current dictionaries. A var. from the same root חָבַר, i.e., *Part. f.* חוֹבֶרֶת, is mentioned in KDS 93. A synonym used by Abraham Avigdor is המחיצה המחברת (see entry מְחִיצָה).

[חבש] • *Pi'el* **חִבֵּשׁ** · **to use in a plaster, salve**: Arab. ضمّد · Ibn Sīnā, *K. al-Qānūn fī al-ṭibb* · trans. Nathan ha-Me'ati, *Sefer ha-Qanun* II, fol. 68[a]: באדורד ... מועיל ממורסות הליחה הלבנה מפני שבו מההתך והקבוץ ומחבשים בו ובעקרו לבד (Soldier thistle: ... As it is dissolvent and astringent, it is useful in phlegmatic swellings. Especially the root is used in plasters). Hebr. *Pi'el* חִבֵּשׁ features in the current dictionaries in the sense of 'to bind, bind up [wounds]' in attestations from the Bible (cf. KB 289; BM 1439), medieval Hebrew poetry, and modern Hebrew literature (cf. EM 500). Zeraḥyah Ḥen translates Arab. ضمّد as חָבַשׁ (*Qal* conj.) and Anonymous has חֻבַּשׁ (*Pu'al* conj.).

[חדש] • *Hitpa'el* **הִתְחַדֵּשׁ** • **ההתפשטות המתחדש בעין** → הִתְפַּשְּׁטוּת.

חָדָשׁ · **bleeding (of a wound)**: Arab. طري (Gr. ἔναιμος; cf. UW 240–241)· Ibn Sīnā, *K. al-Qānūn fī al-ṭibb* · trans. Zeraḥyah Ḥen, *Sefer ha-Qanun* II, fol. 254[b]: עֻצָּה הרועה ... והוא מועיל מאד החבלות והנגעים יחייה[90] החבלות החדשות (Common knotgrass: ... It is very

90 יחייה: يدمل a.

beneficial for tumors and ulcers. It heals bleeding wounds). In the sense of 'bleeding,' Hebr. חָדָשׁ is a non-attested semantic borrowing from Arab. طري. Nathan ha-Me'ati translates Arab. طري as טָרִי (see entry).

חולי → חֳלִי.

חולשה → חֲלָשָׁה.

חום → חֹם.

חוש · **to hasten, hurry**: Lat. *festino* (Arab. لا توانى) · Constantinus Africanus, *Viaticum peregrinantis* · trans. Do'eg ha-Edomi, *Sefer Ya'ir Netiv* v.13: ועל כן יאות כי בסבות ובאותות הצמחים אשר בכליות נחוש לרפאתם כי הכליות קשות לעזור וכח הרפואה לא יבא שם בהאפסו באריכות הדרך (Therefore, once we see the causes and symptoms of kidney ulcers, we should hasten to treat them since it is hard to cure the kidneys and the medicine does not reach them with its full strength but only in a weakened form because it has such a long way to go before getting to [the kidneys]). Hebr. חוש is not attested in medieval medical literature. Moses ibn Tibbon translates Arab. لا توانى as לא נתעצל.

חָזֶה • **דוחק בחזה** → דֹּחַק.

• **העצמות מלמטה מן הצואר על החזה** → עֶצֶם.

• **צרות החזה** → צָרוּת.

חֲזָזִית · **scurf; dandruff**: Arab. حزاز (Gr. πίτυρον; cf. UW 530–531) · Ibn Sīnā, *K. al-Qānūn fī al-ṭibb* · trans. Zeraḥyah Ḥen, *Sefer ha-Qanun* II, fols. 182ª–182ᵇ: בֹּוֶרֶק ... יועיל מן החזזית והקצף עם הדבש כשיושם באוזן ינקה ופותח ויועיל מן החרשות (Borax (sodium borate): ... It is useful for dandruff. Ear drops made from its foam [mixed] with honey cleanse and open the ears and are good for deafness). Hebr. חֲזָזִית features in JD 442 in the sense of 'lichen; a cuteneous disease connected with desquamation and sometimes ulceration' (cf. BM 1483), and in Low LIV as 'Egyptian papula.' Nathan ha-Me'ati translates Arab. حزاز as יַלֶּפֶת (see entry).

[חזק] • *Pi'el* חִזֵּק • **חיזק והדביק** · **to close [a wound]**: Lat. *solido* (Arab. غرّى) · Constantinus Africanus, *Viaticum peregrinantis* · trans. Do'eg ha-Edomi, *Sefer Ya'ir Netiv* v.13: כל אלה מבושלים ישקיטו מוקד השתן ויחזקו וידביקו הנגעים (When one cooks any of these ingredients, it alleviates burning urination and closes a wound). Hebr. חיזק והדביק does not feature in the current dictionaries. Moses ibn Tibbon reads Arab. غرّى as غذّى, which he translates as זן.

• **הדביק וחיזק** → [דבק].

• *Hitpa'el* הִתְחַזֵּק · **to be prompted**: Lat. *cogor* (Arab. دعا) · Constantinus Africanus, *Viaticum peregrinantis* · trans. Do'eg ha-Edomi, *Sefer Ya'ir Netiv* v.16: ואם האבן במקוה יהיה הכאב נרגש על גב הערוה והחכוך באמה והוא מתחזק לממש אותה ולגרד אותה בידים (If the stone is in the bladder, [the patient] will feel [so much] pain in the pubes and itching in the penis that he is prompted to touch and rub it with his hands). Hebr. *Hitpa'el* הִתְחַזֵּק does not feature in this sense in the current dictionaries. Moses ibn Tibbon translates Arab. دعا as בקש.

• *Part. Hif'il* מַחְזִיק • **הכח המחזיק** → כֹּחַ.

חַי · **pure**: Lat. *purus* (Arab. صحيح) · Constantinus Africanus, *Viaticum peregrinantis* · trans. Do'eg ha-Edomi, *Sefer Ya'ir Netiv* IV.1: הזלת דם הכבד נעשית בענינים רבים והדם יוצא מתמונות משתנות כי הוא יהיה או מהפרדת החבור כמו כאשר עצומו נגוע או מפתיחת המקורות ואלה מתפרדים בעצמם כי דם המקורות הפתוחים הוא חי ואדום ומהנגעים הוא שחור וגס ובלוי (There are many causes for blood flowing from the liver, and the kinds of blood that streams [from the liver] vary. [Blood] can result either from the dissolution of continuity, as in the case that the substance [of the liver] is ulcerated or that a vein has burst. These [kinds of blood] differ on their own because the blood from a burst vein is pure and red, but [the blood] from an ulcer is black, thick, and putrid). In the sense of 'pure,' Hebr. חַי is only attested in the combination יין חי ('unmixed, pure wine'); cf. BCD 117 (NM 1:55–56), a.o., for an attestation from Moses ibn Tibbon, *Sefer Ṣedat ha-Derakhim* VII.11.1 (cf. IJZ 7:142, l. 13). Here, Moses ibn Tibbon translates Arab. صحيح as בריא.

• סיד חי → סִיד.

חיבור → חִבּוּר.

חִיל · **cramps; colic**: Arab. مغص (Gr. στρόφος; cf. UW 644) · Maimonides, *Maqāla fī al-rabw* (*On Asthma*) · trans. Samuel Benveniste, *Ma'amar 'al ha-Qaṣeret* XII.9 (cf. BMA 2:294, l. 17): ואם ימצאהו כאב וחיל בעד המשקה באצטומכא (If, as a result of [taking] the medicine, one experiences pain and cramps (colic) in the stomach ...): Hebr. חִיל features in the Bible in the sense of '1. labour pains; 2. fear and pain' (cf. KB 1:313; BM 1531–1532). Joshua Shatibi translates Arab. مغص as עקיצה (cf. BCD 212–213 (NM 3:182)) and Anonymous has חִתּוּךְ (see entry). Moses ibn Tibbon translates Arab. مغص as משברים in his *Sefer Ṣedat ha-Derakhim* IV.15 (see entry מִשְׁבָּר) and Do'eg ha-Edomi translates the parallel Lat. term *tortura* as עִוּוּת in his *Sefer Ya'ir Netiv* I.10.10 (cf. NM 5:144–145; IJZ 1–2:612). For still other synonyms, see entries חֵבֶל and עֲקִיצָה.

חיתוך → חִתּוּךְ.

חָכַם · **to proceed skilfully, cleverly; to contrive, devise**: Arab. تلطّف (WKAS 2.2:708) · Ibn al-Jazzār, *Zād al-musāfir wa-qūt al-ḥādir* · trans. Moses ibn Tibbon, *Sefer Ṣedat ha-Derakhim* IV.9: ובעבור מה שהקדמנו ראוי למי שנפסד מאכלו ומי שרצה מן האנשים לשמור הבריאות שישמר מכל מסבבי הפסד המאכל וישתדל כאשר מצאהו זה להקיא קודם שישתנה המאכל ויפסד ואם ימנע הקיא תחכם לשלשל טבעו (Because of what I said before, someone who suffers from indigestion and someone who wants to preserve his health should beware of anything that can cause indigestion; once he is affected, he should hasten to vomit before the food changes and putrefies. If he cannot vomit one should contrive to administer a purgative). Hebr. חָכַם features in the the current dictionaries in the sense of 'to know, be wise' or 'to meet for deliberation' (cf. BDB 314; JD 462; BM 1546). Moses ibn Tibbon also uses *Hitpa'el* הִתְחַכֵּם for Arab. تلطّف (see next entry). Do'eg ha-Edomi translates the parallel Lat. term *studeo* as [שדל], *Hitpa'el* הִשְׁתַּדֵּל.

• *Hitpa'el* הִתְחַכֵּם · **to proceed skilfully, cleverly; to contrive, devise**: Arab. تلطّف (WKAS 2.2:708) · Ibn al-Jazzār, *Zād al-musāfir wa-qūt al-ḥādir* · trans. Moses ibn Tibbon, *Sefer Ṣedat ha-Derakhim* v.17: וראוי להתחכם להוציא שתנם בזיעה והוא שיושיב החולה בכלי חם ויוציא ראשו לחוץ כי זה ממה שיזיע גופו (One should contrive to extract their urine through sweating; one should do so by placing the patient in a hot vessel with his head outside the vessel, for this is one way to make the body sweat). Hebr. *Hitpa'el* הִתְחַכֵּם features in the current dictionaries in the sense of 'to deal wisely, shrewdly,' 'to make (show) oneself wise,' or 'to become wise' (BDB 314; JD 462; BM 1546–1547), and in PESHAT as 'to become wise, acquire wisdom/knowledge in the sciences.'[91] Moses ibn Tibbon also uses *Qal* חָכַם for Arab. تلطّف (see previous entry). Do'eg ha-Edomi translates the parallel Lat. term *studeamus ut sudet* as נזיעהו.

חָכְמָה • חכמת הכריתות · **surgery**: Lat. *chirurgia* · Constantinus Africanus, *Viaticum peregrinantis* · trans. Do'eg ha-Edomi, *Sefer Ya'ir Netiv* IV.19: ואם נעשה כל אשר הזכרנו ולא יועיל יאות להתבונן שאין לא עזר כי אם בחכמת שירורגיא היא חכמת הכריתות (If we do all those things that I mentioned but it does not help, we should understand that the only cure [for hemorrhoids] is surgery). In the sense of 'surgery,' Hebr. כְּרִיתוּת on its own features in BM 2516 in a later attestation from Hillel ben Samuel, *Sefer Keritut* (cf. BCD 132 (NM 1:27)). For כְּרִיתוּת in the sense of 'scarification,' see entry.

חָלָב • מיץ חלב → מִיץ.

• **המיץ היוצא מן החלב** → מִיץ.

חלוחלת • פי החלוחלת → פֶּה.

חַלְחֹלֶת → חלוחלת.

חֳלִי • חולי הזחיר · **tenesmus**: Lat. *tenesmus* · *Sefer ha-Refu'ot le-Ḥakham Qoṣṭa'ntin*, fol. 183b: בחולי הזחיר: אמר פלאטיאריש: חולי טנאשמון הוא פונץ שיוצא לנקביו בכבדות (On tenesmus: Says Platearius: The illness [called in Lat.] ṬN'ŠMWN, i.e., [in Rom.] PWNṢ; [meaning that] someone can only pass stools with difficulty). חולי הזחיר is a non-attested combined term consisting of Hebr. חלי and Arab. زَحير (transcribed as זחיר), meaning 'tenesmus' (cf. UW 669).

• **חולי כליי** · **a functional illness [i.e., an illness that impedes the functioning of an organ]**: a) Lat. *morbus officialis* (cf. DMLBS 2365, s.v. *officialis*: '*1* of or connected with the performance of function, functional: *a*) (of organ or part of body); *b*) (of ailment or sickness)') · Gerard de Solo, *Practica super nono Almansoris* · trans. Abraham Avigdor, *Ha-Ma'amar ha-Teshi'i le-Sefer ha-Mansuri le-Razi*, fol. 36b: שער ט' דֵי טוֹרטוּרָא אוֹרִיש: ראוי שתדע בבאור הרובריקא כי עקום הפה הוא חולי כליי מפסיד תמונת הפנים וצורתם (Chapter 9: *De tortura oris*: Regarding the explanation of the heading you should know that paralysis of the facial nerve is an illness that impedes the functioning of an organ; [i.e.,] corrupts (distorts) the form and shape of the face). Hebrew חולי כליי is not attested in the current dictionaries.

---

91 https://peshat.org/display/peshat_lemmas_00028145 (accessed December 2, 2021).

· b) Arab. المرض الآلي · Ibn al-Jazzār, *Zād al-musāfir wa-qūt al-ḥāḍir* · trans. Moses ibn Tibbon, *Sefer Ṣedat ha-Derakhim* v.1: ואומר כי הכבד יכאב ויחלה על ב׳ פנים אם מעצמו ואם לכאב זולתו על דרך השותפות. ויקרה לו כאב בעצמו בעבור שלשה סוגי החלאים כמו שיקרה לשאר האברים. אחד מהם מזג כמו שיקרה בו חום או קור או לחות או יובש נפרדים או מחוברים וישנו מזגו ויפסידוהו והשני יקרא חלי כליי כמו שיקרו בו סתומים ומורסות והג׳ יקרא פרוד החבור כמו שיקרה בו נגע וחמרמרות וחתוך ומה שדומה לזה (I say that the liver suffers from pain and illness in two ways, either on its own or through a pain that affects it through sympathetic affection [with another organ]. It suffers from pain on its own because of three kinds of illnesses as in the case of the other organs. The first [kind] is the temperament as when it is affected by heat, cold, moisture, or dryness, separately or in combination; they change and corrupt its temperament. The second [kind] is called a 'functional illness' as it happens in the case of obstructions and tumors. The third [kind] is called 'dissolution of continuity' as it happens in the case of an ulcer, abrasion, cut, and the like). Do'eg ha-Edomi transcribes the parallel Lat. term *officiales* as אופיציאלש and also renders the same Lat. term as משרתים (in *Sefer Ya'ir Netiv* v.5; see entry תַּחֲלוּא), while Sing. *morbus officialis* is rendered by him as חולי משרת (in *Sefer Ya'ir Netiv* v.11; see next entry).

• **חולי משרת · a functional illness [i.e., an illness that impedes the functioning of an organ]**: Lat. *morbus officialis* (Arab. مرض آلة) · Constantinus Africanus, *Viaticum peregrinantis* · trans. Do'eg ha-Edomi, *Sefer Ya'ir Netiv* v.11: וחולי הטחול דומה מאד לחולי הכבד וסובל בשלשה ענינים כמו שאמרנו שסובלים שאר איברי הגוף זהו בחבור רע בחולי משרת הוא אופיציאל בהפרדה רבה מהדבקים (A disease of the spleen is very similar to that of the liver; it can be affected by three things, just as we said concerning the other organs, [namely] by a bad temperament, by a functional illness [called] ʾWPYṢYʾL [i.e., Lat. *official*[*is*]] or by a dissolution of continuity). Hebr. חולי משרת is not attested in the current dictionaries. Lat. Plur. *officiales morbi* is translated by Do'eg as תחלואי המשרתים (*Sefer Ya'ir Netiv* v.5; see entry תַּחֲלוּא). Moses ibn Tibbon translates the parallel Arab. term مرض آلة as חלי הכליי (see also entry תַּחֲלוּא and entry above (for Arab. (المرض الآلي)).

• **חולי הנמלה · herpes**: Arab. نملة · Ibn Sīnā, *K. al-Qānūn fī al-ṭibb* · trans. Nathan ha-Me'ati, *Sefer ha-Qanun* ii, fol. 112[a]: עצא אלראעי ... עושין ממנו תחבשת למורסת הפלגמוני ואל האודם הנקרא חמרה בער׳ ולחולי הנמלה ויועיל מאד המכות והנגעים יסגר המכות הטריות (Common knotgrass: ... Its plaster is useful for treating inflamed tumors, erysipelas called *ḥumra* in Arab., herpes, tumors, and ulcers. It heals bleeding wounds). Hebr. חולי הנמלה is attested in BM 157 in a later attestation from Jacob ben Isaac Zahalon, *Ozar ha-Hayyim*. Zeraḥyah Ḥen translates Arab. نملة as הנמלה and Anonymous has נמלה.

• **חולי רעבון · ravenous hunger; bulimia**: Lat. *bulimus* · *Sefer ha-Refu'ot le-Ḥakham Qosṭa'ntin*, fol. 163[a]: בחולי רעבון: אמר פלאטיאריש: בוליסמוס הוא חולי רעבון שאוכל האדם

וכל היום רוצה לאכול יותר מבשיעור ואינו שבע (On ravenous hunger (bulimia): Says Platearius: BWLYSMWS [i.e., Lat. *bulimus*] is a ravenous hunger meaning that a person [suffering from it] eats and wants to eat the whole day more than is proper and yet he is not satiated). Hebr. חולי רעבון does not feature in the current dictionaries. For the synonymous בּוּלְמוֹס, see entry.

• **חולי השחורה** · **melancholy**: Lat. *melancolia* · Gerard de Solo, *Practica super nono Almansoris* · trans. Abraham Avigdor, *Ha-Ma'amar ha-Teshi'i le-Sefer ha-Mansuri le-Razi*, fol. 52[a]: וזה השם יאמר בכלל וביחוד. אמנם בכלל הנה היא תורה על מאניאה קאנינאה ובלשוננו שגעון כלבי ותורה גם כן על מאניאה דִימוֹנִיאַטִיקָאה ובלשוננו שגעון שדיי ועל חולי השחורה ובלשונם מאלאינקוניאה (This term [i.e., melancholy] is used in a general and specific sense. In general, it indicates M'NY'H Q'NYN'H [i.e., *mania canina* ('dog mania')], in Hebr. *shigga'on kalbi*. But it can also indicate M'NY'H DiYM-WoNiY'aṬiYQa'H [i.e., *mania demoniatica* ('demonic mania')], in Hebr. *shigga'on shedi*, and 'black bile illness' (melancholy), in Lat. M'L'YNQWNY'H [i.e., *melanchonia*]). In the sense of 'melancholy,' Hebr. חולי השחורה features in BCD 98 (NM 3:87) in a later attestation from Joseph Delmedigo's trans. of Hippocrates' *Aphorisms* III.14.

• **הנמלטים מחולי** → [מלט].

חֲלִישׁוּת • **חלישות התשמיש** · **impotence**: Arab. الضعف عن الباه · Ibn al-Jazzār, *Zād al-musāfir wa-qūt al-ḥādir* · trans. Abraham ben Isaac, *Sefer Ṣedah la-Oreḥim* VI.1: השער הראשון יזכיר מיעוט זרע התאוה והתשמיש וחלישותו (Ch. 1: On the lack of [sexual lust] and impotence). In the sense of 'impotence,' Hebr. חלישות התשמיש is non-attested loan translation of Arab. الضعف عن الباه. Moses ibn Tibbon translates Arab. الضعف عن الباه as חולשת המשגל (see entry חֻלְשָׁה).

[חלל] • *Hitpolel* **הִתְחוֹלֵל** · **to be dissolved**: Arab. تحلّل · Maimonides, *Maqāla fī al-rabw* (*On Asthma*) · trans. Anonymous, *Sefer ha-Qaṣeret* II.1 (cf. BMA 2:393, ll. 6–8): וסבת זה מבוארת והוא שהמזונות כשיתאכלו באברים והיתה יתרות העיכול השלישי בהן מעוטה לא מודבקת ולא עבה תתחולל חלילות נסתר ותצא באד והזיעה (The reason for this is clear—namely, that when foods are digested in the organs and when the superfluity from the third digestion is minimal and neither sticky nor thick, they are dissolved in a hidden way and leave [the body] through evaporation and perspiration). In the sense of 'to be dissolved,' Hebr. *Hitpolel* הִתְחוֹלֵל is not attested in the current dictionaries. The verb חָלַל features in the *Hitpa'el* conj. in Rabb. literature in the sense of 'to be loose [of bowels];' cf. JD 470. Samuel Benveniste translates Arab. تحلّل as *Nif'al* נִמְחָה (see entry מָחָה) and Joshua Shatibi has נמס.

[חלף] • *Part. Hitpa'el* **מִתְחַלֵּף** • **הכח המתחלף** → **כֹּחַ**.

• *Part. Hif'il* **מַחֲלִיף** • **הכח המחליף** → **כֹּחַ**.

[חלק] • *Part. Hif'il* **מַחֲלִיק** • **דברים מחליקים** → **דָּבָר**.

חָלָק · **mild**: Lat. *lenis* (Arab. أقلّ حدّة) · Constantinus Africanus, *Viaticum peregrinantis* · trans. Do'eg ha-Edomi, *Sefer Ya'ir Netiv* IV.17: ואם הוא מהלבנה יוסר הצמאון והדפק

מעורב[92] והחולי ארוך והכאב חלק אך יש לו מעמס וכובד רב והכאב והמעמס לא יצאו מהמקום (If the colic is caused by phlegm, [the patient] will not be thirsty anymore, the pulse will be slow,[93] the illness will last for a long time, and the pain will be mild. But he will suffer from [a sensation of] great heaviness, while the pain and heaviness will stay in one and the same spot). Hebr. חָלָק features in BM 1596–1597 in the sense of 'bald; smooth; slippery' and in BCD 101 (NM 1:149) as 'soft' (for Arab. لِيِّن) in an attestation from Zeraḥyah Ḥen, *Sefer ha-Peraqim* (*Pirqei Moshe*) I.9 (cf. BMMZ 16, l. 23). Moses ibn Tibbon translates Arab. أقلّ حدّة as חדודו קטן יותר.

חֵלֶק • *Plur.* **חלקים • החלקים האחרונים** · **extremities**: Lat. *extremitates* (Arab. أطراف) · Constantinus Africanus, *Viaticum peregrinantis* · trans. Do'eg ha-Edomi, *Sefer Ya'ir Netiv* IV.16: ואותו שהוא מהליחות הקרות אין לו נפח ולא התפשטות ולא צמאון וקדחת אך המקרים הנכנסים אחרי כן הם קרירות החלקים האחרונים מהגוף והמצוקות והתעורות ושאינו יכול לעמוד במקום אחד ([Ileus] caused by cold humors does not [in the beginning] come with inflation (inflammation), stretching, thirst, or fever; but the subsequent symptoms are: cold of the extremities of the body, distress, sleeplessness, and disturbance (restlessness)). Moses ibn Tibbon translates the parallel Arab. term أطراف as קצוות.

• **החלקים השפלים מהבטן** · **the abdominal wall**: Lat. *inferiores ventris* (Arab. مرّاق البطن) · Constantinus Africanus, *Viaticum peregrinantis* · trans. Do'eg ha-Edomi, *Sefer Ya'ir Netiv* IV.17: ואם הוא מן הצמח נתבונן כי במגע כי יתראה בחוץ בחלקים השפלים מהבטן (When [the colic] originates from an ulcer, it can be identified by [the sense of] touch, for the ulcer appears in the abdominal wall). Hebr. החלקים השפלים מהבטן is not attested in the current dictionaries. Moses ibn Tibbon translates the parallel Arab. term مرّاق البطن as בשר הבטן (see entry בָּשָׂר).

חֶלְקָה · **lightness**: Lat. *levitas* (Arab. خفّة) · Constantinus Africanus, *Viaticum peregrinantis* · trans. Do'eg ha-Edomi, *Sefer Ya'ir Netiv* V.10: ואם יתראה ביום קריטיק כמו ז' או יא' או יד' ואחרי הראותו יהיה אות הבשול וחלקת החולי אז הוא טוב ומבשר הבריאות (But if [jaundice] becomes visible on a critical day—such as the seventh or eleventh or fourteenth—and after its appearance [one can observe that the illness is cocted and light; it is a good sign indicating recovery). Hebr. חֶלְקָה features in BM 1601–1602 in the sense of 'smoothness' only. Moses ibn Tibbon translates the parallel Arab. term خفّة as קלות.

חֲלָקוּת (also: חַלְקוּת) · I. **diarrhea**: Arab. انطلاق · Maimonides, *Maqāla fī al-rabw* (*On Asthma*) · trans. Joshua Shatibi, *Ma'amar 'al ha-Qaṣeret* XIII.5 (cf. BMA 2:370, ll. 17–18): ואם הקדמת בקביצה ועצירת זה החלקות וחזר הטבע להרגלו בסמים (And if you hasten to use astringents and [thus stop] this diarrhea, [your] nature returns to its nor-

92 מעורב: *tardus* L.

93 'slow': Trans. after L.

mal condition by means of medication). Hebr. חַלְקוּת/חֲלָקוּת features, a.o., in BCD 101 (NM 1:150) in the sense of 'softness; softening effect' (for Arab. لين and تليين) in attestations from Zeraḥyah Ḥen, *Sefer ha-Peraqim* (*Pirqei Moshe*) I.11; IX.72 (cf. BMMZ 17, l. 9; 109, l. 12; BMMG nos. 4689, 4693). Samuel Benveniste translates Arab. انطلاق as שִׁלּוּחַ (see entry) and Anonymous has שלשול.

חֻלְשָׁה • חולשת המשגל · **impotence**: Arab. الضعف عن الباه · Ibn al-Jazzār, *Zād al-musāfir wa-qūt al-ḥādir* · trans. Moses ibn Tibbon, *Sefer Ṣedat ha-Derakhim* VI.1: השער הראשון מן המאמר הששי במיעוט המשגל והחולשה ממנו (The first chapter of the sixth treatise: On the lack of sexual intercourse and impotence). In the sense of 'impotence,' Hebr. חולשת המשגל is a non-attested loan translation of Arab. الضعف عن الباه. Abraham ben Isaac translates the Arab. term as חלישות התשמיש (see entry חֲלִישׁוּת).

חֹם • החום העקרי · **the innate heat**: Arab. الحرارة الغريزية · Ibn Sīnā, *K. al-Qānūn fī al-ṭibb* · trans. Nathan ha-Me'ati, *Sefer ha-Qanun* II, fol. 69b: בסר ובלח ... ינפח ויותר כשותין אחריו המים וכשהוא מתוק יוליד רעמים יותר ויוליד האטמים בקרבים ותבשיל הבסר וישקיט להבה עם שמירתו החום העקרי (BSR and BLḤ [i.e., Arab. *busr* and *balaḥ*, 'unripe dates']: ... They are flatulent, particularly when water is taken after their consumption. Sweet dates especially produce intestinal rumblings; they also produce obstructions in the intestines. The decoction of unripe dates alleviates burning and preserves the innate heat). Hebr. החום העקרי is not attested in the current dictionaries. Zeraḥyah Ḥen translates Arab. الحرارة الغريزية as החמימות היסודי (see entry חֲמִימוּת). Synonyms featuring in medieval medical literature are: החום הטבעי (in Moses ibn Tibbon, *Perush Aphorismi shel Apuqraṭ* (*Pirqei Abuqraṭ*) I.14 (41); cf. BCD 102 (NM 3:91); BMCH 1:329, l. 24), חום יסודי (in Hillel ben Samuel, *Aphorismi* I.14; cf. BCD 103 (NM 3:91)), and החמימות העיקרי (see also entry חֲמִימוּת). Anonymous has החום הטבעי, just like Ibn Tibbon in his *Perush Aphorismi shel Apuqraṭ* (*Pirqei Abuqraṭ*).

חֶמְאָה • חמאת בקר · **buttermilk**: Arab. مخيض اللبن · Ibn Sīnā, *K. al-Qānūn fī al-ṭibb* · trans. Nathan ha-Me'ati, *Sefer ha-Qanun* II, fol. 68b: בלאדר ... הוא מכלל הארסים וישרוף התערובים והתריאק שלו חמאת בקר ושמן אגוזים וזה שמשבר כחו (Marking nut: ... It is one of the poisons and burns humors. Buttermilk is its antidote. The oil of walnut breaks its toxic strength). Hebr. חמאת בקר is not attested in the current dictionaries. חֶמְאָה on its own features in BM 1607–1608 in the sense of 'curdled milk; butter.' In his *Sefer ha-Peraqim* (*Pirqei Moshe*) XXIII.107, Nathan translates Arab. مخيض as החלב המשוכשך (cf. BCD 94 (NM 2:63); BMMN 232, l. 18; BMMG no. 4719). Zeraḥyah Ḥen translates Arab. مخيض اللبن as חמאת בקר as well and Anonymous has a combination of both terms: חלב בקר מסוכסך.

חַמָּה · **summer**: Arab. صيف · Maimonides, *Maqāla fī al-rabw* (*On Asthma*) · trans. Samuel Benveniste, *Ma'amar 'al ha-Qaṣeret* VII.2 (cf. BMA 2:266, ll. 8–9): ואם הוצרך לזה מפני צאתו לדרך ימזגהו במים קרים בחמה ובחמים בימות הגשמים (But if it is necessary to mix it [i.e., the remedy] because one has to go on a journey, one should mix it with cold water in the summer and with warm water in the winter). Hebr. חַמָּה stands for ימות החמה ('the sunny season'), which features in BM 1612–1613 in attestations from Rabb. literature. Joshua Shatibi and Anonymous both render Arab. صيف with the Hebr. standard term קיץ. For 'the rainy season' (ימות הגשמים) (i.e., autumn and winter), see entry גֶּשֶׁם.

חִמּוּץ • חמוץ האתרוג · the acidic inner part of the lemon: Arab. حمّاض الأترجّ · Ibn Zuhr, *K. al-Aghdhiya* · trans. Nathan ha-Me'ati, *Sefer ha-Mezonot*, fol. 16ª: ואמנם חמוץ האתרוג קר רטוב (The acidic inner part of the lemon is cold and moist). Hebr. חמוץ האתרוג features also in Nathan's *Sefer ha-Peraqim* (*Pirqei Moshe*) XXII.52 (cf. BMMN 215, l. 21), while Zeraḥyah Ḥen has חימוץ האתרוגים there (cf. BCD 103 (NM 1:150); BMMZ 213, l. 10) (cf. also BMMG no. 1178).

חֲמִימוּת · fever: Arab. حمّى · Maimonides, *Maqāla fī al-rabw* (*On Asthma*) · trans. Anonymous, *Sefer ha-Qaṣeret* XII.1 (cf. BMA 2:429, ll. 29–30): ואם היתה החמימות חלושה אין רוע בתוספת הצמוקים המוסרים הגרעינים או התאנים במורתחין (When the fever is mild, there is no objection to adding seedless raisins or figs to the decoctions). Hebr. חֲמִימוּת only features in the current dictionaries in the sense of 'heat' (cf. BM 1620–1621; EM 553). Samuel Benveniste and Anonymous both translate Arab. حمّى as קדחת.

• החמימות היסודי · the innate heat: Arab. الحرارة الغريزيّة · Ibn Sīnā, *K. al-Qānūn fī al-ṭibb* · trans. Zeraḥyah Ḥen, *Sefer ha-Qanun* II, fol. 183ᵇ: בֹסֶר ובלח ... מנפח וכל שכן כשישתה מיד מים ובהיותו מתוק יחדש קולות יותר ויחדשו הסתימות בקרבים ובשול הבוסר ישכך הלהבת עם שמירת החמימות היסודי (BoSeR and BLḤ [i.e., Arab. *busr* and *balaḥ*, 'unripe dates']: ... They are flatulent, particularly when water is taken immediately [after their consumption]. Sweet dates especially produce intestinal rumblings; they also produce obstructions in the intestines. A decoction of sweet dates alleviates burning but preserves the innate heat). Hebr. החמימות היסודי is not attested in the current dictionaries. Nathan ha-Me'ati translates Arab. الحرارة الغريزيّة as החום העקרי (cf. entry חֹם). For synonyms in medieval Hebr. medical literature, see ibid.

• החמימות העיקרי · the innate heat: Arab. الحرارة الغريزيّة · Maimonides, *Maqāla fī al-rabw* (*On Asthma*) · trans. Samuel Benveniste, *Ma'amar 'al ha-Qaṣeret* VII.1 (cf. BMA 2:265, ll. 9–10): ומכלל תועלותיו שהוא מטיב העכול ויפרה ויצמיח החמימות העיקרי ויוציא הנוספות בזיעה ובשתן ואין יתרון לספור תועלות דבר נמנע להנות בו (One of its benefits [i.e., of wine], is that it improves digestion, increases the innate heat, and expels the superfluities by means of perspiration and urine. But it is useless to enumerate the benefits of something the consumption of which is impossible [for my Master]). Hebr. החמימות העיקרי is not attested in the current dictionaries. For synonyms, cf. entry חֹם.

[חמם] • *Nitpa'el* נִתְחַמֵּם · to suffer from fever: Arab. حمّ · Maimonides, *Maqāla fī al-rabw* (*On Asthma*) · trans. Anonymous, *Sefer ha-Qaṣeret* XIII.33 (cf. BMA 2:447, ll. 12–13): וכבר ראיתי במערב בחור יתר הכח נראה ההתמלאות נתחמם חמימות תמידית של מרה אדומה (In the Maghreb, I [once] saw a young man who was very strong but clearly suffering from overfilling and became afflicted with continuous choleric fever). Hebr. *Nitpaʿel* נִתְחַמֵּם does not feature in this sense in the current dictionaries. Samuel Benveniste translates Arab. حمّ as נקדח and Joshua Shatibi has הוקדח.

חֲמַרְמְרוּת · **dysentery**: Arab. سحوج (cf. SN 1:111 (265), s.v. إسهال وهو سحج: 'dysenteria rheumatica') · Ibn al-Jazzār, *Zād al-musāfir wa-qūt al-ḥāḍir* · trans. Moses ibn Tibbon, *Sefer Ṣedat ha-Derakhim* IV.15: תאר אבק חברתיו לנגע ולחמרמרות המתילד במעים מליחה לבנה מלוחה (Recipe of a powder that I composed for ulcers and dysentery originating in the intestines from salty phlegm). Hebr. חֲמַרְמְרוּת features in BCD 104 (NM 1:56) in the sense of 'abrasion.' In addition to חֲמַרְמְרוּת, Moses ibn Tibbon renders Arab. س(و)ج as עִצּוּר (see entry). Do'eg ha-Edomi transcribes the parallel Lat. term *dysenteria* as דישנטיריאה.

חֲנִיקָה • **חניקת הרחם** · **hysterical suffocation**: Arab. احتناق الرحم · al-Rāzī, *K. al-Manṣūrī fī al-ṭibb* · trans. Shem Tov ben Isaac, *Sefer Almansur*, fol. 4[a]: שער בחניקת הרחם (Chapter on hysterical suffocation). In the sense of 'hysterical suffocation,' Hebr. חניקת הרחם features in BCD 104 (NM 3:94) in a later attestation from Zeraḥyah Ḥen, *Perush Aphorismi shel Apuqraṭ* (*Pirqei Abuqraṭ*) V.35 (255) (cf. BMCH 1:479, l. 14), and also in his *Sefer ha-Peraqim* (*Pirqei Moshe*) XVI.16, 18 (cf. BMMZ 165, l. 23; 166, l. 3; BMMG no. 1601). Abraham Avigdor translates the parallel Lat. term *suffocatio matricis* as החנק הרחם (as does Moses ibn Tibbon in his *Perush Aphorismi shel Apuqraṭ* (*Pirqei Abuqraṭ*) V.35 (255); cf. BCD 104 (NM 3:94); BMCH 1:383, l. 9). See also מְצוֹק and מצוקת האם (entry מְצוּקָה), featuring in Do'eg ha-Edomi, *Sefer Ya'ir Netiv* VI.11; and חֲנִיקוּת, featuring in Abraham ben Isaac, *Sefer Ṣedah la-Oreḥim* VI.11 (see next entry).

חֲנִיקוּת · **hysterical suffocation**: Arab. احتناق الرحم · Ibn al-Jazzār, *Zād al-musāfir wa-qūt al-ḥāḍir* · trans. Abraham ben Isaac, *Sefer Ṣedah la-Oreḥim* VI.11: השער אחד עשר יזכיר חניקות הנק׳ בלשון יון פלגמוני הוא חניקות הנולד ברחם (Ch. 11: On hysterical suffocation called in Greek PLGMWNY [i.e., φλεγμονή, 'inflamed tumour; boil']; i.e, a suffocation originating in the womb). Hebr. חֲנִיקוּת is not attested in the current dictionaries. Moses ibn Tibbon translates Arab. احتناق الرحم as החנק הרחם (as in his *Perush Aphorismi shel Apuqraṭ* (*Pirqei Abuqraṭ*) V.35 (255); cf. BCD 104 (NM 3:94); BMCH 1:383, l. 9) and Do'eg ha-Edomi translates the parallel Lat. term *suffocatio matricis* as מצוקת האם (see entry מְצוּקָה). See also חניקת הרחם (previous entry).

חֶנֶק • *Plur.* **חנקים** · **quinsy**: Arab. خوانيق (cf. UW 654, s.v. συνάγχη: 'Halsentzündung; Diphtherie') · al-Rāzī, *K. al-Manṣūrī fī al-ṭibb* · trans. Shem Tov ben Isaac, *Sefer Almansur*, fol. 3[b]: נ"א בחנקים ([Chapter] 51: On quinsy). Hebr. *Plur.* חנקים is not attested in the current dictionaries. Hebr. *Sing.* חֶנֶק (for Arab. خوانيق and ذبحة ('angina')) features in BCD 104–105 in attestations from Zeraḥyah Ḥen, *Sefer ha-Peraqim* (*Pirqei Moshe*) XXV.11 (cf. NM 1:150–151, corr. 4:229; BMMZ 245, l. 1; BMMG no. 1599) and his *Perush Aphorismi shel Apuqraṭ* (*Pirqei Abuqraṭ*) I.12 (39) (cf. NM 3:94–95; BMCH 1:428, l. 12). Abraham Avigdor also translates the parallel Lat. term *squinantia* as חֶנֶק. A var. featuring in *Sefer Almansur*, fol. 122[b], is חֲנִיקָה; cf. also Shem Tov's use of the same term in his *Sefer ha-Shimmush* XXX.2.95 (cf. BCD 104 (NM 1:194)).

[חסר] • *Hif'il* **הֶחְסִיר** · **to restrain, suppress, subdue, check**: Arab. قمع · Ibn Sīnā, *K. al-Qānūn fī al-ṭibb* · trans. Nathan ha-Me'ati, *Sefer ha-Qanun* II, fol. 122[b]: ... רמאן החמוץ יחסיר המרה האדומה וימנע שפיכת היתרונים אל הקרבים (Pomegranate: ... The sour [pomegranate] checks yellow bile and prevents the flow of superfluous matters towards the intestines). Hebr. [חסר], *Hif'il* הֶחְסִיר, does not feature in this sense in the current dictionaries. Zeraḥyah Ḥen translates Arab. قمع as [סור], *Hif'il* הֵסִיר, and Anonymous has [שקע], *Hif'il* הִשְׁקִיעַ. Shem Tov ben Isaac translates Arab. قمع as [רתע], *Hif'il* הִרְתִּיעַ, in his *Sefer ha-Shimmush* XXVII (cf. BCD 267 (NM 4:197–198)).

חָסֵר · **incompetent**: Arab. مقصّر · Maimonides, *Maqāla fī al-rabw* (*On Asthma*) · trans. Samuel Benveniste, *Ma'amar 'al ha-Qaṣeret* XIII.22 (cf. BMA 2:305, l. 16): אך החסרים לא ימנעו מרפאת ולא יביטו המקומות האלה כלם (On the other hand, the incompetent [physician] never stops rendering medical treatment, although he is ignorant of all these subjects). Hebr. חָסֵר is attested in medieval philosophical literature, a.o., in the sense of 'deficient; lacking in something' (cf. PESHAT[94]). Joshua Shatibi and Anonymous both render Arab. مقصّر as מְקַצֵּר (see entry [קצר]). A synonymous term employed by Samuel Benveniste in the same paragraph is שאינו שלם (cf. also entry [קצר]).

חֵפֶץ · **appetite**: Lat. *appetitus* (Arab. شهوة الطعام) · Constantinus Africanus, *Viaticum peregrinantis* · trans. Do'eg ha-Edomi, *Sefer Ya'ir Netiv* IV.10: ואם תהיינה הליחות קרות החפץ יהיה בפחות צמא (If the humors [in the stomach] are cold, there will be appetite with less thirst). Hebr. חֵפֶץ does not feature in this sense in the current dictionaries. In addition to חֵפֶץ, Do'eg renders Lat. *appetitus* as חפץ המאכל (see entry below). Moses ibn Tibbon translates the parallel Arab. term شهوة الطعام as תאות מאכל.

• **החפץ הכלביי** · **canine appetite**: Lat. *appetitus caninus* (Arab. الشهوة الكلبية) · Constantinus Africanus, *Viaticum peregrinantis* · trans. Do'eg ha-Edomi, *Sefer Ya'ir Netiv* V.17: יש אל הכליות חולי הנקרא דיאביטיש מאפיסת הכח המחזיק באשר הסובל יצמא מאד ולא ישבע מים וישתין המים בצבע ובכמות אשר שתה אותם כמו שנראה בחפץ הכלביי (The kidneys may be affected by an illness called DY'BYṬYŠ [i.e., diabetes] caused by a weakness of the retentive faculty during which the patient suffers from an extreme thirst that cannot be quenched by water and he passes the water [that he drank] in the same color and amount as he drank it. We see the same in the case of canine appetite). Hebr. החפץ הכלביי is not attested in the current dictionaries. A synonymous התאוה הכלבית is used by Moses ibn Tibbon for the parallel Arab. term الشهوة الكلبية and features also in his *Perush Aphorismi shel Apuqraṭ* (*Pirqei Abuqraṭ*) II.21 (73) (cf. BCD 289 (NM 3:238); BMCH 1:339, l. 18).

---

94 https://peshat.org/display/peshat_lemmas_00001915 (accessed March 15, 2022).

• חפץ המאכל · **appetite**: Lat. *appetitus* (Arab. شهوة) · Constantinus Africanus, *Viaticum peregrinantis* · trans. Do'eg ha-Edomi, *Sefer Ya'ir Netiv* VI.9: וכבר אמר גליאנוס בספר אבדימיאה והזכיר המעשה שעשה באשה אחת שאפסה נדתה ח' חדשים והיתה חלושה ונתמעט בשר גופה גם אפסה תאותה (Galen stated in his [*Commentary on Hippocrates'*] *Epidemics* and mentioned his treatment of a woman whose menstrual blood had been retained for eight months, so that she was in a state of emaciation and had no appetite anymore). Hebr. חפץ המאכל features in BCD 106 (NM 4:71–72) in a later attestation from Jacob ibn Tibbon, *Hanhagat ha-Beri'ut le-Abu 'Ali ben Zuhr* (cf. RSA 149). In addition to חפץ המאכל, Do'eg renders Lat. *appetitus* as חֵפֶץ (see entry above). Moses ibn Tibbon and Abraham ben Isaac both translate Arab. شهوة as תאוה.

• הגרת השתן מבלי חפץ → הַגָּרָה.

• כח החפץ → כֹּחַ.

• התנועה אשר מבלי חפץ → תְּנוּעָה.

חָפֵץ • הכח החפץ → כֹּחַ.

חָצָץ · **intestinal stones**: Arab. حصاة · Ibn Zuhr, *K. al-Aghdhiya* · trans. Nathan ha-Me'ati, *Sefer ha-Mezonot*, fol. 4b: ואמנם היענה חמה ויבשה בהפלגה ... ובקלפת קורקבנה יש סגלה המועילה לעלולי האצטומ' ויעשה בפתות החצץ ([The flesh of] ostriches is extremely hot and dry ... the membrane of their crop has the specific property of being beneficial for those who have a stomach illness; it is also used for pulverizing intestinal stones). In the sense of 'intestinal stones,' Hebr. חָצָץ features in BM 1710 in attestations, a.o., from Nathan's *Sefer ha-Peraqim* (*Pirqei Moshe*) VI.92 (cf. BMMN 78, l. 15; BMMG no. 989).

חֹק • בחוק · **with reference to; relating to; according to**: Arab. بحقّ · Maimonides, *Maqāla fī al-rabw* (*On Asthma*) · trans. Samuel Benveniste, *Ma'amar 'al ha-Qaṣeret* V.1 (cf. BMA 2:259, ll. 1–2): ואחרי אמרנו באיכותו ראוי לדבר בכמותו והוא משתנה בחוק האישים מבני האדם (Since I have spoken about the quality [of the food to be ingested], I should also speak about its quantity, which varies according to the [different] individual characteristics of people). In the sense of 'with reference to; relating to; according to,' Hebr. בחוק is a semantic borrowing from Arab. بحقّ, which is attested in medieval Hebr. philosophical literature; cf. BM 1717; EP 54; KTP 1:323. Joshua Shatibi and Anonymous both render Arab. بحقّ as בחוק as well.

חֲרָדָה • חרדת המחשבה · **mental confusion; delirium**: Lat. *alienatio mentis* (Arab. اختلاط الذهن) · Constantinus Africanus, *Viaticum peregrinantis* · trans. Do'eg ha-Edomi, *Sefer Ya'ir Netiv* IV.9: אם הראש יהיה חלוש הוא ירגיש כובד וכאב ותעורה וחרדת המחשבה (When someone's head is weak, it will feel heavy and painful; he will suffer from sleeplessness and mental confusion (delirium)). Hebr. חרדת המחשבה features in NM 5:84 in an attestation from *Sefer Ya'ir Netiv* I.16.1 (cf. IJZ 1–2:617) as a trans. of Lat. *stupor mentis* ('torpor; lethargy'). Moses ibn Tibbon translates the parallel Arab. term اختلاط الذهن as ערבוב שכל (cf. also BCD 213–214 for the use of the same term (for Arab. تخليط) in his *Sefer Ṣedat ha-Derakhim* VII.13.2 (cf. NM 1:65; IJZ 7:145, l. 12) and also (for Arab. اختلاط عقل) in Nathan ha-Me'ati, *Sefer ha-Peraqim* (*Pirqei Moshe*) XXIII.58 (cf. NM 2:73–74; BMMN 226, ll. 3–4; BMMG no. 1529)).

חַרְדַל • צף החרדל → צף.

חַרְחוּר · **marasmus**: Arab. ذبول · Ibn Zuhr, *K. al-Aghdhiya* · trans. Nathan ha-Me'ati, *Sefer ha-Mezonot*, fol. 8[b]: זכרון אלהר יבש סגולתו שאם ייגע האדם הרבה יחדש שדפון וחרחור (Cats are dry; their special property is that if a person touches them a lot, it causes marasmus). Hebr. חַרְחוּר features in the current dictionaries with attestations from the Bible in the sense of 'burning [of a fever]' (cf. BDB 359; CD 3:316) and from medieval medical literature in attestations from the *Sefer ha-Qanun* and Abraham Portaleone, *Shiltei ha-Gibborim* as 'the name of an illness' (cf. BM 1756–1757). Nathan renders Arab. ذبول as צמוק in his *Sefer ha-Peraqim* (*Pirqei Moshe*) XXII.44 (cf. BMMN 215, l. 2: קרבת החתולים ועורותיהם מוריש הצמוק והשדפון (The proximity to cats causes marasmus and phthisis); BMMG no. 1961).

חֲרִיפוּת • חֲרִיפוּת השתן · **(lit., 'sharpness of the urine'); a burning sensation during urination (dysuria)**: Arab. حرقة البول (SN 1:112 (266)) · al-Rāzī, *K. al-Manṣūrī fī al-ṭibb* · trans. Shem Tov ben Isaac, *Sefer Almansur*, fol. 133[b]: שער בחריפות השתן: כשימצא החולה חריפות בעת ההשתנה ראוי להזירו מן המליח והחמוץ והחריף (Chapter on sharpness of the urine (a burning sensation during urination): When the patient has the feeling that his urination is sharp (burning), one should not give him anything salty, sour, or …). Hebrew חריפות השתן does not feature in the current dictionaries. Abraham Avigdor translates the parallel Lat. term *ardor urine* as שרפת השתן (see entry שְׂרֵפָה).

חֲרִיקָה • חריקת שנים · **teeth grinding**: Arab. تصرير الأسنان · Ibn al-Jazzār, *Zād al-musāfir wa-qūt al-ḥādir* · trans. Moses ibn Tibbon, *Sefer Ṣedat ha-Derakhim* IV.18: ומהם מה שיתילד במעים השפלים סמוך לפי הטבעת ורוב מה שיתילדו בזה תולעים קטנים ואם יניחו אותם מה שספרנו ובארנו מבטול תאות המאכל והשתוק[95] וערבוב עד שיגדלו יקרה לחולה מן הרעה השכל והקדחות ופעמים יחדש חריקת השנים בשינה (Some of them [i.e., intestinal worms] originate in the lower intestines close to the anus; they are mostly small and if one leaves them alone until they grow, the patient will suffer from afflictions that are worse than [those in the case of other worms], which I mentioned and explained. [He will suffer] from lack of appetite, apoplexy,[96] mental confusion, fevers, and sometimes from teeth grinding during sleep). Hebr. חריקת שנים only features in the current dictionaries as a modern term (cf. EM 587). Do'eg ha-Edomi translates the parallel Lat. term *stridor dentium* as יחרוק שניו.

חַשְׁמַל • כעין החשמל · **purple**: Arab. فرفري · Ibn Sīnā, *K. al-Qānūn fī al-ṭibb* · trans. Nathan ha-Me'ati, *Sefer ha-Qanun* II, fol. 68[a]: באדורד קרדאלה המהות הוא שוכה אלביצה ידמה אל החצד אלא שהוא יותר חזק הלובן וקוציו יותר ארוכים וידמו עליו לבעלי החמאמה אלא שהם

95 והשתוק: om. a.
96 'apoplexy': om. a.

יותר רקיקים ויותר לבנים ויש שיגיעו שוקיו כמו שני אמות וציציו כעין החשמל ובערבי פרפירי (*Bādhāward* ('soldier thistle'); [Rom.] QRD'LH: What is it (*ha-mahut*)?:[97] It is the white thistle; it resembles tribulus (caltrop) but is whiter in color and has larger spikes. The leaves resemble those of amomum but are thinner and whiter. The stem can be as long as two cubits. The flowers are purple, in Arab. PRPYRY [i.e., *firfirī*]). Hebr. כעין החשמל features in Ez 1:4, 27. The meaning of חַשְׁמַל is uncertain, cf. BDB 365: 'evidently some shining substance.' Ibn Janāḥ interprets the term as كلون نار زرقاء باضمار النار 'like the color of bluish fire, while the fire cannot be seen'.[98] Zeraḥyah Ḥen renders Arab. فرفري as כמו הפּוֹרְפּוֹרָא; cf. also Anonymous: פרפורי.

השתקות · **apoplexy**: Arab. سكتة (Gr. ἀποπληξία; cf. UW 1:152) · Ibn Sīnā, *K. al-Qānūn fī al-ṭibb*, Hebr. trans. Nathan ha-Me'ati, *Sefer ha-Qanun* II, fol. 116ª: פטר ... יוליד בטול ההרגש הנקר' כדר בערבי וההשתקות[99] ובער' סכתה (Mushrooms: ... They cause numbness, called *khadar* in Arab., and apoplexy, i.e., *sakta* in Arab.). Hebr. השתקות is not attested in the current dictionaries. In his *Sefer ha-Peraqim* (*Pirqei Moshe*), Nathan translates Arab. سكتة throughout as שִׁתּוּק (cf. BMMG no. 2426), a term that is also used by Zeraḥyah Ḥen in the *Sefer ha-Qanun*. See also BCD 286 for additional attestations from Zeraḥyah's *Sefer ha-Peraqim* (*Pirqei Moshe*) VI.1 (NM 1:193; cf. BMMZ 59, l. 21; BMMG no. 2426) and Moses ibn Tibbon, *Sefer Ṣedat ha-Derakhim* I.22.1 (cf. NM 4:14; IJZ 1–2:474).

חִתּוּךְ · **cramps; colic**: Arab. مغص (Gr. στρόφος; cf. UW 644) · Maimonides, *Maqāla fī al-rabw* (*On Asthma*) · trans. Anonymous, *Sefer ha-Qaṣeret* XII.9 (cf. BMA 2:435, ll. 18–19): ואם תמצא לרפואה חיתוך ומכאוב (If, as a result of [taking] the medicine, one experiences pain and cramps [in the stomach] ...). Hebr. חִתּוּךְ does not feature in this sense in the current dictionaries. Samuel Benveniste translates Arab. مغص as חִיל (see entry) and Joshua Shatibi has עֲקִיצָה (cf. also BCD 212–213 (NM 3:182) for the same Hebr. term in Zeraḥyah Ḥen, *Perush Aphorismi shel Apuqraṭ* (*Pirqei Abuqraṭ*) V.41 (261) (cf. BMCH 1:480, l. 18)). For other synonyms, see חבלי הבטן (entry חֵבֶל), מַשְׁבֵּר, and עקיצת המעים (entry עֲקִיצָה).

[חתל] *Pi'el* חִתֵּל · **to foment**: Arab. كمّد · Ibn Sīnā, *K. al-Qānūn fī al-ṭibb* · trans. Nathan ha-Me'ati, *Sefer ha-Qanun* II, fol. 123ᵇ: שיח ... יחתלו במימיו האפר הנקר' רמד בערבי ויתיכנו (Wormwood: ... If you foment [the eyes] with its water, it relieves conjunctivitis, called *ramad* in Arab.). Hebr. *Pi'el* חִתֵּל features in BM 1824–1825 in the sense of 'to swaddle' and in the *Pu'al* conj. in BCD 109 (NM 4:73–74) in the sense of 'to be applied as a poultice' (for Arab. ضمّد). Zeraḥyah Ḥen translates Arab. كمّد as משח and Anonymous has הניח הנחה חמה.

---

97 See entry מָהוּת.

98 Ibn Janāḥ, *K. al-Uṣūl*, 258.

99 The term השתקות also features on fol. 78ª: והשתקות הנקרא סכתה as part of the entry דבודאר (DBWD'R [i.e., deodar or Himalayan cedar]).

ט

טַבַּעַת • בְּלִיטָה → בליטת פי הטבעת.
• יְצִיאָה → יציאת פי הטבעת.
• פֶּה → פי הטבעת.

[טהר] • *Piʿel* טִהֵר · **to melt, liquefy, dissolve**: Lat. *liquefacio* (Arab. أذاب) · Constantinus Africanus, *Viaticum peregrinantis* · trans. Do'eg ha-Edomi, *Sefer Ya'ir Netiv* V.15: טרוסיקש אלה מן גיאלינוס מטהרים הדם המקובץ משברון מקורות הכבד והכליות והוא נזול ברוח המקוה (These pastilles compounded by Galen dissolve the blood that has coagulated because of a burst vessel in the liver or kidneys and that has flown into the hollow part of the urinary bladder). Hebr. *Piʿel* טִהֵר does not feature in this sense in the current dictionaries. Moses ibn Tibbon translates Arab. أذاب as [נתך], *Hifʿil* הִתִּיךְ. Do'eg ha-Edomi also uses *Piʿel* טִהֵר to render Lat. *do catarticum* ('to administer a cathartic') in *Sefer Ya'ir Netiv* II.18.5 (cf. NM 5:87; IJZ 1–2:647).

טָחוֹר • *Plur.* טחורים · **polyps (growth or ulcer in the nose)**: Lat. *polipus* (Arab. نواسير) · Gerard de Solo, *Practica super nono Almansoris* · trans. Abraham Avigdor, *Ha-Ma'amar ha-Teshiʿi le-Sefer ha-Mansuri le-Razi*, fol. 89[a]: שער בטחורים המתחדשים בחוטם (Chapter on nasal polyps). In the sense of 'polyps,' Hebr. *Plur.* טחורים features in BCD 112 (NM 2:12 (corr. below)) in an earlier attestation from Shem Tov ben Isaac's glossary to the *Sefer Almansur* (cf. BMZ 70 (Qof 9)). The term is the result of mistakenly reading Arab. نواسير (i.e., polyps) as بواسير (i.e., hemorrhoids).

טִיּוּל · **exercise**: Arab. رياضة · Maimonides, *Maqāla fī al-rabw* (*On Asthma*) · trans. Joshua Shatibi, *Ma'amar ʿal ha-Qaṣeret* V.5 (cf. BMA 2:336, ll. 14–16): וזה שהאדם לא יחלה אם ישגיח בשלא יהיה לו רוע העכול כלל ולא יתנועע אחר האכילה תנועה חזקה. וזה כי כמו שהטיול קודם המאכל יותר מועיל מכל הדברים בהתמדת הבריאות כן התנועה אחר המאכל יותר מזיק מכל הדברים (For a person does not fall ill if he takes care to ensure that bad digestion never befalls him and that he does not move vigorously after eating. This is because—just as exercise before a meal is more beneficial than anything else for the preservation of health—movement after a meal is worse than anything else …). Hebr. טִיּוּל only features in the current dictionaries as a modern term in the sense of 'walk; trip' (cf. BM 1868; EM 620). Samuel Benveniste translates Arab. رياضة as עמל and Anonymous has יגיעה.

[טיל] • *Piʿel* טִיֵּל · **to exercise**: Arab. راض · Maimonides, *Maqāla fī al-rabw* (*On Asthma*) · trans. Joshua Shatibi, *Ma'amar ʿal ha-Qaṣeret* X.7 (cf. BMA 2:355, l. 3): ואין ראוי שיטייל האברים החלושים מן הזקנים בשום עת מן העתים (One should never exercise the weak limbs of old people). Hebr. *Piʿel* טִיֵּל only features in the current dictionaries in the sense of 'to walk;' cf. BM 1869–1870. Samuel Benveniste and Anonymous both render Arab. راض as יגע.

טָלֶה • לָשׁוֹן → לשון טלה.

טמם (*Aram.*) • *Palpel* טַמְטֵם · **to close**: Arab. كثّف · Maimonides, *Maqāla fī al-rabw* (*On

Asthma) · trans. Samuel Benveniste, *Ma'amar 'al ha-Qaṣeret* x.2 (cf. BMA 2:277, ll. 16–17): אך הרחיצה אינה טובה לך אבל המים הקרים מזיק בחולי זה הרבה שמטמטם נקבי הגוף וימנע ההמס שהוא דבר גדול בחולי זה (Taking a bath is not fitting for [my Master]. Cold water is [often] harmful in this disease because it closes the pores of the body and prevents the dissolution [of phlegm], which is the main aim in [treating] this disease). Aram. *Palpel* טַמְטֵם features in Rabb. literature, a.o., in the sense of 'to close [around];'[100] cf. the *Targum* of סָגַר in Ju 3:22 (cf. JD 540, DAN 171). Joshua Shabiti translates Arab. كثّف as סגר and Anonymous renders Arab. كثّف المسامّ as החשיר מקום השער מהגוף. See also NM 5:89–90, entry [טמטם] (corr. below).

[טָעַם] • *Part. Hof'al* **מוּטְעָם** · **good-tasting; delicious:** Lat. *saporatus* (Arab. لذيذ) · Constantinus Africanus, *Viaticum peregrinantis* · trans. Do'eg ha-Edomi, *Sefer Ya'ir Netiv* v.16: ולא ישתו יין כי עם דק וצלול ומוטעם (They [i.e., those suffering from stones in the kidneys or bladder] should only drink wine that is thin, clear, and good-tasting (delicious)). Hebr. מוּטְעָם features in BM 1896 in a later attestation from Maimonides, *Commentary on the Mishnah*. Moses ibn Tibbon translates Arab. لذيذ as ערב.

טָפָה • **השתין טפה טפה** → [שתן].

טֶפֶס · **recipe:** Arab. صفة · Maimonides, *Maqāla fī al-rabw* (*On Asthma*) · trans. Anonymous, *Sefer ha-Qaṣeret* IV.2 (cf. BMA 2:399, ll. 7–9): ומזה צמוקיה היא בתכלית התועלת ועריבת הטעם והיא כרפואה וטופסה: שולקין בשר הצאן או העוף וקולין אותו כמו שקולין כל התבשילין בתבלין שאזכרם אחר כן (Another dish is that prepared from raisins: it is extremely beneficial and very tasty and is like a remedy. Its recipe is: Boil mutton or fowl that has been roasted in the same way as other foods [and] spices that I will describe further on). Hebr. טֶפֶס features in the current dictionaries in the sense of 'formula; frame; mould; cast,' but is not attested in medieval medical literature; cf. JD 525, s.v. טוֹפֶס; HM 105–106, s.v. טפוס; BM 1913; for the Aram. counterpart טוּפְסָא, cf. SDA 498: 'template; formula.' Samuel Benveniste translates Arab. صفة as מַתְכּוֹנֶת (see entry) and Joshua Shatibi has תואר.

טִפְּשׁוּת · **mania; madness:** Arab. جنون · Ibn Sīnā, *K. al-Qānūn fī al-ṭibb* · trans. Nathan ha-Me'ati, *Sefer ha-Qanun* II, fol. 112b: ענב אלתעלב ... אם שותים מאשר המבטל ההרגש יותר מעשרה[101] גרגרים יוליד הטפשות וכשמגמעים מימיו יועיל ממורסות הלשון (Black nightshade: ... The intake of its sedative variety, in a dose exceeding ten[102] grains, produces mania (madness). Gargling with its water is useful in swellings of the tongue (glossitis)). Hebr. טִפְּשׁוּת features in BM 1917 in the sense of 'stupidity' (סגולת הטפש) only. Moses ibn Tibbon translates Arab. جنون as בלבול השכל in his *Perush Aphorismi shel Apuqraṭ* (*Pirqei Abuqraṭ*) v.40 (260) (cf. BCD 35 (NM 3:34, corr. 4:229);

---

100 Cf. the term טִמְטוּם in the sense of 'obstruction' (for Arab. سدّ) in NM 5:89.

101 מעשרה: اثنا عشر a.

102 'ten': twelve a.

BMCH 1:384, l. 10). Zeraḥyah Ḥen and Anonymous both translate the Arab. term as שְׁטוּת (for other meanings in medieval medical literature, see BCD 273).

טרוסישקש · **round tablets; pills; pastilles; trochisks:** Lat. *trociscos* (Arab. أقراص) · Constantinus Africanus, *peregrinantis* · trans. Do'eg ha-Edomi, *Sefer Ya'ir Netiv* v.4: ומהרפואה המורכבת נתן לו אלה הטרוסישקש (From the compound medicines, we administer him the following pastilles). Hebr. טרוסישקש is a non-attested loan word from Lat. *Plur. Acc. trociscos*. In addition to this loan word, Do'eg renders Lat. *trociscos* as Hebr. *Plur.* עוגות (cf. NM 5:144, s.v. *Sing.* עוּגָה). The latter term is also used by Moses ibn Tibbon for the parallel Arab. term أقراص (see also Hebr. *Sing.* עוּגָה for Arab. قرص in *Sefer Ṣedat ha-Derakhim* VII.18.4, cf. BCD 197 (NM 1:63–64; IJZ 7:156, l. 22)).

טָרִי · **bleeding (of a wound):** Arab. طري (Gr. ἔναιμος; cf. UW 240–241)· Ibn Sīnā, *K. al-Qānūn fī al-ṭibb* · trans. Nathan ha-Me'ati, *Sefer ha-Qanun* II, fol. 112[a]: עצא אלראעי ... עושין ממנו תחבשת למורסת הפלגמוני ואל האודם הנקרא חמרה בער׳ ולחולי הנמלה ויועיל מאד המכות והנגעים יסגר המכות הטריות (Common knotgrass: ... Its plaster is very useful for treating inflamed tumors, erysipelas, called *ḥumra* in Arab., herpes, tumors, and ulcers. It closes (heals) bleeding wounds). In the sense of 'bleeding,' Hebr. טָרִי is a non-attested semantic borrowing from Arab. طري. Zeraḥyah Ḥen translates Arab. طري as חָדָשׁ (see entry) and Anonymous has טָרִי, just like Nathan.

טריתא (*Aram.*) · **soup; broth:** Arab. حسو (cf. NA 607: 'light, smooth, and thin soup made with water, flour, or fine bread crumbs, and light soups, which can be sipped;' L 572, s.v. حساء: 'A well-known kind of food; soup; i.e., what is supped or sipped; thin cooked food, that is supped or sipped, made of flour and water and oil or grease, and sometimes sweetened') · Ibn Zuhr, *K. al-Aghdhiya* · trans. Nathan ha-Me'ati, *Sefer ha-Mezonot*, fol. 3[b]: הטריתה הלקוחה מלחם חמץ עצמו אחר האפותו הנה היותר הטוב הטריתא מלחם חטים חמץ לבריאים ולחולים אין בו רוע (For healthy persons, the best leavened bread soup (broth) once the bread has been baked is that prepared from leavened wheat bread; it is also not bad for sick people). Aram. טריתא (< M. Ir. **tarīt* [perh. < N. Pers. *tarīt/d*, 'bread crumbled into milk or broth') (cf. SDA 472) features in Rabb. literature in the sense of 'a sort of pastry; fritters; etc.' (JD 554) or 'type of bread' (SDA 472). Shem Tov ben Isaac renders Arab. حسو as שֶׁרֶף in his *Sefer ha-Shimmush* XXVII (cf. BCD 286 (NM 4:213)).

• *Plur.* **טריתות** · **dishes consisting of broken pieces of bread sopped in broth with meat and/or vegetables:** Arab. ثريدة, *Plur.* ثرائد (cf. FL 1:214; L 334–335; NA 618) · Ibn Zuhr, *K. al-Aghdhiya* · trans. Nathan ha-Me'ati, *Sefer ha-Mezonot*, fols. 3[b]–4[a]: והטריתות כלם יהיו מהם לחות לבנות עבות ונאות (All dishes consisting of broken pieces of bread sopped in broth with meat and/or vegetables produce thick, crude, phlegmatic humors). Shem Tov ben Isaac translates Arab. ثرائد as רביכות in his *Sefer ha-Shimmush* XXVII (cf. BCD 257 (NM 4:192–193), s.v. רְבִיכָה).

יָבֵשׁ • קלפות יבשות → קלפה.

יוֹם • **יום גבול** · (lit., 'day of crisis'); **crisis**: Lat. *crisis* (Arab. بحران) · Constantinus Africanus, *Viaticum peregrinantis* · trans. Do'eg ha-Edomi, *Sefer Ya'ir Netiv* V.18: קרישיש זהו יום גבול אשר בו התולדת יגרש חוץ הטבע ויעבור דרך הכליות והמקוה (QRYŠYŠ [i.e., Lat. *crisis*], i.e, [Hebr.] *yom gevul*, during which nature expels the [putrid] matter [that caused the illness] so that it passes through the kidneys and urinary bladder). In the sense of 'crisis,' Hebr. יום גבול does not feature in the current dictionaries. In the sense of 'a day of prognostic indication,' Do'eg uses it also for Lat. *dies prenunciata* in *Sefer Ya'ir Netiv* III.12 (cf. NM 5:92–93). The term גְבוּל on its own is used in the sense of 'crisis' in Nathan ha-Me'ati, *Sefer ha-Peraqim* (*Pirqei Moshe*) N (cf. BCD 42 (NM 2:33); BMMN 20, l. 20; BMMG no. 186). Moses ibn Tibbon translates Arab. بحران as נִקָּיוֹן (also in *Sefer Ṣedat ha-Derakhim* VII.7.1; cf. BCD 180 (NM 1:62–63); IJZ 7:135, l. 2).
• *Plur.* **ימים** • עול ימים → עול.

יוֹנָה • *Plur.* **יונים** • תרנגלי יונים → תַּרְנְגוֹל.

יוֹצֵא (*Part.*) → יָצָא.

יוֹתֵר · **especially**: Arab. خصوصا · Ibn Sīnā, *K. al-Qānūn fī al-ṭibb* · trans. Nathan ha-Me'ati, *Sefer ha-Qanun* II, fol. 68ª: באן ... יפסיק רעיפת דם הנחירים ויקבצהו[103] והוא נאות לכאב האוזן ואל הצליל אשר בה ויותר עם שמן אווזות קטנה הנקראת אניד בלעז (B'N [i.e., fruit of the ben oil tree [*Moringa oleifera* Lam.]]: ... It stops nosebleeds because[104] of its astringency. It is good for earache and tinnitus, especially with the fat of a little duck, called in Rom. *aneda*[105]). Hebr. יוֹתֵר does not feature in this sense in the current dictionaries. A var. reading with the same meaning featuring in Rabb. literature is וביותר (cf. JD 572; EM 666; BM 2008). The Arab. synonym لا سيما is translated by Nathan as קל וחומר (see entry קַל). Zeraḥyah Ḥen and Anonymous both translate Arab. خصوصا as כל שכן; the latter term is also used by Zeraḥyah for the Arab. synonym لا سيما (see entry כֹּל).

[יחד] • *Part. Pu'al* **מְיֻחָד** · **simple**: Arab. مفرد · Ibn al-Jazzār, *Zād al-musāfir wa-qūt al-ḥādir* · trans. Abraham ben Isaac, *Sefer Ṣedah la-Oreḥim* VI.13: וקח מאילו הסמים מיוחדים או מורכבים אך אם יהיו מורכבים ערבם במי פלנטייני או עם מי שעורים ועשה ארגליון ברחם (These drugs should be taken simple or compound; if compound, they should be mixed with waybread juice or with barley juice and injected with a tube in the uterus). Hebr. *Part. Pu'al* מְיֻחָד does not feature in this sense in the current dictionaries. Moses ibn Tibbon translates Arab. مفرد as [פרד], *Part. Nif'al* נִפְרָד.

---

103 ויקבצהו: يقبضه a.

104 'because of its astringency': Trans. after a.

105 See entry אנידא.

• *Hitpa'el* הִתְיַחֵד · **to be peculiar, special, specific**: Arab. اختصّ · Ibn al-Jazzār, *Zād al-musāfir wa-qūt al-ḥādir* · trans. Moses ibn Tibbon, *Sefer Ṣedat ha-Derakhim* v.5: וכבר זכר יודע חכמת הרפואה והפילוסוף שלה ר״ל גלינוס הנכבד שאי אפשר שיתחדש השקוי מבלתי שיחלה הכבד כי הוא אמנם יתילד מחולי הכח המבשל שחלה אשר הוא מוליד הדם שמתיחד עמו הכבד (The expert in the science of medicine, the philosopher; i.e., the honourable Galen, has said that it is impossible for dropsy to occur without an illness of the liver. For [dropsy] originates from an affliction of the digestive faculty that produces the blood that is peculiar to the liver). Hebr. *Hitpa'el* הִתְיַחֵד does not feature in this sense in the current dictionaries. In medieval philosophical literature it features as 'unite; unify; specify' (see PESHAT[106]). Do'eg ha-Edomi translates the parallel Lat. term *proprius sum* as קָרוֹב (cf. NM 5:180).

יַיִן • יין מבושל · I. **inspissated (thickened) grape juice**: Arab. ربّ عنب · Ibn al-Jazzār, *Zād al-musāfir wa-qūt al-ḥādir* · trans. Moses ibn Tibbon, *Sefer Ṣedat ha-Derakhim* IV.14: יקובץ זה על אש ויבושל עד שישוב לחצי ואח״כ יסננהו בנפה וישיבהו על האש וישים עליו ג׳ ליט׳ סוכר קשה או יין מבושל (Put all these ingredients on a fire and boil them until one half remains; filter this and again put it on a fire and add three liters[107] of candy sugar or inspissated grape juice to it). The same Arab. term ربّ عنب is translated by Moses ibn Tibbon as יין מבושל עד ששב כדבש ('grape juice boiled down to a syrup') in his *Sefer Ṣedat ha-Derakhim* II.17.6 (cf. BCD 117 (NM 4:77); IJZ 1–2:506). Do'eg ha-Edomi transcribes the parallel Lat. term *sapa* as שפא (cf. NM 5:198).

· II. **syrup**: Arab. ميبختج[108] · [*Synonima*], Ms Vatican, Biblioteca Apostolica, ebr. 550, fol. 124ᵇ: מי בכתג שפא הוא יין מבושל (MY BKTG [i.e., Arab. *maybakhtaj*]; ŠP' [i.e., Lat. *sapa*[109]]; i.e., [lit.,] 'boiled wine'). In the sense of 'syrup,' Hebr. יין מבושל features in NM 5:93 in an attestation from Moses ibn Tibbon, *Sefer Ṣedat ha-Derakhim* III.1.

יַלֶּפֶת · **scurf; dandruff**: Arab. حزاز (Gr. πίτυρον; cf. UW 530–531) · Ibn Sīnā, *K. al-Qānūn fī al-ṭibb* · trans. Nathan ha-Me'ati, *Sefer ha-Qanun* II, fol. 69ᵃ: בורק ... איברי הראש: יועיל מהילפת הנקרא חזאז בערבי ומהזעף הנקרא רעוה[110] בערבי עם דבש וכשמטיפים ממנו באזן ינקה ויועיל מהחרשות (Borax (sodium borate): ... The parts of the head: It is useful for dandruff, called *ḥazāz* in Arab. Ear drops made from its foam, called *raghwa* in Arab., mixed with honey cleanse the ears and are good for deafness). Hebr. יַלֶּפֶת features

106 https://peshat.org/display/peshat_lemmas_00016161 (accessed Nov 2, 2021).

107 'liters': Arab. *arṭāl*. The weight of a *raṭl* is varying according to region and period; from the twelfth century on, its general weight in Egypt is 450 grams.

108 Arab. ميبختج: From Pers. مى پخته; cf. VL 2:1246: 'syrupus, et sec. al. vinum cum aliis medicamentis bullitum et defaecatum' (syrup, according to others: wine boiled and purified with other medications); MSh no. 566: 'syrup made of must' (cf. no. 84, and MIG 227).

109 Lat. *sapa*; cf. DMLBS 3283, s.v. *sapa* [CL], '1 sapus, new wine boiled down to a fraction of its original volume.'

110 רעוה (رغوة a): emend. ed. רעונה Ms.

in KB 2:413 as 'Egyptian lichen,' and as identical with חֲזָזִית; see also JD 579: 'lichen; a cutaneous disease;' BM 2054: 'a skin disease, such as: Egyptian lichen;' and Low LIV: 'Egyptian papula.' R. Sa'adya Gaon translates Hebr. יַלֶּפֶת, as it features in Lev 21:20 as Arab. حزاز (cf. S 176: חזאז; SHS 1:259–260 (Yod 19)), the same term used by Ibn Sīnā. Zeraḥyah Ḥen translates Arab. حزاز as חֲזָזִית (see entry) and Anonymous has only the transcribed Arab. term חזאז.

יְסוֹדִי • **החמימות חיסודי** → **חֲמִימוּת**.

[יסף] • *Part. Nif'al* **נוֹסָף** • *Plur.* **נוספים** · **residues; superfluities**: Arab. أخلاط · Maimonides, *Maqāla fī al-rabw* (*On Asthma*) · trans. Samuel Benveniste, *Ma'amar 'al ha-Qaṣeret* II.1 (cf. BMA 2:247, ll. 19–21): כי הכונה שיהיו העורקים כלם והנקבים פתוחים והשבילים נקיים שלימים מן הסתום והמצוקה כדי שירוצו בהם הרוחות והליחות ויצאו מהם הנוספים (One's intention should be that all the veins and passages are open and clean and free from obstruction and constriction so that the pneumas and humors stream through them [freely] and the superfluities are expelled). In the sense of 'residue,' Hebr. [יסף], *Part. Nif'al* נוֹסָף (*Sing.*) is attested in BCD 117 (NM 3:151–152) in an earlier attestation from Do'eg ha-Edomi, *Sefer Agur* I.2. Benveniste also translates Arab. فضول (a synonym of أخلاط) as *Part. Hof'al* מוּסָף, *Plur.* מוספים in *Ma'amar 'al ha-Qaṣeret* XIII.25 (see entry below). Joshua Shatibi translates Arab. أخلاط as מותרות and Anonymous has יתרונות (see entry יִתְרוֹן). For *Part. Nif'al* נוֹסָף, functioning as *Adj.* in the sense of 'superfluous,' see NM 5:94.

• **בשר נוסף** → **בָּשָׂר**.

• *Part. Hif'il* **מוֹסִיף** • **הנגעים המוסיפים** → **נֶגַע**.

• *Part. Hof'al* **מוּסָף** • *Plur.* **מוּסָפִים** · **residues, superfluities**: Arab. فضول · Maimonides, *Maqāla fī al-rabw* (*On Asthma*) · trans. Samuel Benveniste, *Ma'amar 'al ha-Qaṣeret* XIII.25 (cf. BMA 2:306, ll. 9–13): אמר ג'אלינוס במאמר ממאמריו הידועים וזה נסחת דבריו אמר: היונים אם נסתפק להם חולי הניחוהו בין הטבע ובינו והוא [כלה] יגרשהו. והביאו טענה לדבריהם שהטבע ממונה ופקיד על החי בבריאותו וסועד אותו במחלתו ויודע מזג האיברים וישלח לכל אבר הראוי לו מן המסעד אחרי שהכין מקומות למוספי המסעד ולחות מקובלות לגוף (In one of his well-known treatises, Galen said the following: When the Greeks were in doubt about a disease, they left it to nature to expel it. Their argument for this was that nature is in charge of the health of living beings and treats them in the case of disease, and that it knows the temperament of their organs and sends to every individual organ the appropriate kind of nourishment, after first preparing sites for the superfluities of the food and humors appropriate to the body). In the sense of 'residue; superfluity,' Hebr. *Part. Hof'al* מוּסָף, *Plur.* מוספים, is not attested in the current dictionaries. Samuel Benveniste also translates Arab. أخلاط (a synonym of فضول) as *Part. Nif'al* נוֹסָף, *Plur.* נוספים, in *Ma'amar 'al ha-Qaṣeret* II.1 (see entry above). Joshua Shatibi translates Arab. فضول as מותרים and Anonymous has יתרונות (see entry יִתְרוֹן).

[יסר] • *Nif'al* **נוֹסַר** · **to be educated**: Arab. تأدّب · Maimonides, *Maqāla fī al-rabw* (*On

Asthma) · trans. Anonymous, *Sefer ha-Qaṣeret* XIII.23 (cf. BMA 2:444, ll. 14–15): ואמר ⟨ש⟩הטבע יעשה מה שראוי לעשות שהוא בעל מוסר טוב המוסר שבו נלמד ונוסר (And he further said: Nature does what should be done because it is well trained and educated. Consequently, through nature we learn and are educated). Hebr. נוֹסַר features in the current dictionaries in the sense of 'to be corrected, admonished, chastened' in attestations from Biblical literature only (cf. BDB 416; BM 2079). Samuel Benveniste translates Arab. تأدّب as למד מוסר and Joshua Shatibi has קיבל מוסר.

יַעֲרִי • *Plur.* **יעריים** • **favus**: Arab. الأورام الشهدية (cf. UW 344, s.v. κηρίον; LS 948: 'honeycomb; *II.* a cutaneous disease; μελικηρίς;' cf. LS 1097, s.v. μελικηρίς: 'a kind of cyst or wen, from its resembling a honeycomb') · Ibn Sīnā, *K. al-Qānūn fī al-ṭibb* · trans. Anonymous, *Sefer ha-Qanun* II, fol. 52ᵇ: בקלה ימאניה ... יחובש בשרשו ליעריים (Amaranth: ... A poultice of its root is put on favus). Hebr. *Sing.* יַעֲרִי is attested in the current dictionaries as *Adj.* derived from יַעַר in the sense of 'forest' (cf. BM 2092; NM 5:95: 'wild'), not from יַעַר ('honey') or יַעֲרָה ('honeycomb'). Nathan ha-Me'ati translates Arab. الأورام الشهدية as המורסות הדבשיות (see entry מֻרְסָה) and Zeraḥyah Ḥen has מור׳ הנקרא דבשיית.

יִפּוּי · **cosmetic**: Arab. زينة · Ibn Sīnā, *K. al-Qānūn fī al-ṭibb* · trans. Zeraḥyah Ḥen, *Sefer ha-Qanun* II, fol. 167ᵇ: אֶס הדס ... ביפוי: שמנו ובשולו ומיצו מחזק שרשי השער וימנע השרתו ויאריכנו וישחירנו וכל שכן השותה אותו ('eS [i.e., Arab. *ās*, i.e., myrtle]; [Hebr.] *hadas* ... As a cosmetic: The oil, decoction, and juice [prepared from it] strengthen the roots of the hair and prevent it from falling out and makes it grow and darkens it; esp. when it is drunken). Hebr. יִפּוּי is not attested in medieval Hebrew medical literature in the current dictionaries. Nathan ha-Me'ati translates Arab. زينة as עֲדִי (see entry) and Anonymous has קִשּׁוּט (see entry).

יָצָא · I. **to be abolished, eliminated, dispelled**: Arab. كان مرتفع · Maimonides, *Maqāla fī al-rabw* (*On Asthma*) · trans. Samuel Benveniste, *Ma'amar 'al ha-Qaṣeret* XIII.22 (cf. BMA 2:304, ll. 19–21): אני יודע שתאמר כי תכלית מה שהגיענו מדבריך לעזוב הרפואות. אם כן כל מה שיגעו בו ויזהירו באומנות הזאת הכל יהיה לריק. אני אוציא הספק. ואם יצא מכח דברי הקודמים אעפ״כ אקיימהו (I know that you could say: The conclusion to be drawn from your words is to abandon medicine, because every effort and attention given to this art is [given] in vain. I will dispel the doubt. And if it has already been dispelled by the force of my words so far, I will nevertheless return to the subject [once again]). Hebr. יָצָא features in the current dictionaries in the sense of 'to be excluded, exempt' in attestations from Rabb. literature only (cf. JD 587; BM 2107). Joshua Shatibi translates Arab. كان مرتفع as *Nif'al* נַעֲלָה (see entry [עלה]) and Anonymous has [סור], *Hof'al* הוּסַר.

· II. **to evacuate the bowels; to relieve oneself**: Lat. *egero* (Arab. تغوّط) · Constantinus Africanus, *Viaticum peregrinantis* · trans. Do'eg ha-Edomi, *Sefer Ya'ir Netiv* IV.19: ואלה הדברים אם יקרו מהליחות הגסות והדבקות יש להם נפח רב וקול והברה במעים ואם הוא מליחות מחודדות יהיה כאב וחכוך בעגבות וכאב גם טינשמוש והחולה ידמה בנפשו לצאת כאשר אין שם מאומה (If they [i.e., hemorrhoids] originate from thick, viscous superfluities, they come with a lot of flatulence and intestinal rumblings. If they originate from sharp, biting superfluities, they come with pain and itching in the buttocks and tenesmus so that the patient thinks that he needs to relieve himself even though he does not have to). In the sense of 'to relieve oneself,' Hebr. יָצָא is attested in Rabb. literature only (cf. JD 587; EM 683). Moses ibn Tibbon translates Arab. تغوّط as יָצָא as well.

• *Part.* **יוֹצֵא** • **חמיץ היוצא מן החלב** → מִיץ.

• *Hifʿil* **הוֹצִיא** · **to abolish, eliminate, dispel**: Arab. رفع · Maimonides, *Maqāla fī al-rabw* (*On Asthma*) · trans. Samuel Benveniste, *Maʾamar ʿal ha-Qaṣeret* XIII.22 (cf. BMA 2:304, ll. 19–21): אני יודע שתאמר כי תכלית מה שהגיענו מדבריך לעזוב הרפואות. אם כן כל מה שיגעו בו ויזהירו באומנות הזאת הכל יהיה לריק. אני אוציא הספק. ואם יצא מכח דברי הקודמים אעפ״כ אקיימהו (I know that you could say: The conclusion to be drawn from your words is to abandon medicine, because every effort and attention given to this art is [given] in vain. I will dispel the doubt. And if it has already been dispelled by the force of my words so far, I will nevertheless return to the subject [once again]). In the sense of 'to abolish, eliminate, dispel,' Hebr. *Hifʿil* הוֹצִיא is not attested in the current dictionaries. Joshua Shatibi translates Arab. رفع as *Hifʿil* הֶעֱלָה (see entry [עלה]) and Anonymous has [סור], *Hifʿil* הֵסִיר.

• *Part. Hifʿil* **מוֹצִיא** · **pressing out**: Arab. عصر · Maimonides, *Maqāla fī al-rabw* (*On Asthma*) · trans. Anonymous, *Sefer ha-Qaṣeret* XII.3 (cf. BMA 2:430, ll. 17–19): אחר חזק זכרו גאלינוס יוקח בצל אחת של ענצל ומוציאין מימיו ומשימים עם המים כמותן דבש ומעמידין אותו משקה ויוקח ממנו אוקיה קודם האכילה וכמו כן אחריה (Another strong [linctus] mentioned by Galen: Take squill, press it out, add to the juice a similar amount of honey, thicken it until it becomes a syrup, and take one ounce of it before and after meals). In the sense of 'to press, squeeze,' Hebr. *Hifʿil* הוֹצִיא, *Part.* מוֹצִיא, is not attested in the current dictionaries. Samuel Benveniste translates Arab. عصر as שָׁחַט (see entry) and Joshua Shatibi has עָצַר (see entry [2]עָצַר).

יְצִיאָה · **stools; excrements**: Arab. براز · Ibn al-Jazzār, *Zād al-musāfir wa-qūt al-ḥādir* · trans. Moses ibn Tibbon, *Sefer Ṣedat ha-Derakhim* IV.15: ומזה כי אנחנו נקח ראיה על מקום החמרמרות והעצור בהרגש הכאב במעים ומאיכות הדבר אשר יתערב ביציאה (For we conclude to the site of the abrasion and dysentery from the feeling of pain in the intestines and from the quality of the matter that is mixed with the excrements). In the sense of 'stools; excrements,' Hebr. יְצִיאָה features in BCD 118 in attestations from Hillel ben Samuel, *Aphorismi* IV.83 (for Lat. *secessus*) (cf. NM 3:107) and Nathan ha-Me'ati, *Sefer ha-Peraqim* (*Pirqei Moshe*) V.1 (cf. NM 2:50; BMMN 62, ll. 15–16; BMMG no. 254). Do'eg ha-Edomi translates the parallel Lat. term *digestio* as בִּשּׁוּל (see entry).

• **יציאת פי הטבעת** · **prolapse of the anus (procidentia ani)**: Arab. خروج المقعدة · Ibn al-Jazzār, *Zād al-musāfir wa-qūt al-ḥādir* · trans. Moses ibn Tibbon, *Sefer Ṣedat ha-Derakhim* IV.20: ואם היתה סבת יציאת פי הטבעת העצור כמו שזכרנו ימצא החולה עם העצור כאב חזק וראוי שנרפא הסבה שמעוררת החולי ויושיבו החולה במים שנתבשלו בהם הסמים

הקובצים (If the prolapse of the anus is caused by the tenesmus, as we mentioned, the patient will, in addition to the tenesmus, suffer from severe pain. We should treat the cause of the illness by letting him sit in water in which astringent remedies have been cooked). Hebr. **יציאת פי הטבעת** does not feature in the current dictionaries. Masie (MD 601, s.v. 'prolapsus ani') has **צניחת פי הטבעת**.

• **יציאת הרחם** · **prolapse of the uterus**: Arab. نتوء الرحم · Ibn al-Jazzār, *Zād al-musāfir wa-qūt al-ḥādir* · trans. Abraham ben Isaac, *Sefer Ṣedah la-Oreḥim* VI.14: והראוי תחילה לרפאות ביציאת הרחם צוה לאשה ותישן על גבה (To treat prolapse of the uterus, one should first of all tell the woman to sleep on her back). Hebr. **יציאת הרחם** is not attested in this sense in the current dictionaries. Moses ibn Tibbon translates Arab. نتوء الرحم as בליטת הרחם in *Sefer Ṣedat ha-Derakhim* I.0.4 (cf. BCD 36 (NM 4:27); IJZ 1–2:441).

• **יציאת השתן** · **polyuria; diabetes**: Lat. *lubrica urina* (Arab. سلس البول; cf. FL 2:340, s.v. سَلَسٌ: 'profluvium urinae; diabetes;' SN 1:112 (266): 'Krampfhafte Harnruhr (*Diabetes spasticus*)') · Constantinus Africanus, *Viaticum peregrinantis* · trans. Do'eg ha-Edomi, *Sefer Ya'ir Netiv* V.18: אחר זה טוב אל יציאת השתן (Another [remedy] beneficial for polyuria (diabetes)). Hebr. **יציאת השתן** does not feature in the current dictionaries. Moses ibn Tibbon translates Arab. سلس البول as התרת השתן (cf. also BCD 78 for the use of the same term (for Arab. استطلاق البول) in *Sefer ha-Peraqim* (*Pirqei Moshe*) XXIV.39 by both Nathan ha-Me'ati (cf. NM 2:43; BMMN 239, l. 4) and Zeraḥyah Ḥen (cf. NM 1:143; BMMZ 238, l. 25) (cf. also BMMG no. 3187)). See also הגרת השתן מבלי חפץ (entry הַגָּרָה) and **יציאת השתן מבלי הרגש** (next entry).

• **יציאת השתן מבלי הרגש** · **urinary incontinence (unvoluntary urination, polyuria)**: Arab. سلس البول (cf. FL 2:340, s.v. سَلَسٌ: 'profluvium urinae; diabetes'; SN 1:112 (266): 'Krampfhafte Harnruhr (*Diabetes spasticus*)') · al-Rāzī, *K. al-Manṣūrī fī al-ṭibb* · trans. Shem Tov ben Isaac, *Sefer Almansur*, fol. 4[a]: ע"ה ביציאת השתן מבלי הרגש ([Chapter] 75: On urinary incontinence (unvoluntary urination, polyuria)). Hebr. **יציאת השתן מבלי הרגש** does not feature in the current dictionaries. In addition to this term, Shem Tov ben Isaac translates Arab. سلس البول as הגרת השתן מבלי חפץ (see entry הַגָּרָה). See also **יציאת השתן** (entry above).

יְצִירָה · **intelligence; natural disposition to understand**: Arab. فطرة (cf. GL 509 (274–275): 'esprit; intelligence au sens de disposition naturelle à comprendre') · Maimonides, *Maqāla fī al-rabw* (*On Asthma*) · trans. Joshua Shatibi, *Ma'amar 'al ha-Qaṣeret* XIII.11 (cf. BMA 2:372, ll. 12–13): אמנם הבן זה כלו מן הספרים קל מאד על כל שלם היצירה אמנם העשיה בהם אצל האישים יקשה מאד על היודע המיושב (Understanding all this from books is very easy for everyone who is in full possession of his faculties (intelligence), but applying it in an individual case is very difficult for a conscientious scholar). Hebr. יְצִירָה features in KTP 2:46–48 in the sense of 'creature; nature; virtue' and in PESHAT[111] as '(1) nature; disposition; (2) innate characteristic; (3) char-

111 https://peshat.org/display/peshat_lemmas_00002104 (accessed April 2, 2022).

acter trait; (4) nature; (5) creature; something formed; (6) forming; act of creation; (7) form; shape.' Samuel Benveniste translates Arab. كامل الفطرة as בעל שכל.

יְרִיעָה ‣ I. **diaphragm**: Arab. حجاب · Ibn al-Jazzār, *Zād al-musāfir wa-qūt al-ḥādir* · trans. Moses ibn Tibbon, *Sefer Ṣedat ha-Derakhim* v.3: וכשיתנשם או יתמלא מן המאכל או המשקה או ילך מהר ויקרה לו קושי הנשימה כי עליון הכבד דבק ביריעה המבדלת בין כלי המזון וכלי הנשימה וישעול שעול יבש בזולת רקיקה כי החומר חוץ מן האברים אשר ילך בהם רוח הנשימה (When he [i.e. someone suffering from an ulcer in the liver] breathes, or fills himself with food or drink, or walks fast, he will suffer from dyspnea because the upper part of the liver is attached to the diaphragm that divides between the digestive organs and the respiratory organs. He will suffer from a dry cough without expectoration because the [superfluous] matter is outside the organs through which breath passes). Hebr. יְרִיעָה does not feature in this sense in the current dictionaries. Synonyms featuring in medieval medical literature are: חצר הכבד (cf. BCD 107 (NM 3:96)); יֹתֶרֶת (cf. BCD 122 (NM 3:105–106)); המכסה המבדיל (cf. BCD 130 (NM 1:29–30)); and קֶרֶב (BCD 249 (NM 3:207)); see also MD 221. Do'eg ha-Edomi transcribes the parallel Lat. term *diaphragma* as דיאפרגמא.

‣ II. **peritoneum**: Arab. صفاق · Ibn al-Jazzār, *Zād al-musāfir wa-qūt al-ḥādir* · trans. Moses ibn Tibbon, *Sefer Ṣedat ha-Derakhim* v.5: ואם ימצא מיץ המזון הכח המבשל כלו מתעצל ולואה מהשיבו דם כלל יתחדש ממנו לחות כרכומי מלוח רע וכאשר יחלש הכבד ולא יוכל לברור אותו ולשלחו אל האברים אי אפשר[112] בהכרח שיתיכהו חום הכבד וישיבהו ועל כל בני המעים אדים ואז ישליכם אל יריעת הבטן ההנקרא ציפאק הנמשכת עליו (When the digestive faculty is too slow and weak to change the juice of the food into blood, a bilious, salty, bad moisture is the result. And when the liver is so weak that it cannot clean [this moisture] and send it to the organs, the heat of the liver turns[113] it necessarily into vapors and then expels them to the peritoneum, which is called ṢYP'Q [i.e., Arab. *ṣifāq*], that covers the stomach and all the [other] intestines). Hebr. יְרִיעָה does not feature in this sense in the current dictionaries. Synonyms featuring in medieval medical literature are: זיפק (Lat. *siphac*; in Hillel ben Samuel, *Sefer Keritut*; cf. BCD 83–84 (NM 1:43)) and קְרוּם (in David Caslari, *Sefer Ro'a Mezeg Mitḥallef* III.3; cf. BCD 249 (NM 2:169)). Do'eg ha-Edomi translates the parallel Lat. term *pelliculas as* דַּף (see entry).

• *Plur.* **יריעות** ‣ **membranes (of the eye)**: Lat. *tunicae* · Gerard de Solo, *Practica super nono Almansoris* · trans. Abraham Avigdor, *Ha-Ma'amar ha-Teshi'i le-Sefer ha-Mansuri le-Razi*, fol. 69b: ודע שסבת הנגע לפעמים תהיה חיצונית ופעמים תהיה פנימית והסבה החיצונית אם הכאה או חתוך והסבה הפמימית היא ליחה חדה עוקצת ומאכלת יריעות העין (Know that the cause of ulcers [in the eye] is sometimes external and sometimes internal;

112 אי אפשר בהכרח: ولابدّ ضرورة a.

113 'turns it necessarily': Trans. after a.

the external cause is a blow or a cut, and the internal cause is a sharp ḥumor that bites into the membranes of the eye and corrodes them). In the sense of 'membrane (of the eye),' Hebr. *Sing.* יְרִיעָה features in KDS 86 (cf. the term היריעה הלבנה ('conjunctiva') in BCD 121 (NM 4:77) for an attestation from Moses ibn Tibbon, *Sefer Ṣedat ha-Derakhim* II.1.1 (cf. IJZ 1–2:485)).

יָרְקוֹן → הִדְרָקוֹן.

[ירש] • *Hif'il* **הוֹרִישׁ** · **to produce, cause**: Arab. أورث · Ibn Sīnā, *K. al-Qānūn fī al-ṭibb* · trans. Nathan ha-Me'ati, *Sefer ha-Qanun* II, fol. 70ᵇ: באדנגאן ... מה שהוא קטן מהבדנגאן ראוי לאכלו מקולף ויוריש הכתם הנקרא כלף (Eggplant: ... Small eggplants should be eaten peeled, but they cause freckles called *kalaf* [in Arab.]). In the sense of 'to produce, cause,' Hebr. [ירש], *Hif'il* הוֹרִישׁ, is a non-attested semantic borrowing from Arab. أورث. Zeraḥyah Ḥen and Anonymous both translate Arab. أورث as *Hif'il* הוֹרִישׁ as well.

יַשְׁנוּת • **שב לישנות** → [שוב].

יִתְרָה · **superfluity**: Arab. فضلة · Maimonides, *Maqāla fī al-rabw* (*On Asthma*) · trans. Anonymous, *Sefer ha-Qaṣeret* XI.2 (cf. BMA 2:426, ll. 2–3): והוא ⟨ש⟩הוא יתכן בשום עת שתהיה היתרה הנמצאת באבר משונה ממזג האבר עצמו העיקרי והמקרי (This can occur at any time—that is to say that the superfluity in an organ is contrary to the temperament of the essential or incidental organ itself). Hebr. יִתְרָה is only attested in the Bible in the sense of 'abundance; riches' (cf. BDB 452). For a var. reading, cf. entry יִתְרוֹן below. Samuel Benveniste translates Arab. فضلة as *Part. Nif'al* נוֹסָף (cf. entry [יסף]) and Joshua Shatibi has מותר.

יִתְרוֹן · **excess**: Arab. إفراط · Maimonides, *Maqāla fī al-rabw* (*On Asthma*) · trans. Samuel Benveniste, *Ma'amar 'al ha-Qaṣeret* X.8 (cf. BMA 2:279, ll. 19–20): אבל המשגל נודע ואף בכל המון שמזיק מאד לרב בני אדם והיתרון ממנו מזיק לכל בני האדם (As for sexual intercourse, it is well known—even to the masses—that it is very harmful to most people and that excessive indulgence in it is harmful to all people). Hebr. יִתְרוֹן does not feature in this sense in the current dictionaries. Joshua Shatibi and Anonymous both render Arab. إفراط as הרבות.

• *Plur.*¹ **יתרונות** · **superfluities**: Arab. فضلات · Maimonides, *Maqāla fī al-rabw* (*On Asthma*) · trans. Anonymous, *Sefer ha-Qaṣeret* II.1 (cf. BMA 2:393, ll. 20–21): שהכונה שיהיו הגידים כולם והפילושים פתוחי השביל נקיים מהאוטם והצוק עד שירוצו בהם הרוחות והלחות ונדחים מהם היתרונות (One's intention should be that all the veins and passages are open and clean and free from obstruction and constriction so that the pneumas and humors stream through them [freely] and the superfluities are expelled). In the sense of 'superfluity,' Hebr. יִתְרוֹן, *Plur.* יתרונות, features in BM 2206, a.o., in an attestation from Meir Aldabi, *Shevilei Emunah*. For var. readings, cf. *Plur.*² יתרונים below, and also entries יִתְרָה and יְתֵרוּת. Samuel Benveniste translates Arab. فضلات as נוספים (see entry [יסף]) and Joshua Shatibi has מותרות.

• *Plur.*² **יתרונים** · **superfluities**: Arab. فضول · Ibn Sīnā, *K. al-Qānūn fī al-ṭibb* · trans.

Nathan ha-Me'ati, *Sefer ha-Qanun* II, fol. 88[a]: חגר אל לבן ... יכחלו כאשר מחככים ממנו במים וימנע הגרת היתרונים לעין (The milky stone [i.e., a stone that, when rubbed with water, yields a milky substance (chalk)]: ... If it is rubbed and used as *kohl* (collyrium) with water, it prevents (stops) the flow of superfluities towards the eyes). In the sense of 'superfluity,' Hebr. *Sing.* יִתְרוֹן is only attested in the current dictionaries with *Plur.*[1] יתרונות (see previous entry). Zeraḥyah Ḥen and Anonymous both translate Arab. فضول as מותרות.

יִתְרוֹנִי · **superfluous**: Arab. فضلي · Ibn Sīnā, *K. al-Qānūn fī al-ṭibb* · trans. Nathan ha-Me'ati, *Sefer ha-Qanun* II, fol. 99[a]: לוביא ... האדום יותר טוב מכלם ובן מאסויה וארמניס[114] אמרו שהוא קר ויבש ולפי דעתי כי הוא יבש ובו רוטבה יתרונית (Black-eyed pea: ... The red variety is the best. Both, Ibn Māsawayh and Archigenes, state that it is cold and dry, but in my opinion it is dry and has superfluous moisture). Hebr. יִתְרוֹנִי does not feature in the current dictionaries. Zeraḥyah Ḥen translates Arab. فضلي as עודף.

יְתֵרוּת · **superfluity**: Arab. فضلة · Maimonides, *Maqāla fī al-rabw* (*On Asthma*) · trans. Anonymous, *Sefer ha-Qaṣeret* II.1 (cf. BMA 2:393, ll. 6–8): וסבת זה מבוארת והוא שהמזונות כשיתאכלו באברים והיתה יתרות העיכול השלישי בהן מעוטה לא מודבקת ולא עבה תתחולל חלילות נסתר ותצא באד והזיעה (The reason for this is clear—namely, that, when foods are digested in the organs and when the superfluity from the third digestion is minimal and is not sticky or thick, they are dissolved in a hidden way and leave [the body] through evaporation and perspiration). Hebr. יְתֵרוּת is not attested in the current dictionaries. Samuel Benveniste translates Arab. فضلة as שארית and Joshua Shatibi has מותר.

---

114 וארמניס: أرنجانس a.

כ

כְּאֵב • כאב צדי הצלעות · **pleuralgia**: Arab. وجع الجنبين · Ibn Sīnā, *K. al-Qānūn fī al-ṭibb* · trans. Nathan ha-Me'ati, *Sefer ha-Qanun* II, fol. 74[a]: גואשיר ... והגואשיר כמו כן יועיל מכאב צדי הצלעות והשעול מקרירות (Opopanax: ... Opopanax is also useful for pleuralgia and for cough caused by cold). Hebr. כאב צדי הצלעות does not feature in the current dictionaries. Zeraḥyah Ḥen translates Arab. وجع الجنبين as כאבי הצד and Anonymous has כאב הצדדים.

כאגד · **papyrus**: a) Lat. *carta bombicina* · Constantinus Africanus, *Viaticum peregrinantis* · trans. Do'eg ha-Edomi, *Sefer Ya'ir Netiv* IV.15: ארסניקי סנדראקא שמרי חומץ שרופים אכאסיא גומי דרכמ' וחצי סיד חי כאגד שרופה ב' דרכמ' אלום אופי חצי דרכ' ותשחוק: לאבק ותמזוג ביין אדום ותעשה משם עוגות ([Recipe for pastilles]: [Take] one and a half *dirham* [each] of red and yellow arsenic, burnt vinegar sediment, and acacia gum; two *dirhams* [each] of quicklime and burned papyrus; half a *dirham* of alum and opium; pulverize [these ingredients], mix this with red wine, and make pastilles of it). The term כאגד is a transcription of Arab. كاغد or كاغذ ('paper,' from Pers.; cf. SCP 1006), cf. WKAS 1:10. Moses ibn Tibbon transcribes the parallel Arab. term قرطاس as כאגד as well.[115]

· b) Arab. قرطاس · Ibn al-Jazzār, *Zād al-musāfir wa-qūt al-ḥādir* · trans. Moses ibn Tibbon, *Sefer Ṣedat ha-Derakhim* IV.15:[116] תואר עוגות אחרות מארסיניקום ואורופימנט יועילו כמו אשר לפניהם והם חזקות מנוסות ערובם: יקח ארסיניקום ואורופימינט ושמרי חומץ יין מנוגב שרוף ואכסיא וגומא ארביקא מ"א שקל וסיד בלתי מכובה וכאגד שרוף מ"א ב' דר' אלום לבן דר' אופי חצי דר' יודקו הסמים וינופו ויולשו ביין אדום ריחני ויעשה עוגות וינגבם בצל וירגילם (A recipe for other pastilles with red and yellow arsenic that are beneficial just like the ones [mentioned] before and that are strong and tested: Take one *sheqel*[117] each of red and yellow arsenic, of dried, burned vinegar sediment, of acacia gum, and of gum Arabic; two *dirhams* each of quicklime and burned papyrus; one *dirham* of white alum; half a *dirham* of opium. Pound the ingredients, sieve them, knead them with fragrant red wine, make pastilles, dry them in the shade, and apply them). The term כאגד also features for Arab. قرطاس in [*Synonima*], Ms Vatican, Biblioteca Apostolica, ebr. 550, fol. 128[b]: קרטאס הוא כאגד (QRṬ'S [i.e., Arab. *qirṭās*]; i.e., [Arab.-Pers.] K'GD). Do'eg ha-Edomi renders the parallel Lat. term *carta bombicina* as כאגד as well (see previous entry).

---

115 The faulty entry בֶּגֶד for Arab. قرطاس in BCD 30 (NM 4:24) (in an attestation from Moses ibn Tibbon, *Sefer Ṣedat ha-Derakhim* I.7.1 (cf. IJZ 1–2:451)) should be corrected as כאגד.

116 The faulty entry בֶּגֶד for Arab. قرطاس in BCD 30 (NM 4:24) (in an attestation from Moses ibn Tibbon, *Sefer Ṣedat ha-Derakhim* I.7.1 (cf. IJZ 1–2:451)) should be corrected as כאגד.

117 Hebr. *sheqel* stands forn Arab. *mithqāl*; one *mithqāl* is 4.46 grams; cf. HIM 4–7.

כֹּבֶד • כובד הנשימה ׳ shortness of breath; dyspnea: Arab. عسر النفس · Ibn Sīnā, *K. al-Qānūn fī al-ṭibb* · trans. Anonymous, *Sefer ha-Qanun* II, fols. 237ª–237ᵇ: שיח ... מועיל מכובד הנשימה (Wormwood: ... It is beneficial for dyspnea). Hebr. כובד הנשימה features in BM 2230 in an attestation from the *Sefer ha-Qanun*. Nathan ha-Me'ati translates Arab. عسر النفس as קצר הנשימה (see entry קֹצֶר) and Zeraḥyah Ḥen has עוצר הניפוש (see also the use of the same term in his *Sefer ha-Peraqim* (*Pirqei Moshe*) XXIII.79; cf. BCD 212 (NM 1:178); BMMZ 227, l. 23; BMMG no. 3344).

[כבה] • *Part. Pu'al* **מְכֻבֶּה • סיד בלתי מכובה** → סִיד.

כָּבַשׁ • *Part.* **כּוֹבֵשׁ • הכח הכובש** → כֹּחַ.

כֶּבֶשׁ • לשון הכבש → לָשׁוֹן.

כַּדּוּר • *Plur.* **כדורים ׳ hazelnuts:** Arab. بندق · *Shinnui ha-Shemot ha-Niqra'im Synonimi*, fol. 73ᵇ: בנדאק[118] פי׳ כדורים (BND'Q [read: BNDQ, i.e., Arab. *bunduq*]; i.e., *kaddurim*). Hebr. *Sing.* כַּדּוּר only features in the current dictionaries in the sense of 'globe; ball' (cf. BM 2259–2261) In the sense of 'hazelnut,' it is a non-attested semantic borrowing from Arab. بندق.

כובד → כֹּבֶד.

כּוֹבַע ׳ aril: Arab. جفت · Ibn al-Jazzār, *Zād al-musāfir wa-qūt al-ḥādir* · trans. Moses ibn Tibbon, *Sefer Ṣedat ha-Derakhim* VI.10: תאר עוגות יעצרו הדם היוצא מחתוך העורקים ברחם או בכליות וישחקו ויכניסום מלמטה לפנים ואחור בפתילה ערובן יקח בלושטיאש וקוקילא מרינה שרופה ואכסיא מ״א ב׳ שקלים עפצים שרופים מכובים בחומץ יין וכאגד שרופה ודם תנין וסומאק וכובע גלנץ (Prescription for pills, which retain the blood bursting forth from a rupture of the veins in the uterus or in the kidneys: They should be pounded and enserted as a pessary [in the vagina] and as a suppository [in the anus]: Take two *sheqels*[119] each of flower of the pomegranate, burned cowrie, and acacia gum, burned gallnut smothered in wine vinegar, burned papyrus, dragon's blood (resin of *Dracaena cinnabari* Balf. f.), sumac, and aril of the acorn). Hebr. כּוֹבַע is not attested in this sense in the current dictionaries. Moses ibn Tibbon also translates Arab. جفت as Rom. קפלץ and Do'eg ha-Edomi translates the parallel Lat. term *cupulae* as כותנות (also in *Sefer Ya'ir Netiv* IV.15, see entry כֻּתֹּנֶת).

כּוֹבֵשׁ (*Part.*) → כָּבַשׁ.

כָּוָה • *Part.* **כּוֹוֶה ׳ caustic:** Arab. كاو · Ibn Sīnā, *K. al-Qānūn fī al-ṭibb* · trans. Nathan ha-Me'ati, *Sefer ha-Qanun* II, fol. 67ᵇ: באן ... ויש באילנו מרירות יותר וקבוץ וזה יוליד בו כח כווה וקלפתו קובצת יותר ולא תכלה משיחתו מהקבוץ ובכלו יש תמרוק וחתוך (B'N [i.e., fruit of the ben oil tree [*Moringa oleifera* Lam.]]: ... The tree is more bitter and astringent, which gives it its caustic property. The peel is more astringent, the oil is also not free from

---

118 בנדאק: Ms¹ בנסאק Ms.

119 Hebr. *sheqel* stands for Arab. *mithqāl*; one *mithqāl* is 4.46 grams; cf. HIM 4–7.

astringency. All of them have detergent and cutting potency). Hebr. *Part.* כּוֹוֶה is not attested in this sense in the current dictionaries. As הסם הכווה ('the caustic remedy'), it features in BCD 187 (NM 4:123) in Anonymous, *Sammim Libbiyim*. Zeraḥyah Ḥen and Anonymous both translate Arab. كاو as כּוֹוֶה as well.

כּוֹוֶה (*Part.*) → **כָּוָה**.

כּוֹחֵל (*Part.*) → **כָּחַל**.

כֹּחַ • הכח החפץ · the appetitive faculty: Lat. *virtus desiderabilis* (Arab. القوّة الشهوانية) · Constantinus Africanus, *Viaticum peregrinantis* · trans. Do'eg ha-Edomi, *Sefer Ya'ir Netiv* IV.2: ואם הוא מאפיסת הכח החפץ ומכבויו יחרד אליו המאכל אשר אהב כבר ויחרד אליו כל טעם ואינו רוצה לקבל מאומה ולא יתאוה לשום מאכל (If [someone's lack of appetite] is caused by a weak and deficient appetitive faculty, he abhors any tasty food he liked, he does not want to take anything, and has no appetite). Hebr. הכח החפץ does not feature in the current dictionaries. Moses ibn Tibbon translates the parallel Arab. term القوّة الشهوانية as הכח המתאוה.

• כח החפץ · the appetitive faculty Lat. *virtus appetitiva* (Arab. شهوة الغذاء) · Constantinus Africanus, *Viaticum peregrinantis* · trans. Do'eg ha-Edomi, *Sefer Ya'ir Netiv* IV.2: אם הוא סובל צמאון רב ואם אפס כח החפץ ממנו ואם צבעו מכורכם והשתן אדום נתבונן מזה כי האפיסה היא מחום (If the patient suffers from severe thirst, his appetitive faculty is weak, his complexion is yellow, and urine is red, we conclude that the weakness hails from heat). Hebr. כח החפץ does not feature in the current dictionaries. Moses ibn Tibbon translates the parallel Arab. term شهوة الغذاء as תאות המזון.

• הכח הכובש · the retentive faculty: Arab. القوّة الماسكة · Maimonides, *Maqāla fī al-rabw* (*On Asthma*) · trans. Samuel Benveniste, *Ma'amar 'al ha-Qaṣeret* XIII.5 (cf. BMA 2:299, ll. 4–5): ופעמים יהיה סבת הרפיון חולשת הכח הכובש (At other times, that softness [of the stools] is caused by the weakness of the retentive faculty). Hebr. הכח הכובש is not attested in the current dictionaries. The standard term is הכח המחזיק, featuring in the trans. by both Joshua Shabiti and Anonymous (and also in Do'eg ha-Edomi, *Sefer Ya'ir Netiv* V.17 (for Lat. *virtus contentiva*), see entry below). Yet another Hebr. term for Arab. القوّة الماسكة is כח התופס (see also entry below).

• הכח המבשל · the[120] digestive faculty [also called 'the transforming faculty']: Arab. القوّة الهاضمة · Ibn al-Jazzār, *Zād al-musāfir wa-qūt al-ḥādir* · trans. Moses ibn Tibbon, *Sefer Ṣedat ha-Derakhim* V.5: ויתחייב ג"כ שיהיה השקוי מחולשת הכח המבשל כי הנה הפסד הדם אמנם יתילד מחולי הכח הזה כמו שבארנו (Dropsy is necessarily also caused by the weakness of the digestive faculty because the corruption of the blood arises from the affliction of this faculty as I have explained). In the sense of 'the digestive fac-

120 'the digestive faculty [also called 'the transforming faculty']': Cf. M. Ullmann, *Islamic Medicine* (Edinburgh 1978), 61: 'the second transforming faculty is also called the digestive faculty. It turns the nourishment suitable for an organ into the substance of this organ by means of heat and moisture.'

ulty,' Hebr. הכח המבשל is attested in KTP 2:75. Do'eg ha-Edomi translates the parallel Lat. term *virtus mutabilis* as הכח המחליף (see entry below).

• **הכח המחזיק · the retentive faculty**: Lat. *virtus contentiva* (Arab. القوّة الماسكة) · Constantinus Africanus, *Viaticum peregrinantis* · trans. Do'eg ha-Edomi, *Sefer Ya'ir Netiv* v.17: יש אל הכליות חולי הנקרא דיאביטיש מאפיסת הכח המחזיק באשר הסובל יצמא מאד ולא ישבע מים וישתין המים בצבע ובכמות אשר שתה אותם כמו שנראה בחפץ הכלביי (The kidneys may be affected by an illness called 'diabetes' caused by a weakness of the retentive faculty during which the patient suffers from an extreme thirst that cannot be quenched and passes the water in the same color and amount as he drank it. We see the same in the case of canine appetite). Hebr. הכח המחזיק features in KTP 2:75 and in PESHAT.[121] Moses ibn Tibbon translates the parallel Arab. term القوّة الماسكة as הכח המחזיק as well. Other Hebr. terms for Arab. القوّة الماسكة are הכח הכובש and כח התופס (see entries above and below).

• **הכח המחליף · the[122] transforming faculty [also called 'the digestive faculty']**: Lat. *virtus mutabilis* (Arab. القوّة الهاضمة) · Constantinus Africanus, *Viaticum peregrinantis* · trans. Do'eg ha-Edomi, *Sefer Ya'ir Netiv* v.5: אם כן אידרופיסים הוא מאפיסת הכח המחליף לבד כי השחתת הדם יחול מחלישות הכח הזה (For this reason, dropsy is especially caused by the weakness of the transforming (digestive) faculty, for the corruption of the blood is caused by the weakness of this faculty). Hebr. הכח המחליף does not feature in the current dictionaries. A var. reading featuring in *Sefer Ya'ir Netiv* IV.2 is הכח המתחלף (see next entry). Moses ibn Tibbon translates the parallel Arab. term القوّة الهاضمة as הכח המבשל (see entry above).

• **הכח המתחלף · the[123] transforming faculty [also called 'the digestive faculty']**: Lat. *virtus mutabilis* (Arab. القوّة المغيّرة) · Constantinus Africanus, *Viaticum peregrinantis* · trans. Do'eg ha-Edomi, *Sefer Ya'ir Netiv* IV.2: אם הזלת הדם תהיה מאפיסת הכח המתחלף בכבד ומאפיסת השחתת חבורו נראה אם הוא סובל צמאון רב ואם אפס כח החפץ ממנו ואם צבעו מכורכם והשתן אדום נתבובן מזה כי האפיסה היא מחום (If the flow of blood is caused by weakness of the transforming faculty in the liver and by the weakness [and] corruption of its temperament, we should pay attention: If the patient suffers from severe thirst, his appetitive faculty is weak, his complexion is yellow, and urine is red, we conclude that the weakness hails from heat). Hebr. הכח המתחלף does not feature in

121 https://peshat.org/display/peshat_lemmas_00033459 (accessed December 1, 2021).

122 'the transforming faculty [also called 'the digestive faculty']': Cf. Ullmann, *Islamic Medicine*, 61: 'the second transforming faculty is also called the digestive faculty. It turns the nourishment suitable for an organ into the substance of this organ by means of heat and moisture.'

123 'the transforming faculty [also called 'the digestive faculty']': Cf. Ullmann, *Islamic Medicine*, 61: 'the second transforming faculty is also called the digestive faculty. It turns the nourishment suitable for an organ into the substance of this organ by means of heat and moisture.'

the current dictionaries. A var. reading featuring in *Sefer Ya'ir Netiv* v.5. is הכח המחליף (see previous entry). Moses ibn Tibbon translates Arab. القوّة المغيّرة as הכח המשנה (see entry below, also for *Sefer Ṣedat ha-Derakhim* v.5).

• **הכח הפולטת** · **the expulsive faculty**: Lat. [*virtus*] *expulsiva* (Arab. القوّة الدافعة) · Constantinus Africanus, *Viaticum peregrinantis* · trans. Do'eg ha-Edomi, *Sefer Ya'ir Netiv* IV.17: ורבים מהקדמונים אמרו להיות זה החולי מאפיסת הכח הפולטת במעי (Many earlier physicians said that this illness [i.e., a colic] is caused by the weakness of the expulsive faculty in the intestines). In addition to *Part. f.* פּוֹלֶטֶת, Do'eg uses *Part. m.* פּוֹלֵט in his *Sefer Ya'ir Netiv* IV.19: ויגרש אותם הכח הפולט (They are expelled by the expulsive faculty). Hebr. הכח הפולטת is not attested in the current dictionaries. Moses ibn Tibbon translates Arab. القوّة الدافعة with the standard term הכח הדוחה.

• **הכח המשנה** · **the[124] transforming faculty [also called 'the digestive faculty']**: Arab. القوّة المغيّرة · Ibn al-Jazzār, *Zād al-musāfir wa-qūt al-ḥādir* · trans. Moses ibn Tibbon, *Sefer Ṣedat ha-Derakhim* v.5: ונאמר כי גדר השקוי היא טעות יפול בפועל הכח המשנה והוא המבשל אשר בכבד (I say that the definition of dropsy is a defect affecting the activity of the transforming faculty, i.e., the digestive faculty, in the liver). Hebr. הכח המשנה features in KTP 2:76 in the sense of 'assimilierende Kraft.'

• **כח התופס** · **the retentive faculty**: Arab. القوة الماسكة · Ibn al-Jazzār, *Zād al-musāfir wa-qūt al-ḥādir* · trans. Abraham ben Isaac, *Sefer Ṣedah la-Oreḥim* VI.3: דע כי יציאת הזרע וזיבתו תדיר בלא רצון ולא תאוה ולא עינוג יהיה מחמת כחישות כח התופס לדפוסי[125] הזרע (A constant involuntary flow and excretion of sperm, without enjoyment, is caused by weakness of the retentive faculty in the seminal vesicles). Hebr. כח התופס is not attested in the current dictionaries. Moses ibn Tibbon translates Arab. القوة الماسكة as הכח המחזיק and Do'eg ha-Edomi also translates the parallel Lat. term *virtus contentiva* with the standard term הכח המחזיק (see entry above). Another Hebr. term for Arab. القوة الماسكة is הכח הכובש (see also entry above).

כְּחוֹל • *Plur.* **כחולים** · **eye powders; collyria**: Arab. كحل, *Plur.* أكحال · Ibn Zuhr, *K. al-Aghdhiya* · trans. Nathan ha-Me'ati, *Sefer ha-Mezonot*, fol. 5b: ואמנם מרורותיהם הנה הם ימרקו העין ויחזקוהו בבאם בכחולים (But their gallbladder [i.e, of crow, vulture, and kite] cleanses and strengthens the eye when applied as a collyrium). Hebr. *Sing.* כְּחוֹל features in BM 2320 in attestations from the *Sefer ha-Qanun*. Nathan uses the same term, both as *Sing.* כְּחוֹל and *Plur.* כחולים, in his *Sefer ha-Peraqim* (*Pirqei Moshe*) IX.30 (*Sing.*); XXII.48 (*Plur.*) (cf. BMMN 107, l. 3; 215, l. 12; BMMG nos. 4343–4344).

כְּחִישׁוּת · **weakness**: Arab. ضُعْف · Ibn al-Jazzār, *Zād al-musāfir wa-qūt al-ḥādir* · trans.

---

124 'the transforming faculty [also called 'the digestive faculty']': Cf. Ullmann, *Islamic Medicine*, 61: 'the second transforming faculty is also called the digestive faculty. It turns the nourishment suitable for an organ into the substance of this organ by means of heat and moisture.'

125 לדפוסי: emend. ed. דפסי Ms.

Abraham ben Isaac, *Sefer Ṣedah la-Oreḥim* VI.3: דע כי יציאת הזרע וזיבתו תדיר בלא רצון ולא תאוה ולא עינוג יהיה מחמת כחישות כח התופס לדפוסי[126] הזרע (A constant involuntary flow and excretion of sperm, without lust or enjoyment, is caused by weakness of the retentive power in the seminal vesicles). Hebr. כְּחִישׁוּת is not attested in this sense in the current dictionaries. Moses ibn Tibbon translates Arab. ضعف as חולשה and Do'eg ha-Edomi translates the parallel Lat. term *defectio* as אֲפִיסָה (see also *Sefer Ya'ir Netiv* I.25.1 (cf. NM 5:21–22; IJZ 1–2:631)).

כָּחַל • *Part.* **כּוֹחֵל** • *Plur.* **כוחלים** · **(pseudo-)oculists**: Arab. كحّالون ('trained or pseudo-oculists;' cf. WKAS 1:175 and D 2:446) · Maimonides, *Maqāla fī al-rabw* (*On Asthma*) · trans. Samuel Benveniste, *Ma'amar 'al ha-Qaṣeret* XIII.32 (cf. BMA 2:309, ll. 2–3): ואתה רואה דרך בני אדם הבריאים והחולים היאך יסמכו על הספרים להוציא הדם ועל נערים כוחלים לשתות המשלשלים (Nevertheless, you find people, both healthy and sick, who rely on barbers for bloodletting and on young pseudo-oculists for the ingestion of purgatives). Hebr. כָּחַל, *Part.* כּוֹחֵל, only features in the current dictionaries in the sense of 'someone who paints the eyelids' (cf. JD 629; BM 2322–2323). Anonymous renders Arab. كحّالون as כוחלים as well.

כִּיס • **כיס השתן** · **urinary bladder**: Arab. مثانة · Ibn Sīnā, *K. al-Qānūn fī al-ṭibb* · trans. Nathan ha-Me'ati, *Sefer ha-Qanun* II, fol. 74[a]: גואשיר ... ויועיל מההדרוקן הנקרא קולנג וישלשל התערוב הנא ויועיל מחכוך כיס השתן (Opopanax: ... It is useful for colic called QWLNG [i.e., Arab. *qūlanj*] and purges raw humors; it is also good for prurigo of the urinary bladder). Hebr. כיס השתן features in MD 104, s.v. 'bladder.' Zeraḥyah Ḥen translates Arab. مثانة as שלפוחית and Anonymous has מקוה. Synonyms featuring in Hebr. medieval medical literature are כיס המים (cf. BCD 126 (NM 4:80)) and כיס מקוה המים (cf. BCD 127 (NM 1:97)).

• *Plur.* **כיסים** • **כיסי הזרע** · **seminal vesicles**: Arab. أوعية المني · Ibn al-Jazzār, *Zād al-musāfir wa-qūt al-ḥāḍir* · trans. Moses ibn Tibbon, *Sefer Ṣedat ha-Derakhim* VI.3: אולם יציאת הזרע והתמדת הגרתו בלי רצון ובלא הנאה יהיה מחולשת הכח המחזיק בכיסי הזרע (A constant involuntary flow and excretion of sperm, without lust or enjoyment, is caused by weakness of the retentive faculty in the seminal vesicles). Hebr. *Sing.* כיס הזרע features in MD 772, s.v. 'vesicle; seminal;' for other meanings of כִּיס in a medical context, see BCD 126–127. Abraham ben Isaac translates Arab. أوعية المني as דפוסי הזרע (see entry דְּפוּס) and Do'eg ha-Edomi translates the parallel Lat. term *vasa spermatis* as כלי הזרע (see entry כְּלִי).

כיעור → **כִּעוּר**.

כַּךְ • *Plur.* **ככים** · **gums**: Lat. *gingivae* (Arab. لثة) · Gerard de Solo, *Practica super nono Almansoris* · trans. Abraham Avigdor, *Ha-Ma'amar ha-Teshi'i le-Sefer ha-Mansuri le-Razi*, fol. 93[b]: שער בככים הנגר מהם דם (Chapter on bleeding gums). In the sense of

126 לדפוסי: emend. ed. דפסי Ms.

'gums,' Hebrew ככים features in BCD 127 (NM 4:81) in an attestation from Moses ibn Tibbon, *Sefer Ṣedat ha-Derakhim* II.18.1 (for Arab. لثة) (cf. IJZ 1–2:508). Shem Tov ben Isaac translates the same parallel Arab. term لثة as דרדני (see entry).

כֹּל • כל שכן · **especially**: a) Arab. لا سيما · Ibn Sīnā, *K. al-Qānūn fī al-ṭibb* · trans. Zeraḥyah Ḥen, *Sefer ha-Qanun* II, fol. 186[b]: בֶּאדַרוּג' ... מיצו כשיוטף[127] מועיל להגרת דם מן האף כל שכן עם חומץ יין וכמפרא (Sweet basil: ... When one drips its juice [into the nose] it is useful for nosebleeds, especially with wine vinegar and camphor). Hebr. כל שכן is not attested in this sense in the current dictionaries. Nathan ha-Me'ati translates Arab. لا سيما as קל וחומר (see entry קַל).

· b) Arab. خصوصا · Ibn Sīnā, *K. al-Qānūn fī al-ṭibb* · trans. Zeraḥyah Ḥen, *Sefer ha-Qanun* II, fol. 180[a]: בֵּין ... ייפסיק הגרת דם הנחירים בקיבוצו ויהיה נאות לכאב האוזן והקול הנשמע בה כל שכן עם שומן האווז (BeYN [i.e., fruit of the ben oil tree [*Moringa oleifera* Lam.]]: ... It stops nosebleeds because of its astringency. It is good for earache and tinnitus, especially with duck fat). Nathan ha-Me'ati translates Arab. خصوصا as יוֹתֵר (see entry).

כַּלְבִּי • החפץ הכלביי → חֵפֶץ.

• שגעון כלבי → שִׁגָּעוֹן.

כְּלִי • *Plur.* **כלים • כלי הזרע** · **seminal vesicles**: Lat. *vasa spermatis* (Arab. أوعية المني) · Constantinus Africanus, *Viaticum peregrinantis* · trans. Do'eg ha-Edomi, *Sefer Ya'ir Netiv* VI.3: הכח המחזיק העומד בכלי הרע (The retentive faculty in the seminal vesicles). Moses ibn Tibbon translates the parallel Arab. term أوعية المني as כיסי הזרע (see entry כִּיס) and Abraham ben Isaac has דפוסי הזרע (see entry דְּפוּס).

כִּלָּיוֹן · **phthisis**: Arab. سلّ · Ibn Sīnā, *K. al-Qānūn fī al-ṭibb* · trans. Nathan ha-Me'ati, *Sefer ha-Qanun* II, fol. 70[a]: ביץ ביצים ... והמבושל במים הנקרא נמרשת יועיל מהשעול וממורסת הקרום הנקרא שוצה ומהכליון הנקרא צל בערבי (Eggs: ... A [soft] boiled egg called NMRŠT [i.e, Pers. *nīmbirisht*; cf. VL 1393: 'ovum sorbile; semicoctum;' IG 626] is useful for cough, pleurisy called ŠWṢH [i.e., Arab. *shawṣa*], and for phthsis called ṢL [*sill*] in Arab.). In the sense of 'phthisis,' Hebr. כִּליוֹן (and a var. reading כְּלָיָה) features in Anonymous, *Perush Aphorismi shel Apuqraṭ* (*Pirqei Abuqraṭ*) III.29 (135) (BMCH 1:548, l. 19) (resp. I.12 (39) (BMCH 1:523, l. 11)); cf. BCD 128 (NM 3:117–118). A synonymous term for 'phthisis' used by Nathan in his *Sefer ha-Peraqim* (*Pirqei Moshe*) XXII.44 is שִׁדָּפוֹן (cf. BCD 269–270 (NM 2:87); BMMN 215, l. 2; BMMG no. 2442). Zeraḥyah Ḥen translates Arab. سلّ as טיציש (i.e., M. Fr. *tisis*; cf. ND 820, 1105) and Anonymous has טיסי.

כִּלְיִי • חולי כליי → חֹלִי.

127 כשיוטף: emend. ed. למטיף? Ms.

כַּמִּיּוּת · **quantity**: Arab. كمّيّة · Ibn al-Jazzār, *Zād al-musāfir wa-qūt al-ḥādir* · trans. Abraham ben Isaac, *Sefer Ṣedah la-Oreḥim* VI.10: ותהיה הירידה או מחמת כמיותה או מחמת אכיותיה ([Loss of blood occurring to women] can be either caused by its quantity or by its quality). Hebr. כַּמִּיּוּת is a non-attested var. of the standard term כַּמּוּת, which is used by Moses ibn Tibbon and also by Do'eg ha-Edomi for the parallel Lat. term *quantitas*.

כֶּסֶף • סיג הכסף → סִיג.

כִּעוּר · **tattoo(s)**: Arab. وشم · Ibn Sīnā, *K. al-Qānūn fī al-ṭibb* · trans. Nathan ha-Me'ati, *Sefer ha-Qanun* II, fol. 68ᵇ: בלאדר ... העדי: יעקור היבלות ובערבי תאליל ויסיר הצרעת ויעקור הכיעור הנקרא ושם בערבי וירפא מחולי השועל הנולד מליחה לבנה (Marking nut: ... [Its use in] cosmetics: It removes warts called in Arab. T'LYL [i.e., *tha'alīl*] and *baraṣ*,[128] eliminates tattoos, called WŠM [i.e., *washm*] in Arab., and cures alopecia originating from phlegm). Hebr. כִּעוּר is not attested in this sense in the current dictionaries. Zeraḥyah Ḥen translates Arab. وشم as סִמָּן (see entry) and Anonymous has כֶּתֶם (see entry).

כַּף • העורק אשר על הכף בין האצבע הקטן ושכנו → עֹרֶק.

כִּפָּה · **umbel**: Arab. إكليل (Gr. στέφανος; cf. UW 638) · Ibn Sīnā, *K. al-Qānūn fī al-ṭibb* · trans. Nathan ha-Me'ati, *Sefer ha-Qanun* II, fol. 74ᵃ: גואשיר ... והשוק[129] העומד עליו כמו שוק הקשואים ועליו שערות דקות כהות ובערבי זגאב ועליו קטנים מאד ובקווציו כפה עגולה דומה לכפת השבת (Opopanax: ... Its stem is similar to that of a cucumber; it has fine pale hair [called] ZG'B [i.e., *zaghab*] in Arab.; its leaves are very small; its ends have round umbels similar to that of dill). Hebr. כִּפָּה does not feature in this sense in the current dictionaries. Zeraḥyah Ḥen transcribes Arab. إكليل as אכליל (lit., 'crown'), while a marginal gloss reads Hebr. נזר (also lit., 'crown'). The latter term features also in the *Sefer ha-Qanun* by Anonymous (see entry נֵזֶר).

כְּרִיתוּת · **scarification**: Lat. *scarificatio* (Arab. شرط) · Constantinus Africanus, *Viaticum peregrinantis* · trans. Do'eg ha-Edomi, *Sefer Ya'ir Netiv* VI.10: ונניח כוסות המציצה על הדדים ונמשוך הדם בלא כריתות (We apply cupping glasses to the breasts and draw forth blood without scarification). Hebr. כְּרִיתוּת is not attested in this sense in the current dictionaries. Moses ibn Tibbon translates Arab. شرط as סְחִיטָה (see entry).

• חכמת הכריתות → חָכְמָה.

כַּרְכֻּמִי · **bilious; choleric**: Arab. صفراوي · Ibn al-Jazzār, *Zād al-musāfir wa-qūt al-ḥādir* · trans. Moses ibn Tibbon, *Sefer Ṣedat ha-Derakhim* IV.17: והסבות הסוגיות אשר יתילד מהם החולי הזה בזה המעי יחלקו על ז' סבות. הא' שירבה חום אשי כרכומי על הזבל וינגב לחותו עד שייבש ויתאבן ויסתבך וימנע מרדת (There are seven generic causes of this illness. The

---

128 '*baraṣ*' (cf. البرص a): A skin disease that has two varieties, namely white and black. The white variety is perh. identical with *sclerodermia circumscripta*, while the black variety may be *psoriasis vulgaris* or *ichthyosis vulgaris*. Arab. *baraṣ* stands for Gr. λέπρα; cf. UW 97; see also IJZ 7:108–113, esp. 108, n. 195.

129 והשוק העומד עליו כמו שוק: وساقه كالقثاء a.

first is when the fiery, choleric heat increases over the feces and dries it so much that it turns hard, gets stuck, and cannot be passed). In the sense of 'bilious; choleric,' Hebr. כַּרְכְּמִי features in BM 2521 in later attestations only, a.o., from the *Sefer ha-Qanun*. Do'eg ha-Edomi translates the parallel Lat. term *colericus* as אָדֹם (see entry).

כָּרַת · **to scarify, apply scarification**: Lat. *scarifico* · Constantinus Africanus, *Viaticum peregrinantis* · trans. Do'eg ha-Edomi, *Sefer Ya'ir Netiv* VI.9: וכאשר נקיז או נכרות נוציא מעט מהדם וביום האחר נוציא מן הרגל האחר (When we bleed or scarify, we draw only a small amount of blood. The next day, we draw [an equal amount of] blood from the other foot). Hebr. כָּרַת does not feature in this sense in the current dictionaries. A synonymous term used by Do'eg for Lat. *scarifico* is עשה גרשא (in *Sefer Ya'ir Netiv* II.22.4; cf. NM 5:157; IJZ 1–2:651). Actually, Ibn al-Jazzār does not recommend 'scarification' (Arab. شرط), but 'bleeding' (Arab. فصد), which is rendered by Moses ibn Tibbon and Abraham ben Isaac as [נקז], *Hifʿil* הִקִּיז.

כשך · **groats**: Arab. كشك (cf. WKAS 1:221: 'bruised grain soaked in milk and later dried; groats') · Ibn Zuhr, *K. al-Aghdhiya* · trans. Nathan ha-Me'ati, *Sefer ha-Mezonot*, fol. 2b: ואמנם כשך[130] השעורים יקרר בשווי וירטיב וימרק וינקה ויועיל מהקדחות החדות (Barley groats have a moderately cooling effect; they moisten, cleanse, and purify and are good for acute fevers). Hebr. כשך is a non-attested calque of Arab. كشك (*kashk*). In a marginal gloss, the Arab. term is rendered as סב, *Plur.* סובין ('bran') (for the Hebr. term סובין שבראש ('scurf; dandruff; favus'), see entry סב). Nathan also uses כשך in his *Sefer ha-Peraqim* (*Pirqei Moshe*) XXI.9; XXIII.107 (cf. BMMN 196, l. 21; 232, l. 18; BMMG no. 4389).

[כשר] • *Hifʿil* הִכְשִׁיר · **to improve**: Arab. طيّب · Ibn Sīnā, *K. al-Qānūn fī al-ṭibb* · trans. Nathan ha-Me'ati, *Sefer ha-Qanun* II, fol. 96a: כולאנגאן ... העדי יכשיר ריח הפה (Galangal: ... [Its use in] cosmetics: It improves the smell of breath). Hebr. [כשר], *Hifʿil* הִכְשִׁיר, does not feature in this sense in the current dictionaries. In their *Sefer ha-Peraqim* (*Pirqei Moshe*) XXII.68, Nathan and Zeraḥyah Ḥen both translate the same Arab. term طيّب النكهة ('to improve the smell of breath') as ייטיב ריח הפה (cf. BMMN 217, l. 19; BMMZ 215, l. 10; BMMG no. 3199), i.e., use [יטב], *Hifʿil* הֵיטִיב, for Arab. طيّب.

כַּת • *Plur.* כתות · **layers**: Arab. طبقات · Maimonides, *Maqāla fī al-rabw* (*On Asthma*) · trans. Anonymous, *Sefer ha-Qaṣeret* IX.12 (cf. BMA 2:418, ll. 18–20): וכשתנקה האצטומכא בקיא כמו שזכר גאלינוס או במשלשל או בדברים שמטבלים בהם שמתיכים הלחה הלבנה מחללה [או] כשלא יהיו שם לחויות מסובבות בכתותיה היא אז לא תכסף דבר מאותם המאכלים הרעים כולם (And when the stomach is cleansed through vomiting—as Galen mentioned—or through a purgative or through [remedies] that [saturate the stomach] and dissolve the phlegm from its innermost parts when there are no humors stuck in its

130 כשך: סובין Ms1.

layers, it will not crave any of those bad foods). In the sense of 'layers,' Hebr. כַּת, *Plur.* כתות, features in BCD 132 (NM 1:160) in an attestation from Zeraḥyah Ḥen, *Sefer ha-Peraqim* (*Pirqei Moshe*) I.43 (cf. BMMZ 22, l. 22; BMMG no. 3104). Samuel Benveniste translates Arab. طبقات as חלקים and Joshua Shatibi has מפרשים (see entry מִפְרָשׂ).

כְּתִישָׁה · **bruise; contusion:** Arab. رضّ (Gr. θλάσμα; cf. UW 297) · Ibn al-Jazzār, *Zād al-musāfir wa-qūt al-ḥādir* · trans. Moses ibn Tibbon, *Sefer Ṣedat ha-Derakhim* V.3: ואם יקרה לחולה עם המורסא חום בכבד נשקהו בלבשטיאש ובול ארמיני במיץ פלנטאגי או במיץ מורילא. וכל מיני בול יועילו למורסות אשר מדם יקרו בתוך הגוף והרצוץ והחבטה והכתישה ויחבוש בתחבושת צנדל ומה שדומה לזה (If, in addition to the tumor, the patient suffers from heat in the liver, we should give him rose or blossom of the wild pomegranate, Armenian earth, with juice of plantain or of black nightshade. All kinds of earth are good for bodily tumors in the body that originate from blood; [they are also good for] a bruise, shock, and contusion. [The patient] should apply a poultice of sandalwood and the like). Hebr. כְּתִישָׁה features in the current dictionaries in the sense of 'crushing; pounding' (cf. JD 681; BM 2554). In addition to כְּתִישָׁה (for Arab. رضّ) in the sense of 'bruise; contusion,' Moses ibn Tibbon uses the term רִצּוּץ (see entry), which he also uses to translate Arab. وثء.

כֶּתֶם · I. **freckles:** Arab. كلف · Ibn Sīnā, *K. al-Qānūn fī al-ṭibb* · trans. Nathan ha-Me'ati, *Sefer ha-Qanun* II, fols. 69b–70a: בטיך ... העדי: ינקה העור ויותר זרעו ותוכו כמו כן יועיל מהכתם הנקרא כלף ובהק וילפת וקל וחומר כשלשים אותו עם מה שבתוכו כמות שהוא עם שמן חטה ומיבשים אותו בשמש (Melon: ... [Its use in] cosmetics: Particularly, its pulp and seeds clear the skin. It is useful for freckles called KLP [i.e., Arab. *kalaf*], for BHQ [i.e., Arab. *bahaq*[131]], and for dandruff, especially when the pulp is mixed, as it is, in the oil of wheat and warmed up in the sun). Hebr. כֶּתֶם is not attested in the sense of 'freckle(s)' in the current dictionaries. Zeraḥyah Ḥen translates Arab. كلف as סַפַּחַת (see entry) and Anonymous has עדשי הפנים, just like Moses ibn Tibbon in his *Sefer Ṣedat ha-Derakhim* I.0.4 (cf. BCD 197 (NM 4:142); IJZ 1–2:440; see also entry עֲדָשָׁה). A synonym featuring in medieval medical literature, e.g., in Shem Tov ben Isaac's glossary to the *Sefer Almansur*, is נֶתֶק (cf. BCD 182 (NM 2:15); BMZ 18 (Bet 7)).

· II. **tattoo(s):** Arab. وشم · Ibn Sīnā, *K. al-Qānūn fī al-ṭibb* · trans. Anonymous, *Sefer ha-Qanun* II, fol. 50b: בלאדר ... קישוט: מחכך[132] יבלות ומסיר נגע[133] צרעת ועוקר הכתם הנקרא ושם ומבריא מחולי השועל הלבניי (Marking nut: ... [Its use in] cosmetics: It removes[134] warts and *baraṣ*,[135] eliminates tattoos, called WŠM [i.e., Arab. *washm*],

131 '*bahaq*': A skin affection causing white or black spots; the white variety is poss. identical with vitiligo and the black is poss. a kind of melanoderma; cf. IJZ 7:108, n. 196.

132 מחכך (מחתך*): يقطع a.

133 נגע צרעת: البرص a.

134 'removes': Trans. after a.

135 '*baraṣ*' (cf. البرص a): A skin disease that has two varieties, namely white and black. The

and cures alopecia originating from phlegm). Hebr. כֶּתֶם is not attested in this sense in the current dictionaries. Nathan ha-Me'ati translates Arab. وشم as כְּעוֹר (see entry) and Zeraḥyah Ḥen has סִמָּן (see entry).

כֻּתֹּנֶת • *Plur.* **כתנות** · **arils:** Lat. *cupulae* (Arab. جفت) · Constantinus Africanus, *Viaticum peregrinantis* · trans. Do'eg ha-Edomi, *Sefer Ya'ir Netiv* IV.15: ואם יהיה לו טינסמון נרחוץ הנקב בדבר עוצר כמו קלפת רמון בלושטיאש כתנות גלנץ (If he suffers from tenesmus, we wash the anus with astringent ingredients such as pomegranate peels, rose (or blossom) of the wild pomegranate, acorn arils …). Hebr. כֻּתֹּנֶת, *Plur.* כתנות, features in BCD 133 in the sense of 'membranes; tunics,' a.o., for Arab. صفاقات in an attestation from Nathan ha-Me'ati, *Sefer ha-Peraqim* (*Pirqei Moshe*) XXIII.25 (cf. NM 2:55; BMMN 221, l. 11; BMMG no. 2909). Moses ibn Tibbon translates the parallel Arab. term جفت as Rom. קפלץ. A synonymous Hebr. term used by him in his *Sefer Ṣedat ha-Derakhim* VI.10 is כּוֹבַע (see entry).

---

white variety is perh. identical with *sclerodermia circumscripta*, while the black variety may be *psoriasis vulgaris* or *ichthyosis vulgaris*. Arab. *baraṣ* stands for Gr. λέπρα; cf. UW 97; see also IJZ 7:108–113, esp. 108, n. 195.

ל

לֵב • מגנת לב → מְגִנָּה.

לָבָן · **phlegmatic:** Lat. *flegmaticus* (Arab. بلغماني) · Constantinus Africanus, *Viaticum peregrinantis* · trans. Do'eg ha-Edomi, *Sefer Ya'ir Netiv* IV.15: ואם הדישנטריאה תהיה מליחות קרות וגסות ולבנות (If the dysentery originates from cold coarse phlegmatic humors …). In the sense of 'phlegmatic,' Hebr. לָבָן is not attested in the current dictionaries. Moses ibn Tibbon translates the parallel Arab. term بلغماني as לְבָנִי (see entry).

• אלום לבן → אֲלוּם.

לְבָנָה • אבן הלבנה → אֶבֶן.

לְבָנִי · **phlegmatic:** Arab. بلغماني · Ibn al-Jazzār, Zād al-musā*fir wa-qūt al-ḥādir* · trans. Moses ibn Tibbon, *Sefer Ṣedat ha-Derakhim* IV.15: ואם נתילד החמרמרות והנגעים במעים העליונים מליחה עבה לבניית (If the abrasion and the ulcers in the upper intestines originate from a thick phlegmatic humor …). In the sense of 'phlegmatic,' Hebr. לְבָנִי features in BM 2626 in later attestations, a.o., from the *Sefer ha-Qanun* and from Nathan ha-Me'ati, *Sefer ha-Peraqim* (*Pirqei Moshe*) X.24 (as part of the Hebr. term הקדחת הלבניית ('the phlegmatic fever'); cf. BMMN 126, ll. 11–12, 16–17; BMMG no. 1100); see also MD 568, s.v. 'phlegmatic': לְבָנִי. Do'eg ha-Edomi translates the parallel Lat. term *flegmaticus* as לָבָן (see entry).

[להב] • *Hif'il* הִלְהִיב · **to burn:** Lat. *incendo* · Constantinus Africanus, *Viaticum peregrinantis* · trans. Do'eg ha-Edomi, *Sefer Ya'ir Netiv* IV.6: ואם שנוי האסטומכא יהיה מחום לבדו יכבה הצמאון בשתיית המים הקרים ואם יהיה מהליחות האדומות נסגרות באסטומכא ירגיש החולה אחרי שתיית המים מרירות הפה ועשן מלהיב הגרון (If a change in the stomach is caused by heat only, the thirst is quenched by drinking cold water, if it is caused by yellow bile that is retained in the stomach, the patient will—after drinking water—suffer from a bitter taste in the mouth and a burning vapor in the throat). Hebr. *Hif'il* הִלְהִיב features in NM 5:105 in the sense of 'to inflame, cause an inflammation' in the anonymous trans. of Isḥāq ibn Imrān, *Treatise on Melancholy*. In the *Pi'el* conj. לִהֵב, the verb [להב] features in the same sense in Shem Tov ben Isaac, *Sefer ha-Shimmush* XXVII (cf. BCD 135 (NM 4:89)).

לוּז · 1. **pill; suppository (that is shaped like a hazelnut):** Arab. بندقة, *Plur.* بنادق (cf. FAQ 181–182) · Ibn al-Jazzār, *Zād al-musāfir wa-qūt al-ḥādir* · trans. Moses ibn Tibbon, *Sefer Ṣedat ha-Derakhim* VI.11: ויעשה ממנו לוזים בשעור פולים מצריים הלקיחה ממנו לוז עם שלשה אונק' יין מתוק (Make pills [of the mentioned ingredients] weighing one Egyptian[136] bean, and the dose to be taken is one pill with three ounces of sweet wine). Hebr. לוּז (here as *Plur.* לוזים) is not attested in this sense in the current dictionaries. Abraham ben Isaac translates Arab. بنادق as גלולות.

---

136 'Egyptian bean': I.e., 2.34 grams, cf. HIM 10.

‣ I. **the weight of a hazelnut (ca. 3.4 grams)**: Arab. بندقة (cf. MIG no. 164) · Ibn Sīnā, *K. al-Qānūn fī al-ṭibb* · trans. Nathan ha-Me'ati, *Sefer ha-Qanun* II, fol. 74a:[137] גואשיר ... ירכך קשי הרחם ויועיל להזלת השתן וישתה ממנו שיעור לוז במים חמים לשלשול השתן (Opopanax: ... It softens the hardness of the uterus and is useful for strangury. A dose of one hazelnut[138] is taken orally with warm water for diuresis). In the sense of 'the weight of a hazelnut,' Hebr. לוז is not attested in the current dictionaries. Zeraḥyah Ḥen translates Arab. بندقة as לוזה and Anonymous has לוז, just like Nathan.

• **לוז אינדי** ‣ **betel nut** [*Areca catechu* L.]: Arab. فوفل; cf. MIG no. 130: البندق الهندي هو الفوفل (*al-bunduq al-hindī* (lit., 'Indian hazelnut') is the betel nut (*fawfal*)) · Ibn al-Jazzār, *Zād al-musāfir wa-qūt al-ḥādir* · trans. Moses ibn Tibbon, *Sefer Ṣedat ha-Derakhim* V.3: וזה תאר שני השנדלוש המועיל בע"ה מרוחות הכבד המתלהבות ומורסות האצטו׳ החמות יקח ורדים ששה דר׳ זעפראן ושנדל אדום מ"א ב׳ דר׳ שנדל לבן ד׳ דר׳ כאנפור חצי דר׳ והנה יושם בו לוז אינדי ומלוישקל (Recipe of the two kinds of sandalwood that is beneficial, God willing, for blazing hot winds in the liver and hot tumors of the stomach: Take six *dirhams* of roses, two *dirhams* each of saffron and red sandalwood, four *dirhams* of white sandalwood, half a *dirham* of camphor and put into this [mixture] betel nut and common marshmallow). Hebr. לוז אינדי is not attested in the current dictionaries. A var. reading לוז הודי, *Plur.* לוזים הודיים, features in Shem Tov ben Isaac, *Sefer ha-Shimmush* XXIX, list 1 (cf. NM 5:106; SHS 1:300 (Lamed 30)).

לוּלָב • *Plur.* **לולבים** ‣ **shoots**: Arab. عساليج · Maimonides, *Maqāla fī al-rabw* (*On Asthma*) · trans. Samuel Benveniste, *Ma'amar 'al ha-Qaṣeret* IV.4 (cf. BMA 2:256, ll. 3–5): ואם תקח לולבי השומר אחרי שגדלו[139] ורבו ונתקלפו ונתחתכו לבותם ובשל בהם לפי מה שזכרנו יהיה מטעם טוב עוזר לרקק (And if one takes the shoots of fennel once they have[140] grown large and peels them and cuts their hearts and cooks them with it as we have described, it is a dish beneficial and helpful for expectoration). Hebr. לוּלָב is attested in Rabb. literature in the sense of 'sprout,' and esp. *lulav*, i.e., the traditional festive palm branch that is carried and waved during the festival of Sukkoth (cf. JD 698–699; BM 2644). Joshua Shatibi translates Arab. عساليج as שריגים and Anonymous has קלחים (see entry קֶלַח).

לְחִיכָה ‣ **linctus**: Arab. لعوق · Maimonides, *Maqāla fī al-rabw* (*On Asthma*) · trans. Samuel Benveniste, *Ma'amar 'al ha-Qaṣeret* XII.3 (cf. BMA 2:288, ll. 19–21): וזכרו האחרונים אחריו הרכבה אחרת והוא פניגריג ותאנים יבשלו ויסננו המים ויצרף לזה דבש ויעשהו משקה לחיכה (Later physicians mention another compound drug: Cook fenugreek and figs, strain the water, add honey to it, so that the potion becomes a linctus).

---

137 השתן: emend. ed. השעור Ms.

138 'hazelnut' (Arab. *bunduqa*): I.e., 3.4 grams, cf. IG 164.

139 שגדלו ורבו: كبرت وعظمت a.

140 'have grown large': Trans. after a.

In the sense of 'linctus,' Hebr. לְחִיכָה features in NM 5:106–107 in an attestation from Moses ibn Tibbon, *Sefer Ṣedat ha-Derakhim* III.7. Joshua Shatibi translates Arab. لعوق as גְּמִיעָה (see entry) and Anonymous has לְעִיטָה (see entry).

[לחלח] • *Part. Pilpel* **מְלַחְלֵחַ** · **laxative:** Lat. *laxativus* (Arab. مسهّل) · Constantinus Africanus, *Viaticum peregrinantis* · trans. Do'eg ha-Edomi, *Sefer Ya'ir Netiv* V.7: עוגות מלחלחות טובות לכאב הכבד ולסובלי איקטריציאה ולחדוד האדומה ולמוקד העצום ולצמח ([A recipe for] laxative pills, which are good for pain in the liver, for those suffering from jaundice, for sharp yellow bile, for severe burning, and for tumors). Hebr. [לחלח], *Part. Pilpel* מְלַחְלֵחַ, does not feature in this sense in the current dictionaries. For the *Hitpalpel* and *Pulpal* conjs. in the sense of 'to be loose [of bowels],' see BCD 136 (NM 3:121). Moses ibn Tibbon translates Arab. مسهّل as משלשל.

לַיְלָה • **מקרה לילה** → מִקְרֶה.

לִילִית · **nightmare:** Lat. *incubus* (DMLBS 1626) · Gerard de Solo, *Practica super nono Almansoris* · trans. Abraham Avigdor, *Ha-Ma'amar ha-Teshi'i le-Sefer ha-Mansuri le-Razi*, fol. 50ª: שער י״ב בקאבוץ הנקרא משק⟨ר⟩א ולילית (Chapter 12: On Q'BWṢ [i.e., Arab. *kābūs*, 'nightmare'] called MŠQ⟨R⟩' [i.e., Lat. *mascara*[141]] and *lilit*). Hebr. לִילִית does not feature in this sense in the current dictionaries. As a medical term, it features (for Arab. عشا) (corr.) in BCD 137 (NM 4:91) in the sense of 'night blindness' in an attestation from Moses ibn Tibbon, *Sefer Ṣedat ha-Derakhim* II.5.0 (cf. IJZ 1–2:491). For a Hebr. synonym for לִילִית in the sense of 'nightmare,' featuring in Shem Tov ben Isaac, *Sefer Almansur*, cf. entry הסת above.

לְעִיטָה · **linctus:** Arab. لعوق (cf. WKAS 2.2:844: 'medicine to be licked with the tongue; linctus; medicine one allows to melt in the mouth') · Maimonides, *Maqāla fī al-rabw* (*On Asthma*) · trans. Anonymous, *Sefer ha-Qaṣeret* XII.3 (cf. BMA 2:430, ll. 14–16): וכבר זכרו האחרונים אחריו הרכבה אחרת והיא חולבה ותאנים יבשים מבשלין אותן ומסננין המים ומוסיפין אליהן דבש של דבורים ומעמידין אותה לעיטה (Later physicians mention another compound drug: Cook fenugreek and dry figs, strain the water, add bee honey to it, and thicken this until it becomes a linctus). Hebr. לְעִיטָה features in BM 2713 in the sense of 'the ingestion of a medicine' (לקיחת רפואה) in an attestation from the *Sefer ha-Qanun*. Samuel Benveniste translates Arab. لعوق as לְחִיכָה (see entry) and Joshua Shatibi has גְּמִיעָה (see entry). Another synonym, featuring in Zeraḥyah Ḥen, *Sefer ha-Qanun* II is לְקִיקָה (see entry).

לְפִיפָה • *Plur.* **לפיפות** · **membrane (capsule) [of the liver]:** Arab. لفافة (WKAS 2.2: 944) · Ibn Sīnā, *K. al-Qānūn fī al-ṭibb*[142] · trans. Nathan ha-Me'ati, *Sefer ha-Qanun*, Ms Oxford, Bodleian Library, Poc. 353, Uri Heb. 314 (Neubauer 2111), fol. 246ᵇ: לפעמים יהיה מחולשה שלא יסבול מה שיגיע אליו מן המזון ויוזקו בו לפיפותיו וגם יתחדש בתנועות הליחות הגבוליות ויחדשו כובד וכאב בצדדי הכבד (Sometimes [pain in the liver] occurs from

141 '*mascara*': Latin treatises sometimes used the word *mascara* when referring to witches; cf. B.G. Walker, *The Woman's Encyclopedia of Myths and Secrets* (San Francisco 1983), 1077.

142 Cf. ed. Bulaq 1877, 2:367.

weakness as it cannot endure the food that reaches it and that harms its membrane (capsule). Pain can also be caused by the movements of the humors that bring the illness to a crisis and that cause heaviness and pain in the parts of liver).[143] Hebr. לְפִיפָה features in BM 2719 in attestations from the *Sefer ha-Qanun* and is explained by Ben Yehuda as a noun derived from the verb לפף ('to swathe').

לְפִיתָה • לפיתת העצבים · **twisted nerves**: Arab. التواء العصب (Gr. στρέμμα; cf. UW 643) · Ibn Sīnā, *K. al-Qānūn fī al-ṭibb* · trans. Zeraḥyah Ḥen, *Sefer ha-Qanun* II, fol. 191[a]: גֶּוֶז ... עם דבש ורוטה ללפיתת העצבים (Walnut: ... [Walnut mixed] with honey and rue [is beneficial] for twisted nerves). Hebr. לפיתת העצבים is not attested in the current dictionaries. Nathan ha-Me'ati translates Arab. التواء العصب as עוות העצבים (see entry עִוּוּת) and Anonymous has רצוץ העצבים (see entry רְצוּץ).

לָקוּת • לקות הפה · **paralysis of the facial nerve**: Arab. لقوة · Ibn Sīnā, *K. al-Qānūn fī al-ṭibb* · trans. Nathan ha-Me'ati, *Sefer ha-Qanun* II, fol. 68[b]: בלאדר ... יועיל מקור העצב ורפיונו ומההדרוקן[144] הנקרא קולינג׳ ומלקות הפה הנקרא לקוה בערבי (Marking nut: ... It is beneficial for cold and laxity of the nerves, for[145] a colic, called QWLYNĞ [i.e., Arab. *qūlanj*], and for paralysis of the facial nerve, called LQWH [i.e., *laqwa*] in Arab.). In the sense of 'paralysis of the facial nerve,' Hebr. לקות הפה features in BM 2728 in an unexplained attestation from Ibn Zabara, *Sefer ha-Sha'ashu'im*. Zeraḥyah Ḥen translates Arab. لقوة as העוות שבפנים (see entry עִוּוּת) and Anonymous has only לקוה, i.e., the transcription of Arab. لقوة, that is additionally also used by Nathan as an explanation for his Hebr. term. Other synonyms featuring in medieval Hebr. medical literature are: נְטִיָּה (see entry), נטי(י)ת הפה (cf. BCD 174 (NM 1:105–106; 4:112) for attestations from Shem Tov Ben Isaac, *Sefer ha-Shimmush* XXVII and XXX.1.6), עוות הפה (cf. NM 5:145 for an attestation from Abraham ben Isaac, *Sefer Ṣedah la-Oreḥim* I.23.3 (cf. IJZ 1–2:576)), and עקום הפה (see entry עִקּוּם)

לְקִיחָה · **dose**: Arab. شربة (cf. FL 2:407: 'dosis una medicamenti; c.c.g. Avicenn.') · Ibn Sīnā, *K. al-Qānūn fī al-ṭibb* · trans. Zeraḥyah Ḥen, *Sefer ha-Qanun* II, fol. 183[b]: בֵּזֶר קַטוֹנָה שֶׁלִּיו המהות הוא שתי מראים חורפי וקייצי והלקיחה מאיזה מהם שיהיה הוא משקל ב׳ דראהם (Fleawort seed: What is it (*ha-mahut*)?:[146] It is of two types: one growing in summer and another in winter. The dose of each type is two *dirhams*). Hebr. לְקִיחָה is attested in the sense of 'taking; seizing' in Rabb. literature only (cf. JD 719; BM 2735). Nathan ha-Me'ati translates Arab. شربة as מַשְׁקֶה (see entry) and Anonymous has שתייה.

143 The same text is quoted by the copyist of Moses ibn Tibbon, *Sefer Ṣedat ha-Derakhim*, in the same manuscript (Ms Oxford, Bodleian Library, Poc. 353, Uri Heb. 314 (Neubauer 2111), fol. 43[b]).

144 מההדרוקן הנקרא קולינג׳: ومن الفالج a.

145 'for a colic, called QWLYNĞ [i.e., Arab. *qūlanj*]': 'for paralysis' a.

146 See entry מָהוּת.

לְקִיקָה · linctus: Arab. لعوق (FAQ 223–224) · Ibn Sīnā, *K. al-Qānūn fī al-ṭibb* · trans. Zeraḥyah Ḥen, *Sefer ha-Qanun* II, fols. 271ᵇ–272ᵃ: רַאסָן ... יועיל על הרקיקה לקיקה עם דבש (Elecampagne: ... As a linctus with honey it is useful for expectoration). In the sense of 'linctus,' Hebr. לְקִיקָה is attested in BM 2735 in attestations from the *Sefer ha-Qanun*. Nathan ha-Me'ati translates Arab. لعوق as כשמלחכים and Anonymous has לְקִיקָה, just like Nathan. For other synonyms, see entry לְעִיטָה.

לָשׁוֹן • לשון טלה · (lit., 'lamb's tongue'); broadleaf plantain [*Plantago major* L.]: Arab. لسان الحمل (MIG no. 507) · Shem Tov ben Isaac, *Sefer ha-Shimmush* XXIX, list 1 (cf. SHS 1:290–291 (Lamed 12)): לשון טלה ב״ה לסאן אלחמל וב״ל פלנטאג׳י ([Hebr.] *leshon ṭaleh*; Arab. LS'N 'LḤML [i.e., *lisān al-ḥamal*]; o.l. PLNṬ'ǦY [i.e., O. Occ./O. Cat. *plantage*]). In the sense of 'broadleaf plantain,' Hebr. לשון טלה is a non-attested calque of Arab. لسان الحمل. In addition to לשון טלה, we find לשון הכבש (see next entry) and לשון השה (see entry below).

• לשון הכבש · (lit., 'sheep's tongue; lamb's tongue'); broadleaf plantain [*Plantago major* L.]: Arab. لسان الحمل (MIG no. 507) · Maimonides, *K. al-Fuṣūl fī al-ṭibb* (*Medical Aphorisms*) · trans. Zeraḥyah Ḥen, *Sefer ha-Peraqim* (*Pirqei Moshe*) XXI.78 (cf. BMMZ 204, ll. 9–10; BMMG no. 4599): הרפואות הקרות היבשות בשנייה: ... לשון הכבש (Remedies that are cold and dry in the second degree: ... broadleaf plantain). In the sense of 'broadleaf plantain,' Hebr. לשון הכבש is a non-attested calque of Arab. لسان الحمل. The same term occurs in *Shinnui ha-Shemot ha-Niqra'im Synonimi*, fol. 76ᵇ: ולסאן[147] חמל ה׳ לשון הכבש (and LS'N ḤML [i.e., Arab. *lisān* [*al-*]*ḥamal*]; i.e., *leshon ha-keves*). In addition to לשון הכבש, we find לשון טלה (see previous entry) and לשון השה (see entry below).

• לשון עוף · **fruit of the European ash** [*Fraxinus excelsior* L.]: Lat. (Rom.) *lingua ocelli* (*ucelli*) (Arab. لسان العصافير; 'lit., 'sparrow's tongue,' the common Arabic name of the fruit of the ash tree' (MIG no. 505)) · Constantinus Africanus, *Viaticum peregrinantis* · trans. Do'eg ha-Edomi, *Sefer Ya'ir Netiv* VI.1: מרקחת יוחנן מדמשק זה עוזר להרבות המשגל מאד: זנגביל פלפל ארוך ה׳ דרכמ׳ זרע בצלים ... העשב הנקרא לשון עוף (An electuary composed by Ibn Māsawayh, which greatly strengthens sexual lust: Take five *dirhams* each of ginger and long pepper, onion seed, ... the fruit of the tree called 'European ash' ...). Hebr. לשון עוף is not attested in the current dictionaries. Moses ibn Tibbon translates Arab. لسان العصافير as לינגא אויס (i.e., O. Occ.-Lat. *linga/lenga avis*, from L. *lingua avis*) and Abraham ben Isaac has לשון צפורים הנק׳ בלשון ישמעאל לישן אלעצפיר והוא בושם נקרא בושם השם ([Hebr.] *leshon* [*ha-*]*ṣipporim*; called in Arab. LYŠN 'L'ṢPYR [i.e., *lisān al-'aṣāfīr*; cf. MIG no. 505]; i.e., a fragrant herb called *bosem ha-Shem*). For Hebr. לשון הצפורים, cf. BCD 139 (NM 4:93) and for לשון הצפור (and the O.Occ.-Lat. var. לנגא אויס), cf. NM 5:108–109 for an attestation from Shem Tov ben Isaac, *Sefer ha-*

147 ולסאן: emend. ed. ולבן Ms.

Shimmush XXIX, list 1 (SHS 1:286–287 (Lamed 3)). For the Hebr. synonym בושם השם, see entry בֹּשֶׂם.

• **לשון השה · (lit., 'lamb's tongue'); broadleaf plantain [*Plantago major* L.]**: Arab. لسان الحمل (MIG no. 507) · Maimonides, *K. al-Fuṣūl fī al-ṭibb* (*Medical Aphorisms*) · trans. Nathan ha-Me'ati, *Sefer ha-Peraqim* (*Pirqei Moshe*) IX.105 (cf. BMMN 118, ll. 16–18; BMMG no. 4599): מה שיהיה מן הנמלה שיהיה עמה אכול אז יהיו רפואותיה מקרירות ולא מרטיבות כשאר מיני הנמלה אבל יהיה בהם עם קרורם נגוב. והניח עליה תחלה ענפי הגפן וענפי הסנה ולשון השה (The kind of shingles that is associated with corrosion should be treated with remedies that are cooling but not moistening, just like the other kinds of shingles. But next to their cooling [properties], they should have drying [properties]. One should initially apply vine tendrils and offshoots of bramble and broadleaf plantain). Hebr. לשון השה features in BM 2743 in an attestation of this aphorism. In addition to לשון השה, we find לשון טלה and לשון הכבש (see entries above).

מַאֲכָל • תעב מאכל → תָּעַב.
 • תיעוב המאכל → תִּעוּב.
מְאַסֵּף (*Part. Pi'el*) → [אסף].
מְבַטֵּל (*Part. Pi'el*) → [בטל].
מְבֹרָךְ (*Part. Pu'al*) → [ברך].
מְבַשֵּׁל (*Part. Pi'el*) → [בשל].
מְבֻשָּׁל (*Part. Pu'al*) → [בשל].
מְבֻשָּׂם (*Part. Pu'al*) → [בשם].
מְגַדֵּל (*Part. Pi'el*) → [גדל].
מַגִּיעַ (*Part. Hif'il*) → נָגַע.
מְגִנָּה · **fainting**: Arab. غشي · Maimonides, *Maqāla fī al-rabw* (*On Asthma*) · trans. Samuel Benveniste, *Ma'amar 'al ha-Qaṣeret* XIII.33 (cf. BMA 2:310, ll. 1–3): וכבר מנע גאלינוס להקיז מי שזאת תכונתו וכל מי שזה דרכו ⟨ש⟩תקדמנו המגנה בעת ההקזה (Galen has forbidden bloodletting [in the case] of someone in this condition or anyone in a similar condition, because the patient will quickly faint during the act of bloodletting). In the sense of 'fainting,' Hebr. מְגִנָּה is a non-attested semantic borrowing from Arab. غشي; cf. the Biblical term מגנת לב (Lam 3:65) ('covering of heart, i.e., a hard shell about the heart = obstinacy;' BDB 171). Samuel Benveniste explicitly uses the biblical term מגנת לב in his *Ma'amar 'al ha-Qaṣeret* XIII.36 (see next entry). Joshua Shatibi translates Arab. غشي as עלוף and Anonymous has התעלפות.
 • **מגנת לב** · **fainting**: Arab. غشي · Maimonides, *Maqāla fī al-rabw* (*On Asthma*) · trans. Samuel Benveniste, *Ma'amar 'al ha-Qaṣeret* XIII.36 (cf. BMA 2:310, ll. 18–19): ואדע שני אנשים שהיתה מיתתם על ידי רופאים בשביל מגנת לב מצאתם בעד ההרקה (I know of two men whose deaths were caused by physicians on account of fainting that overcame them due to [bleeding]). Hebr. מגנת לב features in the Bible (Lam 3:65) in the sense of 'covering of heart, i.e., a hard shell about the heart = obstinacy' (BDB 171). See also the previous entry מְגִנָּה. In both paragraphs, Joshua Shatibi translates Arab. غشي as עלוף.
מַדְבִּיק (*Part. Hif'il*) → [דבק].
מַדְוֶה • *Plur.* מדוים • הרפואות המתנגדות למדוים → רְפוּאָה.
מַדְרֵגָה • *Plur.* מדרגות • **במדרגות** · **gradually**: Arab. على تدريج · Maimonides, *Maqāla fī al-rabw* (*On Asthma*) · trans. Anonymous, *Sefer ha-Qaṣeret* IX.16 (cf. BMA 2:420, ll. 12–14): ומי שהורגל להקיז או לשתות המשלשל בעתים ידועים צריך לשאת פני הרגלו וירחיק בין העתים ההם מעט מעט וימעט בשיעורי הנקוי במדרגות עד שלא יגיע לימי הזקנה אלא וכבר נפסק הרגל ההקזה והשלשול (If someone is accustomed to bloodletting or to the ingestion of purgatives at fixed times, he should watch his habits [and see] if he can gradually increase the intervals between the fixed times and gradually decrease the evacuated amounts, so that when he reaches old age his habit of bloodletting and using purgatives has ceased). Hebr. במדרגות is not attested in the current dictionaries. A var.

reading על מדרגות features in BCD 142 (NM 4:95) in an attestation from Moses ibn Tibbon, *Sefer Ṣedat ha-Derakhim* I.22.5 (cf. IJZ 1–2:476). Samuel Benveniste translates Arab. على تدريج as דרגה דרגה (see entry דַּרְגָּה) and Joshua Shatibi has בהדרגה (see entry הַדְרָגָה).

מָהוּת · **'what is it?'**: Arab. ماهية · Ibn Sīnā, *K. al-Qānūn fī al-ṭibb* · trans. Nathan ha-Me'ati, *Sefer ha-Qanun* II, fol. 61[a]: אניסון המהות הוא זרע השומר הרומי (Anise: What is it (*ha-mahut*)? It is the seed of Roman fennel). The term מָהוּת is a translation of Arab. ماهية, which in philosophical literature refers to the essence of the thing. It recurs throughout Ibn Sīnā's alphabetical list of plants and their properties, followed by هو. It seems that in this context a literal interpretation ('what is it?') is called for.[148] The literal trans. *quid est* can also be found throughout Gerard de Cremona, *Liber Canonis* (ed. Venice 1507). Zeraḥyah Ḥen and Anonymous both translate Arab. ماهية as מָהוּת as well.

מוֹהַל · **juice; sap**: Lat. *sucus* · *Shinnui Shemot ha-Niqra Ṣinonimas* (Ms Leiden, Universiteitsbibliotheek, Cod. Or. 4732/1 (SCAL 15)),[149] fol. 8[a]: סוקוש לקרוצי הוא מוהל שלו (SWQWŠ LQRWṢY [i.e., Lat. *sucus licorucie* (read: *licoricie*)]; i.e., its juice [i.e., juice of licorice]). Hebr. מוֹהַל is only attested in Rabb. literature (cf. JD 739; LW 3:39: 'Saft; das Flüssige, Ausgeschwitzte, das aus Früchten fliesst;' BM 2830) and in medieval literature in the sense of 'moist cheese' (BM 2830).

מוח → מֹחַ.

מוֹךְ · **vaginal suppository (pessary)**: Arab. صوفة (lit., 'wool') (Gr. πέσσος; cf. the definition in Paul of Aegina, *Epitomes iatrikes biblia hepta* III.61 (cf. PAE 1:276, l. 17): πέσσος δέ ἐστιν ἔριον διεξασμένον ('a pessary consists of carded wool')) · Ibn al-Jazzār, *Zād al-musāfir wa-qūt al-ḥādir* · trans. Moses ibn Tibbon, *Sefer Ṣedat ha-Derakhim* VI.9: ג"כ כשיעצר נדותה חצי דר׳ קשטורן עם מי פוליג קרה או תשתה חצי דר׳ קלפת קשיא ליניא שחוקה במי פולייג או תכניסה במוך מלמטה (When the menstrual blood of a woman is retained, one can also administer her half a *dirham* of castor with cold mint juice, or let her take rinds of cinnamon pounded with mint juice. She may also insert it with a vaginal suppository (pessary)). Hebr. מוֹךְ is attested in Rabb. literature (cf. JD 741: 'a soft, spongy substance; hackled wool; rag; lint; etc.'); inserted into the vagina, it was used as a sort of tampon to prevent pregnancy (cf. ShMM 488–489). In his commentary on bShab 47, Rashi remarks that the term applies to anything soft as, e.g., cotton (כל דבר רך קרוי מוכין כגון צמר גפן) (cf. KA 5:132). In the *Sefer Ahavat Nashim* it is, a.o.,

148 Cf. S.M. Afnan, *A Philosophical Lexicon in Persian and Arabic* (Beirut 1968), 274: s.v. ما هو: 'what is it?'.

149 For the Ms and entry מוֹהַל, see G. Bos and Kl.-D. Fischer (eds.), *A Glimpse into Medical Practice among Jews around 1500: Latin-German Pharmaceutical Glossaries in Hebrew Characters extant in Ms Leiden, Universiteitsbibliotheek, Cod. Or. 4732/1 (SCAL 15), fols. 1[a]–17[b]* (Leiden 2021), 3–4, and esp. 30 (entry 269).

used in a magical procedure to prevent a man from having intercourse with another woman besides his wife (CN 114–115). Ibn Tibbon also uses Hebr. מוֹךְ in the sense of 'a piece of cotton' (for Arab. قطنة) in his *Sefer Ṣedat ha-Derakhim* I.17.6 (cf. NM 5:113; IJZ 1–2:468). Abraham ben Isaac translates Arab. صوفة as צֶמֶר (see entry).

• **תשומת מוך** → תשוּמָה.

מוֹסִיף (*Part. Hifʿil*) → [יסף].

מוּסָף (*Part. Hofʿal*) → [יסף].

מוֹצָא • **anus:** Arab. مخرج • Ibn al-Jazzār, *Zād al-musāfir wa-qūt al-ḥāḍir* • trans. Moses ibn Tibbon, *Sefer Ṣedat ha-Derakhim* IV.15: ואם יהיה במעים השפלים נרפא החולה בקלוחים וזה לקורבת אלו המעים מהמוצא (If it [i.e., the cause of dysentery] is in the lower intestines, we treat the patient with clysters because of the proximity of these intestines to the anus). In the sense of 'anus,' Hebr. מוֹצָא features in BCD 143 (NM 1:28) in an attestation from Hillel ben Samuel, *Sefer Keritut*. Do'eg ha-Edomi translates the parallel Lat. term *anus* as נֶקֶב (see entry).

מוֹצִיא (*Part. Hifʿil*) → יָצָא.

מוֹקֵד • **burning:** Lat. *arsura* (Arab. لذع) • Constantinus Africanus, *Viaticum peregrinantis* • trans. Do'eg ha-Edomi, *Sefer Ya'ir Netiv* V.13: ואם המוקד מתארך בשתן אחרי שנטהר הבלוי והנגע נתן לו חלב הפרה (When there is still a burning [feeling] during urination once we removed the pus and cleaned the wound, we give [the patient] cow's milk). Hebr. מוֹקֵד is also used by Do'eg in the sense of 'fire; heat' (for Lat. *ardor*) in his *Sefer Ya'ir Netiv* II.4.4 (cf. NM 5:113; IJZ 1–2:637) Moses ibn Tibbon translates the parallel Arab. term لذع as עקיצה.

מוקדם → מֻקְדָּם.

מורגל → מֻרְגָּל.

מורקא (*Aram.*) • **shreds (of intestinal tissue):** Arab. خراطة • Ibn al-Jazzār, *Zād al-musāfir wa-qūt al-ḥāḍir* • trans. Moses ibn Tibbon, *Sefer Ṣedat ha-Derakhim* IV.15: ואח"כ תצא הצואה נקיה מן הדם והגרידה הוא מורקא (Then the excrements will come out free from blood and intestinal shreds). Aram. מורקא features in KA 5:261, s.v. מרוקא, in the sense of 'unripe dates' and 'dregs; lees; sediment' (foll. Perles); in LF 2:340 as 'date kernel (used for smoothing pergament)' (foll. R. Ḥananel); and as מוריקא or מרוקא in LW 3:260 in the sense of 'Dattelkern' or 'Crocus.' Sokoloff (SDA 667) states that its meaning is uncertain. The term מורקא also features in Shem Tov ben Isaac, *Sefer ha-Shimmush* XXIX, list 2 (SHS 2, forthcoming (Mem 34)): מורקא או פגלאדא וב"ה דרדי וב"ח דורדיא (MWRQ' or PGL'D' and in Arab. DRDY [i.e., *durdī*; 'dregs; lees; sediment'] and in Bibl. Hebr. DWRDY').

מורתח → מֻרְתָּח.

מושלג → מֻשְׁלָג.

מְזוּיָּף (*Part. Puʿal*) → [זיף].

מִזְרָק • *Plur.* **מזרקים** • **arteries:** Arab. شريان, *Plur.* شرايين • Maimonides, *Maqāla fī al-rabw* (*On Asthma*) • trans. Anonymous, *Sefer ha-Qaṣeret* XIII.1 (cf. BMA 2:437, ll. 6–7): ואד

הדם המצוי בלב ובמזרקים שלו יקרא הרוח החיוני (The vapor of the blood found in the heart and the arteries is called 'vital pneuma'). Hebr. מִזְרָק, *Plur.* מזרקים, features in BCD 144 (NM 4:96–97) (corr. in PESHAT[150]) for Arab. مجار in the sense of 'passages (blood vessels)' in an attestation from Shem Tov ben Isaac's *Sefer ha-Shimmush* XXVII. Samuel Benveniste transcribes Arab. شرايين as שריאן, as does Joshua Shabiti, but with an additional Hebr. *Plur.* ending (-ים): שריינים.

מֹחַ • מורסות קרומי המוח → מֻרְסָה.

מַחֲבוֹא • *Plur.* **מחבואים** · **cavity**: Arab. فضاء · Maimonides, *Maqāla fī al-rabw* (*On Asthma*) · trans. Joshua Shatibi, *Ma'amar 'al ha-Qaṣeret* IX.13 (cf. BMA 2:350, ll. 13–14): ואני לא אדע הרגלו בזה ואם הוא נקל עליו יעשהו כפי הרגלו והאופן המפורסם אצלינו לנקות מחבואי האצטומכה והקיא מזה המותר הוא זה (I do not know the habit of [my Master concerning vomiting]. If it is easy for you, do it in your usual manner. Our common way of purifying the cavity of the stomach and vomiting the superfluity it contains is this ...). Hebr. מַחֲבוֹא, *Plur.* מחבואים, does not feature in this sense in the current dictionaries. Samuel Benveniste and Anonymous both render Arab. فضاء as חָלָל (cf. BCD 99 (NM 3:87) for an attestation from Moses ibn Tibbon, *Perush Aphorismi shel Apuqraṭ* (*Pirqei Abuqraṭ*) VII.38 (390) (cf. BMCH 1:412, l. 1)).

מְחַבֵּר (*Part. Pi'el*) → [חבר].

מָחָה • *Inf. Qal* **לִמְחוֹת** · **to dissolve**: Arab. تحليل · Maimonides, *Maqāla fī al-rabw* (*On Asthma*) · trans. Samuel Benveniste, *Ma'amar 'al ha-Qaṣeret* II.1 (cf. BMA 2:247, ll. 13–14): ואם ירצה הרופא לדקקם שמה ולמחותם הוצרך לרפואות חזקות או זמן מרובה או כלם (When a physician wants to dilute and dissolve [the superfluities that are stuck in a weak organ], he needs strong drugs or a long period [of time for treatment] or both). In the sense of 'to dissolve,' Hebr. מָחָה is only attested in Rabb. literature (cf. JD 759; BM 2900–2901). Cf. NM 5:115 for the *Hif'il* conj. הִמְחָה in the sense of 'to dissolve' (for Arab. حلّ) in Moses ibn Tibbon, *Sefer Ṣedat ha-Derakhim* III.6. Joshua Shatibi translates Arab. تحليل as לחולל.

• *Nif'al* **נִמְחָה** · **to be dissolved**: Arab. تحلّل · Maimonides, *Maqāla fī al-rabw* (*On Asthma*) · trans. Samuel Benveniste, *Ma'amar 'al ha-Qaṣeret* II.1 (cf. BMA 2:247, ll. 6–8): וסבת זה מבוארת והוא שהמסעדים אם נתעכלו באברים והיה שארית העכול השלישי בהם מעט לא מדבק ולא עבה נמחה מחוי קל[151] ויצא בהבלי⟨ם⟩ ובזיעה (The reason for this is clear—namely, that, when foods are digested in the organs and when the superfluity from the third digestion is minimal and is not sticky or thick, they are easily[152] dissolved and leave [the body] through evaporation and perspiration). In the sense of 'to be dissolved,' Hebr. *Nif'al* נִמְחָה is only attested in Rabb. literature (cf. JD 759; BM 2901).

150 https://peshat.org/display/peshat_lemmas_00086310 (accessed April 4, 2022).
151 קל (خفيفا): خفيا a.
152 'easily': 'in a hidden way' a.

Joshua Shatibi translates Arab. تحلّل as נמס, and Anonymous has הִתְחוֹלֵל (see entry [חלל]).

מְחוּי · **dissolution**: Arab. تحليل · Maimonides, *Maqāla fī al-rabw* (*On Asthma*) · trans. Samuel Benveniste, *Ma'amar 'al ha-Qaṣeret* II.1 (cf. BMA 2:247, ll. 6–8): וסבת זה מבוארת והוא שהמסעדים אם נתעכלו באברים והיה שארית העכול השלישי בהם מעט לא מדבק ולא עבה נמחה מחוי קל[153] ויצא בהבלי⟨ם⟩ ובזיעה (The reason for this is clear—namely, that, when foods are digested in the organs and when the superfluity from the third digestion is minimal and is not sticky or thick, they are easily[154] dissolved and leave [the body] through evaporation and perspiration). Hebr. מְחוּי is attested for in Rabb. literature in the sense of 'cleansing' (cf. JD 772; BM 2903). Joshua Shatibi translates Arab. تحليل as התכה and Anonymous has חלילות.

מַחְזִיק (*Part. Hif'il*) → [חזק].

מְחִיצָה • **המחיצה המחברת** · **conjunctiva**: Lat. *coniunctiva* · Gerard de Solo, *Practica super nono Almansoris* · trans. Abraham Avigdor, *Ha-Ma'amar ha-Teshi'i le-Sefer ha-Mansuri le-Razi*, fol. fol. 68[b]: ונאמר כי הנגעים המתהווים במחיצה המחברת הוא לובן העין אינם מפחדים כמו המתהוים בקרנית (Let us say that the tumors that arise in the conjunctiva that [covers] the white of the eye (sclera) are not as frightening as those that arise in the cornea). Hebr. המחיצה המחברת does not feature in the current dictionaries. For the synonymous חוברת, cf. KDS 93. Abraham Avigdor calls the 'conjunctiva' מִתְחַבֶּרֶת (see entry [חבר]).

מַחֲלִיף (*Part. Hif'il*) → [חלף].

מַחֲלִיק (*Part. Hif'il*) → [חלק].

מַחְשָׁבָה • **חרדת המחשבה** → חֲרָדָה.

מַטָּה • **למטה מן** · **less than**: Arab. دون · Ibn Zuhr, *K. al-Aghdhiya* · trans. Nathan ha-Me'ati, *Sefer ha-Mezonot*, fol. 3[a]: ואולם לחם הזרעונים הנה הוא הנכון[155] שבהם אחר החטה והשעורה ויזון מאד מוסיף בזרע בכח חזק וממהר הקושי ורוחותיו הם למטה מרוחות הפולים מאד (Bread from chickpeas is best after wheat bread and barley bread; it is very nutritious, it greatly increases the sperm, it gives a quick erection, and it is much less flatulent than beans). In the sense of 'less than,' Hebr. למטה מן only features in the current dictionaries in attestations from the Bible; cf. BM 2941.

מיוחד → מְיֻחָד.

מְיֻחָד (*Part. Pu'al*) → [יחד].

מַיִם • **המים הנוזלים בעין** · **cataract**: Arab. الماء النازل في العين · al-Rāzī, *K. al-Manṣūrī fī al-ṭibb* · trans. Shem Tov ben Isaac, *Sefer Almansur*, fol. 3[b]: כ״ו במים הנוזלים בעין ([Bk. 9, ch.] 26: On cataract). Hebr. המים הנוזלים בעין does not feature in the current dictionaries. The same term is also used by Abraham Avigdor (for the parallel Lat. term *catharacta*).

---

153 קל (خفيفا): خفيا a.

154 'easily': 'in a hidden way' a.

155 הנכון: أصلح a.

For the synonym מים בעין, featuring in Rabb. literature, cf. BM 2967–2968. Another term, a.o., used by Shem Tov in his glossary to the *Sefer Almansur* (cf. BMZ 54 (Mem 17)) is ירידת המים (cf. BCD 120 (NM 2:13)). Yet another var. ירידת המים בעין features (for Arab. نزول الماء في العين) in the *Sefer ha-Peraqim* (*Pirqei Moshe*) XX.48 by both Nathan ha-Me'ati (cf. BMMN 215, ll. 11–12) and Zeraḥyah Ḥen (cf. BMMZ 213, l. 1) (cf. also BMMG no. 5108 and BCD 121 (NM 1:155–156, corr. 4:229; 4:77) for further attestations).
• סיד שלא נגע בו מים → סִיד.

מִיץ • מיץ חלב · **whey**: Lat. *serum* (Arab. ماء الجبن) · Constantinus Africanus, *Viaticum peregrinantis* · trans. Do'eg ha-Edomi, *Sefer Ya'ir Netiv* IV.17: ונתן לו מיץ חלב עזים הוא שיר עם אלואין רחוץ ועם אשקמוניא מבושלת ונעשה אליו תשומת מוך הוא פשיארי מן ויאולא ומלח ודבש גם אשקמוניא (We administer him [i.e., a colic patient] whey prepared from goat's milk, i.e., [Lat.] ŠYR[WM], with washed aloe and boiled scammony, and we apply a suppository, i.e., [Lat.] PŠY'RY, of violets, salt, honey, and also scammony). In the sense of 'whey,' Hebr. מיץ חלב features in BCD 148 (NM 1:71) in a later attestation from Moses ibn Tibbon, *Sefer Ṣedat ha-Derakhim* VII.9.7 (cf. IJZ 7:140, l. 6). In the paragraph quoted here, Moses ibn Tibbon translates the parallel Arab. term ماء الجبن as חלב. In his *Sefer Ya'ir Netiv* V.5, Do'eg translates the same Lat. term *serum* with a var. reading המיץ היוצא מן החלב (see next entry).
• המיץ היוצא מן החלב · **whey**: Lat. *serum* (Arab. ماء الجبن) · Constantinus Africanus, *Viaticum peregrinantis* · trans. Do'eg ha-Edomi, *Sefer Ya'ir Netiv* V.5: השלישית המטהרת המים האלה היא חלב הגמלים והשתן שלהם והמיץ היוצא מן החלב (The third [kind of remedients] that cleanse the [yellowish water in the case of dropsy] is milk or urine of a camel and whey). Hebr. המיץ היוצא מן החלב is not attested in the current dictionaries. For a var. reading מיץ חלב, see previous entry. Here, Moses ibn Tibbon translates the parallel Arab. term ماء الجبن also as מיץ חלב (cf. BCD 148 (NM 1:71) for an attestation from *Sefer Ṣedat ha-Derakhim* VII.9.7 (cf. IJZ 7:140, l. 6)).

מַכְבֵּד • *Plur.* **מכבדות** · **brooms** · [*Synonima*], Ms Vatican, Biblioteca Apostolica, ebr. 550, fol. 115b: גמאד (*גמאר) הוא חריות הדקל מהם עושים מכבדות (GM'R [i.e., Arab. *jummār*]; i.e., palm branches from which brooms are made). Hebr. מַכְבֵּד, *Plur.* מכבדות, is only attested in Rabb. literature (cf. JD 780–781; BM 2984).

מְכֻבָּה (*Part. Pu'al*) → [כבה].

מכובה → מְכֻבָּה.

מַכְתֶּשֶׁת · **mortar**: Arab. مهراس · Ibn al-Jazzār, *Zād al-musāfir wa-qūt al-ḥādir* · trans. Moses ibn Tibbon, *Sefer Ṣedat ha-Derakhim* V.11: ויכתשהו במכתשת בעלי עם פיניגריג וחרדל וקמח שעורים ויערבם בשמן אניט או שמן קמומילא או שמן זנברי ויניחהו עד שישוב כמו אספלנית ויקח ממנו ויטוח על הטחול ועל מורסות בכל מקום שיהיה מן הגוף הנה הוא מועיל חזק התועלת בע"ה (And [if] one pounds [these ingredients] with a pestle in a mortar with fenugreek, mustard, and barley flour, and mixes it with dill oil, camomile oil, or jasmine oil, and leaves it alone until it turns into a salve and takes some of it and rubs it on the spleen or on a tumor in any spot of the body, it is very beneficial, God willing). Hebr. מַכְתֶּשֶׁת features in the current dictionaries in attestations from Rabb. and modern literature only (cf. BM 3003; EM 940).

[מלא] • *Part. Puʿal* מְמֻלָּא · **solid; compact**: Arab. مكتنز · Ibn Sīnā, *K. al-Qānūn fī al-ṭibb* · trans. Nathan ha-Me'ati, *Sefer ha-Qanun* II, fol. 72ᵃ: בסבאיג ... המשובח שבו הוא אשר כגוון פסתק מבפנים העבה כאצבע קטן הנוטה אל האודם והכרכמות והממולא והטרי אשר בו מרירות ומתיקות עם עפיצות ובטעמו טעם קרנפלי (Polypody: ... The best is that which has the same color as pistachio on the inside, which is as thick as an index finger, somewhat red or saffron-like, compact, fresh, bitter but also sweet and acrid, tasting somewhat like a clove). Hebr. [מלא], *Part. Puʿal* מְמֻלָּא, is not attested in this sense in the current dictionaries. Anonymous has מקשיי (cf. BCD 160 (NM 3:141–142)) for מְקֻשִּׁי in the sense of 'dense' (for Arab. متكاثف) in an attestation from Anonymous, *Perush Aphorismi shel Apuqraṭ* (*Pirqei Abuqraṭ*) V.62 (282) (cf. BMCH 1:580, l. 8).

מִלּוּי • **מלוי הראש** · **rheum**: Arab. زكام · Ibn Sīnā, *K. al-Qānūn fī al-ṭibb* · trans. Nathan ha-Me'ati, *Sefer ha-Qanun* II, fol. 70ᵃ: ביץ ביצים ... ויועיל ממלוי הראש הנקרא זכאם (Eggs: ... They are useful for rheum called ZK'M [i.e., Arab, *zukām*]). Hebr. מלוי הראש is not attested in the current dictionaries. Zeraḥyah Ḥen translates Arab. زكام as רֵיוּמָא (i.e., Lat. *rheuma*) and Anonymous transcribes Arab. زكام as זכאם only.

מֶלַח • **מלח ספירית** · **rock salt**: Arab. الملح الأندراني (cf. IG 568) (O. Occ., O. Cat., or L. Lat. *salgema*/*sal gema*/*salgemma*; cf. SHS 1:331 (Mem 60)) · Ibn Sīnā, *K. al-Qānūn fī al-ṭibb* · trans. Zeraḥyah Ḥen, *Sefer ha-Qanun* II, fols. 274ᵇ–275ᵃ: החבלות: ... שֶׁב אלום עם שמרי היין כמוהו אלום מיבש לנגעים הקשים לרפאת והמתאכלות עם כמוהו מלח ספירית ושרפת האש (ŠeB; [i.e., Arab. *shabb*]; 'LWM [i.e., Rom. *alum*]: ... Ulcers: Alum with an equal amount of the dregs of wine dries ulcers that are hard to cure. With an equal amount of rock salt, it is also beneficial for corroded ulcers and for burns). In the sense of 'rock salt,' Hebr. מלח ספירית is a non-attested calque of O. Occ./O. Cat./L. Lat. *salgema*/*sal gema*/*salgemma*. Nathan ha-Me'ati translates Arab. الملح الأندراني as מלח אנדראני.

• **מלח העסה** · **baking salt; bread salt**: Arab. ملح العجين (cf. NA 586, s.v. ملح العجين: 'salt used in bread making because it has a mild flavor; also called ملح الخبز (bread salt) and ملح سبخي; i.e. gathered from *sabkha* (salt marsh);' see also D 1:625, s.v. ملح سباخي: 'du sel tel qu'on en tire des plaines; marécages ou lacs salés qu'on nomme سبخة;' IBF no. 2164) · Ibn al-Jazzār, *Zād al-musāfir wa-qūt al-ḥādir* · trans. Moses ibn Tibbon, *Sefer Ṣedat ha-Derakhim* IV.17: ויעשה לו פתילות יורידו מרה כרכומית ויהיו על התואר הזה: יקח ויאולש דר' מלח העסה כמוהו וידקו ויעורבו עם כמותם עם דבש קשה הנקפא (One should prepare pastilles for him [i.e., the patient suffering from a colic], which bring down the yellow bile and are prepared as follows: Take one *dirham* of violets and baking salt; pound it and mix it with an equal amount of crystallized solid honey). Hebr. מלח העסה is not attested in the current dictionaries. Do'eg ha-Edomi translates the parallel Lat. term *sal communis* as מלח ('salt') only.

מְלַחְלֵחַ (*Part. Pilpel*) → [**לחלח**].

[מלט] • *Part. Nif'al* **נִמְלָט** • **הנמלטים מחולי** · **convalescents:** Arab. الناقهون · Ibn Zuhr, *K. al-Aghdhiya* · trans. Nathan ha-Me'ati, *Sefer ha-Mezonot*, fol. 4[a]: ובשר התרנגלת מתקן ענין החלושים הנמלטים מחולי (Chicken meat strengthens weak persons [and] convalescents). In the sense of 'convalescent,' Hebr. *Sing.* הנמלט מחולי features in BCD 151 (NM 2:67) in an attestation from Nathan's *Sefer ha-Peraqim* (*Pirqei Moshe*) III.71 (cf. BMMN 50, ll. 7–8; BMMG no. 5275).

מְלִיחוּת · **saltiness:** Lat. *salsugo* (Arab. ملوحة) · Constantinus Africanus, *Viaticum peregrinantis* · trans. Do'eg ha-Edomi, *Sefer Ya'ir Netiv* IV.15: או מהלבנה המלוחה או מחודדת ובמליחותה עושה זה הדבר עצמו למעי כמו שנראה במלאכת הניטרי או בלבנה הזכוכית (It [i.e., excoriation (abrasion) of the intestines] may also be caused by sharp salty phlegm, by the very effect of its saltiness on the intestines, as we can see from the effect of borax (sodium borate). It may also be caused by vitreous phlegm). Hebr. מְלִיחוּת is not attested in medical literature, cf. BM 3039 (featuring attestations from Judah Abrabanel and Nachmanides). Moses ibn Tibbon translates the parallel Arab. term ملوحة as מְלִיחוּת as well.

ממולא → מְמֻלָּא.

מְמֻלָּא (*Part. Pu'al*) → **[מלא]**.

מֶמְשָׁלָה · I. **power; strength:** Lat. *potestas* (Arab. قوّة) · Constantinus Africanus, *Viaticum peregrinantis* · trans. Do'eg ha-Edomi, *Sefer Ya'ir Netiv* IV.6: וצמאון האסטומכא יגדל בשני ענינים כפי איכות כמו אם יסבול המוקד והרתיחה כמו שנראה בסובלי הקדחות ואשר לוקחים המאכלים והמשקים חמים בממשלה (Thirst [originating from] the stomach becomes more severe for two reasons: [one,] because of the quality [of the food], as happens when [the patient] suffers from severe heat as we see in those who suffer from fever and who take food and drink that are strongly heating [lit., 'that have heating power']). Hebr. מֶמְשָׁלָה does not feature in a medical context in the current dictionaries. Moses ibn Tibbon translates Arab. قوّة as כח.

· II. **domination:** Lat. *dominatio* (Arab. غلبة)· Constantinus Africanus, *Viaticum peregrinantis* · trans. Do'eg ha-Edomi, *Sefer Ya'ir Netiv* IV.7: והרוח הוא מאפיסת האסטומכא ואפיסת האסטומכא הוא מחבור רע או ממשלת ליחות רעות ([The cause of the] wind [in the case of eructation] is the weakness of the stomach and the weakness of the stomach is caused by a bad temperament or by the domination of bad humors). Moses ibn Tibbon translates the parallel Arab. term غلبة as התגבר.

מְנַגֵּעַ (*Part. Pi'el*) → **נָגַע**.

מְנֻגָּע (*Part. Pu'al*) → **נָגַע**.

מנוגע → מְנֻגָּע.

מנוקה → מְנֻקֶּה.

מְנֻקֶּה (*Part. Pu'al*) → **[נקה]**.

מְסוּבָּךְ (*Part. Pu'al*) → **[סבך]**.

מִסְנֶנֶת · **ethmoid bone:** Arab. مصفاة (cf. DKT 828) · Ibn Sīnā, *K. al-Qānūn fī al-ṭibb* · trans. Zeraḥyah Ḥen, *Sefer ha-Qanun* II, fol. 223[b]: ומסגולותיו להתיר הרוחות מן הנחירים

ויועיל מסתימת הנשימה שבאף מפני היותו פותח לסתימת המסננת בכח (One of its specific properties is to dissolve winds from the nostrils; it is also useful for the obstruction of breathing through the nose. This is achieved by forcefully removing obstructions from the ethmoid bone). Hebr. מְסַנֶּנֶת features in BCD 153 (NM 4:101) as מסננת האף in the sense of 'lamina cribrosa (the cribriform plate of the ethmoid bone)' in an attestation from Abraham Avigdor, *Pirqei Arnavṭ de-Vila Nova* V.22 (AMP 88). Shem Tov ben Isaac renders Arab. العظام المتخلخلة ('ethmoid bones') as העצמים הספוגיים in his *Sefer ha-Shimmush* XXX.2.24 (cf. BCD 210 (NM 1:107)). Nathan ha-Me'ati renders Arab. مصفاة as העצם המסנן.

מִסְעָד • *Plur.* **מסעדים** • **treatments**: Arab. علاجات • Maimonides, *Maqāla fī al-rabw* (*On Asthma*) • trans. Samuel Benveniste, *Ma'amar 'al ha-Qaṣeret* XIII.18 (cf. BMA 2:303, ll. 6–8): וזרזתי עצמי אחר כן בהשגחה ובחריצות כשארצה לסעד החולה במין ממיני המסעדים החזקים שאתבונן ביני ובין עצמי תחלה באחרית הסעד ההוא (From then on I was extremely careful, whenever I wanted to give a patient a strong kind of treatment, that I myself first understood the effect of such a treatment). In a medical context, Hebr. מִסְעָד, *Plur.* מסעדים, features in BM 3131 in attestations from medieval medical literature in the sense of 'food administered to sick people to strengthen them.' A var. from the same root סעד used by Benveniste is סַעַד (see entry). Joshua Shatibi translates Arab. علاجات as *Plur.* רפואות and Anonymous has *Sing.* רפואה.

מִסְפַּחַת • **scurf; dandruff; favus**: Arab. سعفة (cf. UW 156, s.v. ἀχώρ (cf. LS 298: 'scurf; dandruff') and UW 344, s.v. κηρίον (LS 948: 'honeycomb; *II.* a cutaneous disease; μελικηρίς;' cf. LS 1097, s.v. μελικηρίς: 'a kind of cyst or wen, from its resembling a honeycomb')) • Ibn Sīnā, *K. al-Qānūn fī al-ṭibb* • trans. Nathan ha-Me'ati, *Sefer ha-Qanun* II, fol. 68ª: באן ... כשמערבין אותו באספלנית הנקרא מרהם בערבי עם חומץ יועיל מהקלוף והגרב המנוגע ויועיל מהסמנים[156] הרפים והמספחת הנקרא סעפה[157] בערבי (B'N [i.e., fruit of the ben oil tree [*Moringa oleifera* Lam.]]: ... When it is mixed with vinegar in an ointment, called MRHM [i.e., *marham*] in Arab., it is useful for exfoliating and ulcerating scabies, 'milk-like'[158] pimples and scurf (favus), called S'PH [i.e., *sa'fah*] in Arab.). Hebr. מִסְפַּחַת is a var. reading of סַפַּחַת (see entry), which features in the Bible as 'eruption; scab' (BDB 705), and in Rabb. literature as 'rising on the skin; sore' (JD 1012) or as 'a scaly skin-disease; Pityriasis capitis; psoriasis' (Low LXVII), cf. BM 4155: 'psoriasis' (foll. MD 606). Zeraḥyah Ḥen translates Arab. سعفة as סובין שבראש (see entry סב) and Anonymous has הנתק הנקר' סעפה.

מָעוֹג • **confection; comfit; marmelade; jam**: Arab. مربّى (cf. FAQ 247–249) • Ibn Sīnā, *K. al-Qānūn fī al-ṭibb* • trans. Nathan ha-Me'ati, *Sefer ha-Qanun* II, fol. 73ᵇ: גוז ... הוא קשה העכול רע אל האצטומכא והעשוי ממנו מעוג ובער' מורבא כשהוא רטוב הוא מועיל יותר

---

156 מהסמנים הרפים (= البثور اللينة): البثور اللبنية a.

157 סעפה: emend. ed. סחפה Ms سعفة a.

158 ''milk-like' pimples': Trans. after a.

האצטומכא ופחות הזק (Walnut: … It is difficult to digest and is bad for the stomach. But when it is prepared as a confection, in Arab. MWRB' [i.e., *murabban*], and it is fresh, it is better for the stomach and less harmful). In the sense of 'confection,' Hebr. מָעוֹג features in BM 3151 in an attestation from the *Sefer ha-Qanun*. Ben Yehudah explains the term as 'a kind of small cake' (כעין עוגה קטנה). Zeraḥyah Ḥen translates Arab. مربّى as מרוקח עם דבש and Anonymous has מרוקח only.

מעוכב → **מְעֻכָּב**.

מְעִי • המעי הגס · **large intestine**: Lat. *intestinum crassum* (Arab. الأمعاء الغلاظ) · Constantinus Africanus, *Viaticum peregrinantis* · trans. Do'eg ha-Edomi, *Sefer Ya'ir Netiv* IV.18: והמושלים במעי הדק העליון נקראים לומבריגש והם ארוכים והאחרים נולדים במעי הגס שהוא תחת הטיבור ונקראים אשקרידיש גם קוקורניטין (The [worms] that are dominant in the upper small intestine are called LWMBRYGŠ [i.e., *lumbricos*, 'roundworms']; they are long. The other [worms] that originate in the large intestine beneath the navel are called 'ŠQRYDYŠ [i.e., *ascarides*, 'tapeworms'] or QWQWRNYṬYN [i.e., *cucurbitini*[159]]). Hebrew המעי הגס features in MD 391, s.v. 'intestinum crassum;' as a modern term it features in EM 997. Moses ibn Tibbon translates Arab. الأمعاء الغلاظ as *Plur.* המעים העבים (see next entry).

• *Plur.* **מעים • המעים העבים** · **large intestine**: Arab. الأمعاء الغلاظ · Ibn al-Jazzār, *Zād al-musāfir wa-qūt al-ḥādir* · trans. Moses ibn Tibbon, *Sefer Ṣedat ha-Derakhim* IV.18: ומהם מה שיתילד במעים הדקים העליונים ואלו נקראים נחשים בעבור שהם ארוכים ומהם מה שיתילד במעים העבים אשר למטה מן הטבור ויקראו גרגיר הקרא (Some [worms] originate in the upper small intestine and are called *neḥashim* [lit., 'snakes;' i.e., 'roundworms'] because they are long. Other [worms] originate in the large intestine beneath the navel and are called 'tapeworms'). Hebr. המעים העבים features in BM 3166 in a later attestation from Simeon Ben Zemach Duran, *Magen Avot*. Do'eg ha-Edomi translates the parallel Lat. term *intestinum crassum* as *Sing.* המעי הגס (see previous entry).

• **הפשט המעיים** → **הֶפְשֵׁט**.

• **נגע המעים** → **נֶגַע**.

• **עקיצת המעים** → **עֲקִיצָה**.

מעך (*Qal* מָעַךְ or *Pi'el* מִעֵךְ) · **to rub, massage**: Arab. دلك · Ibn al-Jazzār, *Zād al-musāfir wa-qūt al-ḥādir* · trans. Abraham ben Isaac, *Sefer Ṣedah la-Oreḥim* VI.11: ועל כן ראוי תחלה למעך דדיה[160] גם רגליה בשמן דאוקו הוא פיניקלו ותריח דברים שיש להם ריח רע (For this reason one should first of all rub (massage) her breasts[161] and feet with carrot and fennel oil and let her sniff ingredients that have a bad smell). Hebr. מעך features in BM 3169–3170 in the sense of 'to squeeze, crush, press,' a.o., in an attestation from Shabbetai Donnolo, *Sefer ha-Merqaḥot*. Moses ibn Tibbon translates Arab. دلك as

159 '*cucurbitini*': Cf. DMLBS 699: 'gourdworms.'
160 דדיה (= ثدي Ms Dresden, Sächsische Landesbibliothek, Ea 209): يدي a.
161 'breasts' (= Ms Dresden, Sächsische Landesbibliothek, Ea 209): 'hands' a.

משמש and Do'eg ha-Edomi translates the parallel Lat. term *fricor* as [גרד], *Pi'el* גֵּרֵד (cf. NM 5:42 for an attestation from his *Sefer Ya'ir Netiv* I.19.2 (for Lat. *frico*) (cf. IJZ 1–2:622)). In the *Hitpa'el* conj. הִתְמַעֵךְ, the verb מעך is also attested in NM 5:121 in the sense of 'to rub oneself' (for Arab. تمرّخ) in an attestation from *Sefer Ṣedah la-Oreḥim* I.9.2 (cf. IJZ 1–2:550).

מְעֻכָּב (*Part. Pu'al*) → [**עכב**].

מַעֲמָס ‣ I. **tenesmus**: Lat. *pondus* (does not feature in this sense in the current Lat. dictionaries) (Arab. زحير) · Constantinus Africanus, *Viaticum peregrinantis* · trans. Do'eg ha-Edomi, *Sefer Ya'ir Netiv* IV.15: אבק זה טוב לנגעי המעי מהאדומה והמחודדת ולבשול הדם ולכאב ולמעמס ולעוות (This powder is good for intestinal ulcers caused by sharp yellow bile, for bloody diarrhea, for pain, for tenesmus, and for gripes). Hebr. מַעֲמָס features in BM 3182 in the sense of 'load; burden,' but is not attested in medieval medical literature. Moses ibn Tibbon translates the parallel Arab. term زحير as עִצּוּר (see entry).

‣ II. **[sensation of] heaviness**: Lat. *gravitas* · Constantinus Africanus, *Viaticum peregrinantis* · trans. Do'eg ha-Edomi, *Sefer Ya'ir Netiv* IV.17: ואם הוא מהלבנה יוסר הצמאון והדפק מעורב[162] והחולי ארוך והכאב חלק אך יש לו מעמס וכובד רב והכאב והמעמס לא יצאו מהמקום (If the colic is caused by phlegm, [the patient] will not be thirsty anymore, the pulse will be slow,[163] the illness will last for a long time, and the pain will be mild. But he will suffer from [a sensation of] great heaviness, while the pain and heaviness will stay in one and the same spot).

מַעֲפִיץ (*Part. Hif'il*) → [**עפץ**].

מַעֲצוֹר ‣ **abstention; abstinence**: Lat. *abstinentia* (Arab. حمية) · Constantinus Africanus, *Viaticum peregrinantis* · trans. Do'eg ha-Edomi, *Sefer Ya'ir Netiv* IV.9: ועוד שאל אדם אחד אל גיאלינוס: איזו רפואה היא נכונה ושלמה? השיב מעצור (And another person asked Galen: What is the right and perfect remedy? He answered: abstention). In the sense of 'abstention; abstinence,' Hebr. מַעֲצוֹר features in BCD 155 (NM 1:30; 2:61) in later attestations only. Moses ibn Tibbon translates the parallel Arab. term حمية as שְׁמִירָה (cf. BCD 278 for Arab. حمية in the sense of 'diet,' a.o. in an attestation from his *Sefer Ṣedat ha-Derakhim* VII.17.5 (cf. IJZ 7:155, l. 5)).

מַעֲשֶׂה ‣ **composition [of a remedy]; recipe**: Lat. *Rx* [i.e., recipe] (Arab. تأليف) · Constantinus Africanus, *Viaticum peregrinantis* · trans. Do'eg ha-Edomi, *Sefer Ya'ir Netiv* V.7: עוגות ריוברברום מועילות לעצור הכבד והטחול ולחזק האסטומכא וזה מעשיהם (A recipe for rhubarb pastilles, which are good for obstructions in the liver and spleen and strengthen the stomach). In the sense of 'recipe,' Hebr. מַעֲשֶׂה features in NM 5:121 in

162 מעורב: *tardus* L.

163 'slow': Trans. after L.

a later attestation from Abraham ben Isaac, *Sefer Ṣedah la-Oreḥim* I.23.13 (cf. IJZ 1–2:579). Moses ibn Tibbon translates the parallel Arab. term تأليف as חִבּוּר (see entry).

מַפְטִיר (*Part. Hif'il*) → [**פטר**].

מִפְעָל • *Plur.* **מפעלים** • [**healing**] **effects**: Arab. أفعال · Ibn Sīnā, *K. al-Qānūn fī al-ṭibb* · trans. Nathan ha-Me'ati, *Sefer ha-Qanun* II, fol. 103b: מרזנגוש: הטבע חם ויבש בשלישית המפעלים והסגולות הוא מרקיק ומתיך ומפתח בכח (Marjoram: Its nature: It is hot and dry in the third degree. Its healing effects and specific properties: It thins, dissolves and opens with force). Hebr. מִפְעָל, *Plur.* מפעלים, does not feature in this sense in the current dictionaries. Zeraḥyah Ḥen and Anonymous translate Arab. أفعال as פְּעֻלָּה (see entry).

מִפְרָשׂ • *Plur.* **מפרשים** • **layers**: Arab. طبقات · Maimonides, *Maqāla fī al-rabw* (*On Asthma*) · trans. Joshua Shatibi, *Ma'amar 'al ha-Qaṣeret* IX.12 (cf. BMA 2:350, ll. 10–12): וכשתנקה האצטומכה בקיא כמו שזכר ג'אלינוס או במשלשל בדברים שיתיכו הבלגם ממחבואיה אם לא יהיו שם חלטים מסובכים בין מפרשיה אז לא תתאוה דבר מאלו המאכלים הרעים כלם זולתי אם לא יהיה הרגל לאדון הנשא בקיא (And when the stomach is cleansed through vomiting—as Galen mentioned—or through a purgative or through [remedies] that [saturate the stomach] and dissolve the phlegm from its innermost parts when there are no humors stuck in its layers, it will not crave any of those bad foods, unless my Master is accustomed to vomiting them). Hebr. *Sing.* מִפְרָשׂ features in the Bible in the sense of 'spreading out; a thing spread (canvas; sail)' (cf. BDB 831) and in medieval literature, a.o., in the sense of 'curtain; carpet' (cf. BM 3219–3220). Samuel Benveniste translates Arab. طبقات as חלקים and Anonymous has כתות (see entry כַּת).

מַפְשִׁיט (*Part. Hif'il*) → **פָּשַׁט**.

מָצוֹק • I. **slightness; weakness**: Lat. *angustia* (DMLBS 113) (Arab. سهل) · Constantinus Africanus, *Viaticum peregrinantis* · trans. Do'eg ha-Edomi, *Sefer Ya'ir Netiv* V.14: ובנגעי המקוה הכאב נרגש בנקב והמצוק בשתן (In bladder wounds, one will feel pain in the anus while the urine [flow] will be weak). Hebrew מָצוֹק features in the sense of 'narrowness' (for Lat. *angustia* (Arab. ضيق)) in *Sefer Ya'ir Netiv* III.11 (cf. NM 5:122). Moses ibn Tibbon translates Arab. سهل as נקל.

• II. [**hysterical**] **suffocation**: Lat. *suffocatio* (Arab. خنق) · Constantinus Africanus, *Viaticum peregrinantis* · trans. Do'eg ha-Edomi, *Sefer Ya'ir Netiv* VI.11: ובעבור כי הקרב מחובר עם כלי הקול יקרה זה המצוק משם (And since the diphragm is connected to the vocal organs, [the woman] is affected by [hysterical] suffocation). Hebr. מָצוֹק features in the current dictionaries in the sense of 'straitness; straits; stress; anguish;' in BCD 156–157 (NM 3:136) as 'colic' in an attestation from Anonymous, *Perush Aphorismi shel Apuqraṭ* (*Pirqei Abuqraṭ*) IV.11 (148) (cf. BMCH 1:552, l. 1); and in NM 5:122 as 'obstruction' (for Lat. *constipatio*, in an attestation from *Sefer Ya'ir Netiv* I.23.2 (cf. IJZ 1–2:626). A synonymous term for 'hysterical suffocation' used by Do'eg is מצוקת האם (see entry מְצוּקָה). Moses ibn Tibbon translates the parallel Arab. term خنق as [חנק], *Inf. Nif'al* הֵחָנֵק (cf. BM 1661 and BCD 104 (NM 3:94); for Hebr. החנק הרחם in an attestation from Moses ibn Tibbon, *Perush Aphorismi shel Apuqraṭ* (*Pirqei Abuqraṭ*) v.35 (255), cf. BMCH 1:383, l. 9)); Abraham ben Isaac has חֲנִיקוּת (see entry).

• **מצוק הנשימה** · **shortness of breath; dyspnea:** Arab. ضيق النفس · Maimonides, *Maqāla fī al-rabw* (*On Asthma*) · trans. Samuel Benveniste, *Ma'amar 'al ha-Qaṣeret* XII.3 (cf. BMA 2:288, ll. 15–16): אך הלחיכות המנקות הריאות ומבשלות מה שבהם ויקלו הרקיקה ויועילו מן מצוק הנשימה תועלת מבואר וילקחו כל ימי החולי ובאיזה זמן שיזדמן מן היום והלילה אלה מהם (The following are some of the linctuses that cleanse the lungs, coct [the superfluous humors] in them, ease one's expectoration, are clearly beneficial for shortness of breath, and can be taken throughout the disease and at any time during the day or the night). Hebr. מצוק הנשימה is not attested in the current dictionaries. A var. reading מצוקת הנשימה, in the sense of 'hardness [i.e., difficulty] of breathing [i.e., dyspnea]' (for Arab. عسر النفس), features in Moses ibn Tibbon, *Sefer Ṣedat ha-Derakhim* III.6 (cf. NM 5:122–123). Joshua Shatibi translates Arab. ضيق النفس as צרות הנשימה (cf. BCD 233–234 (NM 4:176)) and Anonymous has קצר הנשימה (see entry קֹצֶר).

מְצוּקָה · **narrowness; constriction:** Arab. ضيق · Maimonides, *Maqāla fī al-rabw* (*On Asthma*) · trans. Samuel Benveniste, *Ma'amar 'al ha-Qaṣeret* II.1 (cf. BMA 2:247, ll. 19–21): כי הכונה שיהיו העורקים כלם והנקבים פתוחים והשבילים נקיים שלימים מן הסתום והמצוקה כדי שירוצו בהם הרוחות והליחות ויצאו מהם הנוספים (One's intention should be that all the veins and passages are open and clean and free from obstruction and constriction so that the pneumas and humors stream through them [freely] and the superfluities are expelled). Hebr. מְצוּקָה does not feature in this sense in the current dictionaries. Joshua Shatibi translates Arab. ضيق as צרות and Anonymous has צוק, which is poss. a corruption of צוקה.

• **מצוקת האם** · **hysterical suffocation:** Lat. *suffocatio matricis* (Arab. اختناق الرحم) · Constantinus Africanus, *Viaticum peregrinantis* · trans. Do'eg ha-Edomi, *Sefer Ya'ir Netiv* VI.11: ממצוקת האם (On hysterical suffocation). Hebr. מצוקת האם is attested in BM 3246 in the sense of 'hysterics' in an attestation from Do'eg ha-Edomi, *Sefer ha-Em*, i.e, his trans. of a treatise called *De passionibus mulierum*, spuriously ascribed to Galen.[164] Moses ibn Tibbon translates Arab. اختناق الرحم as החנק הרחם (as in his *Perush Aphorismi shel Apuqraṭ* (*Pirqei Abuqraṭ*) v.35 (255), cf. BCD 104 (NM 3:94); BMCH 1:383, l. 9) and Abraham ben Isaac has חֲנִיקוּת (see entry). See also entry חֲנִיקָה

164 Cf. Gad Freudenthal, 'Appendix: *Do'eg's List of His Translations*,' in 'The Father of the Latin-into-Hebrew translations: 'Do'eg the Edomite,' The Twelfth-Century Repentant Convert,' in *Latin-into-Hebrew: Texts and Studies*, vol. 1: *Studies*, ed. by R. Fontaine and G. Freudenthal (Leiden 2013), 119, no. 13: 'And *Sefer ha-'Em* [= The Book of the Womb] by Galen, which is very good.' For an ed. of the text, see R. Barkaï, *A History of Jewish Gynaecological Texts in the Middle Ages* (Leiden 1998), 145–180.

for the term חניקת הרחם featuring in Shem Tov ben Isaac, *Sefer Almansur*.

• מצוקת השתן · **dysuria**: Lat. *angustia urine* (Arab. عسر البول) · Constantinus Africanus, *Viaticum peregrinantis* · trans. Do'eg ha-Edomi, *Sefer Ya'ir Netiv* v.16: כי אלה המקרים האין נפרדים יחולו תמיד מן הענין הזה: קחדת מצוקת השתן כאב רב אין מפסיק (The following inseparable afflictions always result from this matter [i.e., bladder stones]: fever, dysuria, severe continuous pain). Hebr. מצוקת השתן is not attested in the current dictionaries. Synonyms featuring in medieval medical literature are: עכוב השתן (cf. BCD 201 (NM 4:145 (corr.))); עיצור השתן (cf. BCD 207 (NM 3:179)); עצירת השתן (cf. BCD 208 (NM 3:179)); עוצר השתן (cf. BCD 212 (NM 3:181)); קושי ההשתנה (cf. BCD 252 (NM 3:211)); קשי יציאת השתן (cf. BCD 252 (NM 3:211)); and קושי השתן (cf. BCD 252 (NM 3:212)). Moses ibn Tibbon translates Arab. عسر البول as עוצר שתן (cf. BCD 212 (NM 3:181) for Ibn Tibbon's trans. of Arab. عسر البول as Hebr. עוצר השתן in his *Perush Aphorismi shel Apuqraṭ* (*Pirqei Abuqraṭ*) VI.36 (328) (cf. BMCH 1:400, l. 6)).

מִצְמוּץ · **mouthwash; mouth rinse**: Arab. مضمضة · Ibn Sīnā, *K. al-Qānūn fī al-ṭibb* · trans. Anonymous, *Sefer ha-Qanun* II, fol. 48b: באדורד ... המצמוץ בשליקתו משקיט כאב השנים (Soldier thistle: ... If one rinses one's mouth with its decoction, it alleviates toothache). Hebr. מִצְמוּץ features in the sense of 'mouthwash' in BM 3252, a.o., in attestations from the *Sefer ha-Qanun*. Nathan ha-Me'ati renders Arab. مضمضة as שכשך (cf. BM 7113–7114) and Zeraḥyah Ḥen has קִשְׁקֵשׁ (see entry).

מְצָרֵב (*Part. Pi'el*) → [**צרב**].

מְקֻבָּץ (*Part. Pu'al*) → [**קבץ**].

מֻקְדָּם (*Part. Hof'al*) → [**קדם**].

מקובץ → מְקֻבָּץ.

מִקְוֶה • **צואר המקוה** → צַוָּאר.

מקוטר → מְקֻטָּר.

מָקוֹר • **המקור שהוא בין הגודל והאצבע** · **salvatella vein**: Lat. *vena que est inter pollicem et indicem* (Arab. أسيلم) · Constantinus Africanus, *Viaticum peregrinantis* · trans. Do'eg ha-Edomi, *Sefer Ya'ir Netiv* v.1: העזר: בהיות סתימת הכבד מחום הקיז דם הבשליקא מן היד הימני או מן המקור שהוא בין הגודל והאצבע (Its treatment: When the obstruction in the liver is caused by heat, one should bleed the basilic vein or salvatella vein from the right hand). Hebr. המקור שהוא בין הגודל והאצבע does not feature in the current dictionaries. A var. reading המקור העומד בין האצבע הקטון חבירו features in *Sefer Ya'ir Netiv* III.7 (cf. NM 5:124). Moses ibn Tibbon translates Arab. أسيلم as העורק אשר על הכף בין האצבע הקטן ושכנו (see entry עֶרֶק).

מְקֻטָּר (*Part. Pu'al*) → [**קטר**].

מְקַצֵּר (*Part. Pi'el*) → [**קצר**].

מִקְרֶה • **מקרה לילה** · **nocturnal pollution; emission of sperm**: a) Arab. جوابة[165] · Mai-

165 Arab. جوابة in the sense of '[nocturnal] emission of sperm' is a semantic borrowing from

monides, *Maqāla fī al-rabw* (*On Asthma*) · trans. Samuel Benveniste, *Ma'amar 'al ha-Qaṣeret* x.8 (cf. BMA 2:280, ll. 18–19): ולא יועילם ההמנע ממנו תועלת גדולה. והוא כי יקרם מקרה לילה ויקרה להם מן ההזק ככל מה שיקרה מן המשגל (Abstinence does not benefit them [i.e., people with an excess of hot sperm] very much. The reason for this is that they suffer from nocturnal emissions, so that the same harm occurs to them as that which results from sexual intercourse). Hebr. מקרה לילה features in the current dictionaries as a biblical term only (Deut 23:11; cf. KB 3:1138; BM 3291). The regular term for 'nocturnal pollution' is קרי (cf. BM 6180–6182) as it is also used by Anonymous. Joshua Shatibi translates Arab. جوابة as (?) רחוק ובוה.

· b) Arab. احتلام · Ibn al-Jazzār, *Zād al-musāfir wa-qūt al-ḥāḍir* · trans. Moses ibn Tibbon, *Sefer Ṣedat ha-Derakhim* VI.4: השער הד' במקרה לילה (Chapter 4: On nocturnal pollution). Abraham ben Isaac translates Arab. احتلام as קרי הנקר' בחלום and Do'eg ha-Edomi translates the parallel Lat. term *effusio spermatis in somno* as גרישת הזרע בתוך השינה (see entry גְּרִישָׁה). In addition, Do'eg uses the term גִּעוּל for the Lat. synonym *pollutio* (see entry).

מֻרְגָּל (*Part. Hof'al*) → [רגל].

מָרוֹחַ • מרוח אשך · scrotal hernia: Arab. أدرة · Ibn al-Jazzār, *Zād al-musāfir wa-qūt al-ḥāḍir* · trans. Abraham ben Isaac, *Sefer Ṣedah la-Oreḥim* VI.8: כתוש ותכביר ולוש ושחוק בשמן שושנים וחומץ וטח במקום ויועיל למרוח אשך הנקרה לנערים (Pound [these ingredients], sieve, and knead [the pounded substance] with rose oil and vinegar and rub it on the spot; it is beneficial for scrotal hernia of boys). Hebr. מרוח אשך is only attested in the Bible in the sense of 'someone with crushed testicles' (Lev 21:20, cf. KB 633) and Rabb. literature (cf. JD 838). Moses ibn Tibbon translates Arab. أدرة as בקיעה.

מרוקא → **מורקא**.

מֻרְסָה • מורסת הצפורן · paronychia; whitlow: Arab. داحس (Gr. παρωνυχία; cf. MIG no. 587) · Ibn Sīnā, *K. al-Qānūn fī al-ṭibb* · trans. Zeraḥyah Ḥen, *Sefer ha-Qanun* II, fols. 208[b]–209[a]: זיתון ... עלי הזתים המדבריים טובים למורס' הצפורן (Olive oil: ... Leaves of wild olive are good for whitlow (paronychia)). Hebr. מורסת הצפורן is not attested in the current dictionaries. In addition to מורסת הצפורן, Zeraḥyah translates Arab. داحس as בקיעות הקורה מן האונגלון (see entry בְּקִיעָה) and as Rom. פַּנֲרִיש (see מורסות ראשי האצבעות below). Nathan ha-Me'ati translates Arab. داحس as מורסות ראשי האצבעות (see also below) and Anonymous has מורסת ראשי האצבעות.

• מורסת הקרום · pleurisy: Arab. شوصة · Ibn Sīnā, *K. al-Qānūn fī al-ṭibb* · trans. Nathan ha-Me'ati, *Sefer ha-Qanun* II, fol. 70[a]: ביץ ביצים ... והמבושל במים הנקרא נמרשת יועיל מהשעול וממורסת הקרום הנקרא שוצה ומהכליון הנקרא צל בערבי (Eggs: ... [Soft] boiled egg called NMRŠT [i.e, Pers. *nīmbirisht*; cf. VL 1393: 'ovum sorbile; semicoctum;' IG 626] is useful for cough, pleurisy called ŠWṢH [i.e., Arab. *shawṣa*], and for phthisis called ṢL [i.e., *sill*] in Arab.). Hebr. מורסת הקרום is not attested in the current dictionaries.

Gr. απόκρισις, which can mean both 'answer' and 'excretion [of sperm];' cf. UWS 1:148–149; LSG 204.

In his *Sefer ha-Peraqim* (*Pirqei Moshe*) IX.83; XII.22, 36; XXI.26, Nathan has no Hebr. equivalent for Arab. شوصة and transcribes it as שוצה only (cf. BMMN 114, l. 24; 141, l. 20; 199, l. 4; BMMG no. 2770). The Arab. synonym ذات الجنب is translated by him as בעלת הצד (cf. entry בַּעֲלָה). Zeraḥyah Ḥen translates Arab. شوصة as החולי שבצד (cf. a var. reading חולי הצד in BCD 98 (NM 3:86), a.o., in an attestation from Zeraḥyah's *Sefer ha-Peraqim* (*Pirqei Moshe*) IV.42 (BMMZ 55, l. 23); for other vars., see BMMG no. 1999).

• *Plur.* **מורסות • המורסות הדבשיות** · **favus**: Arab. الأورام الشهدية (cf. UW 344, s.v. κηρίον (LS 948: 'honeycomb; *II.* a cutaneous disease; μελικηρίς;' cf. LS 1097, s.v. μελικηρίς: 'a kind of cyst or wen, from its resembling a honeycomb')) · Ibn Sīnā, *K. al-Qānūn fī al-ṭibb* · trans. Nathan ha-Me'ati, *Sefer ha-Qanun* II, fol. 69^{a}: בקלה ימאניה ... עושים ממנו תחבשת ומעקרו אל המורסות הדבשיות (Amaranth: ... A poultice of its root is applied on favus). Hebr. המורסה הדבשית, *Plur.* המורסות הדבשיות, is not attested in the current dictionaries. Zeraḥyah Ḥen translates Arab. الأورام الشهدية as מור׳ הנקרא דבשיית and Anonymous has יעריים (see entry יַעֲרִי).

• **מורסות הראש** · **phrenitis**: Lat. *frenesis* (Arab.-Pers. سرسام) · Gerard de Solo, *Practica super nono Almansoris* · trans. Abraham Avigdor, *Ha-Ma'amar ha-Teshi'i le-Sefer ha-Mansuri le-Razi*, fols. 13^{a-b}: שער במורסת הראש בערבי שרסאם: כשיקרה לאדם קדחת תדירה עם כובד בראש והעינים ואדמימות בהם ובראש וכאב הראש ומיאוס האור ומהירות בדפק ותכיפות מופלג הנה אלו הוראות מורסות הראש (Chapter on phrenitis, in Arab. ŠRS'M [i.e., *sirsām*]: If someone regularly suffers from fevers and his head and eyes are heavy and red and he suffers from headache and he detests (cannot stand) light and his pulse is very fast and frequent, it indicates phrenitis). In the sense of 'phrenitis,' Hebr. *Sing.* מורסת הראש features in BCD 162 (NM 4:105) in attestations from Moses ibn Tibbon, *Sefer Ṣedat ha-Derakhim* I.18.1 (cf. IJZ 1–2:468) and *Perush Aphorismi shel Apuqraṭ* (*Pirqei Abuqraṭ*) VII.12 (364) (cf. BMCH 1:408, l. 1).

• **מורסות ראשי האצבעות** · **paronychia; whitlow**: Arab. داحس (Gr. παρωνυχὶα; cf. MIG no. 587) · Ibn Sīnā, *K. al-Qānūn fī al-ṭib* · trans. Nathan ha-Me'ati, *Sefer ha-Qanun* II, fol. 122^{b}: רמאן ... גרגרי הרמונים עם דבש עושין בהם משיחה למורסות ראשי האצבעות ובער׳ דאאס (Pomegranate: ... Pomegranate seeds with honey are applied as a salve for whitlow, called D''S (*D'ḤS) in Arab.). Hebr. מורסות ראשי האצבעות is not attested in the current dictionaries. Zeraḥyah Ḥen translates Arab. داحس as Rom. פנַרִיש (cf. ND 786, s.v. *panaricium*), while Anonymous has the same Hebr. term as Nathan. Shem Tov ben Isaac renders Arab. داحس as צמח בצפורן האצבע in his *Sefer ha-Shimmush* XXIX, list 1 (cf. NM 5:169–170; SHS 1:441 (Ṣade 26)). See also בקיעות הקורה מן האונגלון (entry בְּקִיעָה) and מורסת הצפורן (above).

• **מורסות קרומי המוח** · **meningitis**: Arab. أورام حجب الدماغ · Ibn Sīnā, *K. al-Qānūn fī al-ṭibb* · trans. Nathan ha-Me'ati, *Sefer ha-Qanun* II, fol. 112^{b}: ועינב השועל כששוחקים ממנו היטב ועושים ממנו תחבשת על הראש ירפא מהכאב ובערבי צדאע ויתיך מורסות שרשי האזן ומורסות קרומי המוח (When black nightshade is pounded thoroughly and plastered on the head, it cures headache [called] ṢD'ʿ [i.e., *ṣudāʿ*] in Arab. and dissolves (removes) parotitis and meningitis). Hebr. מורסות קרומי המוח is not attested in the current dictionaries. Zeraḥyah Ḥen translates Arab. أورام حجب الدماغ as מורסות קרום המוח.

• **מורסות שרשי האזן** · **parotitis**: Arab. أورام أصل الأذن (cf. UW 507, s.v. παρωτίς) · Ibn Sīnā, *K. al-Qānūn fī al-ṭib* · trans. Nathan ha-Me'ati, *Sefer ha-Qanun* II, fol. 112[b]: ועינב השועל כששוחקים ממנו היטב ועושים ממנו תחבשת על הראש ירפא מהכאב ובערבי צדאע ויתיך מורסות שרשי האזן ומורסות קרומי המוח (When black nightshade is pounded thoroughly and plastered on the head, it cures headache [called] ṢD'ʿ [i.e., *ṣudāʿ*] in Arab. and dissolves (removes) parotitis and meningitis). Hebr. מורסות שרשי האזן is not attested in the current dictionaries. Zeraḥyah Ḥen translates Arab. أورام أصل الأذن as מורסת שרשי האזנים and Anonymous has מורסות שרשי האזן, just like Nathan.

מֶרְקַחַת • **מרקחת בשמים** · **spice-stomachic**: Arab. جوارشن الأفاويه · Ibn al-Jazzār, *Zād al-musāfir wa-qūt al-ḥādir* · trans. Moses ibn Tibbon, *Sefer Ṣedat ha-Derakhim* v.6: תאר מרקחת בשמים הוא בלטין דיא רומה והוא יועיל בע"ה מעובי הליחה לבנה ויתקן האצטו' וייטיב תאות המאכל (Composition of the spice-stomachic, i.e., in Lat. DY' RWMH [i.e., *diaroma*], which is—God willing—beneficial for thick phlegm, cures the stomachic, and improves the appetite ...). Hebr. מרקחת בשמים does not feature in the current dictionaries. Do'eg ha-Edomi transcribes the parallel Lat. term *diaroma*, which is also mentioned by Ibn Tibbon, as דיא רומא (cf. ND 297, s.v. 'diaromata': 'Electuaries containing aromatic spices').

• **מרקחת יקרא הזהבי** · **electuary called 'the golden one'**: Arab. معجون يسمّى الذهبي · Ibn al-Jazzār, *Zād al-musāfir wa-qūt al-ḥādir* · trans. Moses ibn Tibbon, *Sefer Ṣedat ha-Derakhim* v.6: תאר מרקחת יקרא הזהבי הוא דיאקרישיש ילך מהלך הדביבאת (Composition of the electuary, called 'the golden one', i.e., DY'QRYŠYŠ [i.e., Lat. *diacrisis*], that works as an electuary). Hebr. מרקחת יקרא הזהבי is not attested in this sense in the current dictionaries. Do'eg ha-Edomi transcribes the parallel Lat. term *diacrisis*, which is also mentioned by Ibn Tibbon, as דיא קרישיש.

מַרְקִיק (*Part. Hifʿil*) → [רקק].

מֻרְתָּח (*Part. Hofʿal*) → [רתח].

מַשָּׂא · **gestation; pregnancy**: Arab. حَمْل · Ibn Sīnā, *K. al-Qānūn fī al-ṭibb* · trans. Nathan ha-Me'ati, *Sefer ha-Qanun* II, Ms Paris, BnF, héb. 1136, fol. 88[b]: וחלב כל חיוני משאו[166] יותר כבד ממשא האדם [רע (The milk of any animal whose gestation is longer than that of a human being is inferior). In the sense of 'gestation,' Hebr. מַשָּׂא is a non-attested semantic borrowing from Arab. حمل. Nathan (Ms Oxford, Bodleian Library, Can. Or. 88, fol. 99[b]) renders Arab. حَمْل as עִבּוּר and Anonymous has הריון.

מִשְׁבָּר • *Plur.* **משברים** · **cramps; colic**: Arab. مغص (Gr. στρόφος; cf. UW 644) · Ibn al-Jazzār, *Zād al-musāfir wa-qūt al-ḥādir* · trans. Moses ibn Tibbon, *Sefer Ṣedat ha-*

---

166 רע: رديء a.

Derakhim IV.15: ואולם אותות העצור הכולל העוות הוא המשברים והצער ויציאת הדם מעורב בליחה כרכומית (In general, the symptoms of dysentery are cramps (colic), i.e., [Hebr.] *ha-mishbarim*, pain, loss of blood mixed with yellow bile). Hebr. *Sing.* מִשְׁבָּר features in BM 3355 in the sense of 'severe intestinal pain' in attestations from Pseudo-Ibn Ezra, *Sefer ha-Nisyonot* and the *Sefer ha-Qanun*. See also BCD 197–198 (NM 4:142) for Ibn Tibbon's use of the Hebr. synonym עִוּוּת in his *Sefer Ṣedat ha-Derakhim* I.O.4 (cf. IJZ 1–2:441). Do'eg ha-Edomi translates the parallel Lat. term *tortura* as עִוּוּת as well (cf. NM 5:144–145 for an attestation from *Sefer Ya'ir Netiv* I.10.10 (cf. IJZ 1–2:612)). For other synonyms, see חִיל, חבלי הבטן (entry חֶבֶל), and עקיצת המעים (entry עֲקִיצָה).

מִשְׁגַּל • חולשת המשגל → חֻלְשָׁה.

מָשׁוּחַ (*Part. Pass.*) → **מָשַׁח**.

מִשּׁוּשׁ • **massage**: Arab. دلك • Maimonides, *Maqāla fī al-rabw* (*On Asthma*) • trans. Samuel Benveniste, *Ma'amar 'al ha-Qaṣeret* X.6 (cf. BMA 2:279, ll. 6–7): אמר ג'אלינוס דברים וזה נסחם אמר: אך משוש האברים החלושים יאות להזהר מעשותו בעתות שיסתערו ויתרגשו בהם עלותם (Galen has said the following, and these are his very words: One should beware of applying massage to weak limbs at times when their diseases are stirred up in them). Hebr. מִשּׁוּשׁ features in the current dictionaries in the sense of 'touch' only (cf. BM 3364–3365). Joshua Shatibi translates Arab. دلك as חֲפִיפָה (as it is also used in trans. by Moses ibn Tibbon, Zeraḥyah Ḥen, and Nathan ha-Me'ati, cf. BCD 105–106 (NM 1:57, 151; 2:48; 3:95–96)) and Anonymous has זִלּוּף (see entry).

מָשַׁח • *Part. Pass.* **מָשׁוּחַ** • **greasy; fatty**: Lat. *unctuosus* (Arab. دهني) • Constantinus Africanus, *Viaticum peregrinantis* • trans. Do'eg ha-Edomi, *Sefer Ya'ir Netiv* IV.3: ואם הכח החפץ יתאוה לאכל דברים משוחים יועילו לתתם אליו וטוב לתת לו בכל מאכליו דברים משוחים (If someone [suffering from ravenous hunger caused by a cold temperament] has appetite to eat fatty things, it is good to give them to him and to let him consume fatty things with all his meals). Hebr. מָשׁוּחַ is attested in the Bible in the sense of 'anointed' (cf. KB 603). For the verb מָשַׁח, featuring in medieval medical literature in the sense of 'to salve, smear,' see BM 3366. Moses ibn Tibbon translates Arab. دهني as דשן.

מַשְׁחִין (*Part. Hif'il*) → [שחן].

מְשִׁיחָה • **oil**: Arab. دهن • Ibn Sīnā, *K. al-Qānūn fī al-ṭib* • trans. Nathan ha-Me'ati, *Sefer ha-Qanun* II, fol. 67v: באן ... ויש באילנו מרירות יותר וקבוץ וזה יוליד בו כח כווה וקלפתו קובצת יותר ולא תכלה משיחתו מהקבוץ ובכלו יש תמרוק וחתוך (B'N [i.e., fruit of the ben oil tree [*Moringa oleifera* Lam.]]: ... The tree is more bitter and astringent, which gives it its caustic property. The peel is more astringent, the oil is also not free from astringency. All of them have detergent and cutting potency). Hebr. מְשִׁיחָה is only attested in the sense of 'anointment; ointment' (cf. JD 852; BM 3372; NM 5:127). In his *Sefer ha-Peraqim* (*Pirqei Moshe*), Nathan translates Arab. دهن as שמן throughout (cf. BMMG no. 1796). The latter term is also used by Zeraḥyah Ḥen and Anonymous in this paragraph of the *Sefer ha-Qanun*.

מִשְׁכְּבָא (*Aram.*) • *Plur.* **מִשְׁכְּבִין** · **sexual intercourse; coitus:** Lat. *coitus* (Arab. وطئ) · Constantinus Africanus, *Viaticum peregrinantis* · trans. Do'eg ha-Edomi, *Sefer Ya'ir Netiv* v.13: ואם הבטן עצור נעזור עם קלישטרי משעור ויאולא מלבא שמן ורד ודומיהם ונאכילהו מאכלים לחים וממהרים לבשל כמו טיבשנא וישמר ממשכבי אשה גם מיגיעה וממרכב (If [the patient] suffers from constipation, we administer him a clyster from barley, violets, marshmallow, rose oil, and the like. We feed him with moist foodstuff that is quickly digested, such as barley broth. He should beware of having intercourse with a woman, he should not exert himself nor ride an animal). In the sense of 'sexual intercourse,' Aram. מִשְׁכְּבָא, *Plur.* מִשְׁכְּבִין, is attested in Rabb. literature (*Targum*) on Num 31:17 (cf. DAN 257). Moses ibn Tibbon translates Arab. وطئ as משגל.

מֻשְׁלָג (*Part. Hof'al*) → [שלג].

מַשְׁמָעוּת · **purpose; aim; end; goal:** Lat. *intentio* (Arab. غرض) · Constantinus Africanus, *Viaticum peregrinantis* · trans. Do'eg ha-Edomi, *Sefer Ya'ir Netiv* v.5: ואולם בשני הענינים נעזור האינדרופישים כמו שאמר גיאלינוס ומשמעותנינו להיות האחד להתחזק הכח המבשל ואשר הדברים המזיקים אליו ימנעו ממנו (However, in treating dropsy we should—as Galen said—set ourselves two goals (strive after two things): to strengthen the digestive faculty [of the liver] and to prevent harmful things from reaching it ...). Hebr. מַשְׁמָעוּת does not feature in this sense in the current dictionaries. Moses ibn Tibbon translates Arab. غرض as כונה.

מִשְׁמָר · **attack; paroxysm (of an illness):** Arab. نوبة (Gr. παροξυσμός: cf. UW 505) · Maimonides, *Maqāla fī al-rabw* (*On Asthma*) · trans. Samuel Benveniste, *Ma'amar 'al ha-Qaṣeret* N.3 (cf. BMA 2:242, ll. 17–19): וכבר זכרת לי שאויר אלסכנדריאה יזיק אותך מאד ואתה תשים פניך למצרים בעתות שתירא לבא זמן המשמר מפני שאויר מצרים יבש ושוקט יותר ויקל עליך לסבול אותה משמרה (You told me that the air of Alexandria is very harmful for you and that you go to Cairo whenever you expect the onset of an attack [of asthma] because the air of Cairo is drier and calmer so that it is easier for you to bear that attack). Hebr. מִשְׁמָר does not feature in this sense in the current dictionaries. In addition to מִשְׁמָר, Benveniste translates Arab. نوبة also as מִשְׁמָרָה (see next entry). Joshua Shatibi translates Arab. نوبة as עוֹנָה (cf. BCD 198, a.o., in attestations from the *Sefer ha-Peraqim* (*Pirqei Moshe*) by both Zeraḥyah Ḥen (III.103; cf. NM 1:175; BMMZ 48, l. 1) and Nathan ha-Me'ati (*Plur.* עונות, IV.22; cf. NM 2:70; BMMN 59, l. 3) (cf. also BMMG nos. 5312, 5314)). Anonymous has מִשְׁמֶרֶת (see entry).

מִשְׁמָרָה · **attack; paroxysm [of an illness]:** Arab. نوبة (Gr. παροξυσμός: cf. UW 505) · Maimonides, *Maqāla fī al-rabw* (*On Asthma*) · trans. Samuel Benveniste, *Ma'amar 'al ha-Qaṣeret* N.3 (cf. BMA 2:242, ll. 17–19): וכבר זכרת לי שאויר אלסכנדריאה יזיק אותך מאד ואתה תשים פניך למצרים בעתות שתירא לבא זמן המשמר מפני שאויר מצרים יבש ושוקט יותר ויקל עליך לסבול אותה משמרה. (You told me that the air of Alexandria is very harmful for you and that you go to Cairo whenever you expect the onset of an attack [of asthma] because the air of Cairo is drier and calmer so that it is easier for you to bear that attack). Hebr. מִשְׁמָרָה does not feature in this sense in the current dictionaries. In addition to מִשְׁמָרָה, Benveniste translates Arab. نوبة also as מִשְׁמָר (see previous entry). Joshua Shatibi translates Arab. نوبة as עוֹנָה (cf. BCD 198, see above) and Anonymous has מִשְׁמֶרֶת (see next entry).

מִשְׁמֶרֶת · **attack; paroxysm [of an illness]**: Arab. نوبة (Gr. παροξυσμός: cf. UW 505) · Maimonides, *Maqāla fī al-rabw* (*On Asthma*) · trans. Anonymous, *Sefer ha-Qaṣeret* N.3 (cf. BMA 2:388, l. 13–15): וכבר זכרה לי ירפאה האל שרוח של אסכדריאה מזיק לה ושהיא תכון ללכת אל מצרים בעתות שיראה בהם ביאת זו המשמרת מפני היות אויר מצרים יותר קל ומושקט יקל עליה שאת אותה המשמרת (You told me—may God heal you—that the air of Alexandria is harmful for you and that you go to Cairo whenever you expect the onset of an attack [of asthma] because the air of Cairo is lighter and calmer so that it is easier for you to bear that attack). Hebr. מִשְׁמֶרֶת does not feature in this sense in the current dictionaries. Samuel Benveniste translates Arab. نوبة both as מִשְׁמָר and מִשְׁמָרָה (see previous entries) and Joshua Shatibi has עוֹנָה (cf. BCD 198, see above).

מְשַׁנֶּה (*Part. Piʿel*) → **[שנה]**.

מַשְׁקֶה · **dose**: Arab. شربة (cf. FL 2:407: 'dosis una medicamenti; c.c.g. Avicenn.') · Ibn Sīnā, *K. al-Qānūn fī al-ṭibb* · trans. Nathan ha-Me'ati, *Sefer ha-Qanun* II, fol. 69^{b}: בזר קטונא המהות הוא שני גוונים אחד נולד בימות החמה ואחד בימות הגשמים והמשקה מאיזה מהם שיהיה הוא שני זוזים (Fleawort seed; What is it (*ha-mahut*)?:[167] It is of two types: one growing in summer and another in winter. The dose of each type is two *zuzim*.[168]) In the sense of 'dose,' Hebr. מַשְׁקֶה is a non-attested semantic borrowing from Arab. شربة. Zeraḥyah Ḥen translates Arab. شربة as לְקִיחָה (see entry) and Anonymous has שתייה.

• *Plur.* **משקים** · **decoctions**: Arab. مغليات · Maimonides, *Maqāla fī al-rabw* (*On Asthma*) · trans. Samuel Benveniste, *Ma'amar ʿal ha-Qaṣeret* XII.0 (cf. BMA 2:287, ll. 3–4): אך המשקים אשר הכונה בהם לבשל ולהקל הרקיקה ולנקות הריאה והם אותם הראויים להקדים למשלשלים (Decoctions with which one wishes to coct [the superfluities] and to ease expectoration and to clean the lungs, and which should be used before the purgatives). Hebr. *Sing.* מַשְׁקֶה only features in BM 3414–3415 as 'beverage; liquid; potion.' Joshua Shatibi translates Arab. مغليات as בישולים (see entry בִּשּׁוּל, *Plur.* בשולים, featuring also in Do'eg ha-Edomi, *Sefer Ya'ir Netiv* V.5) and Anonymous has מורתחים.

• **משקה השרשים** · **the roots decoction**: Lat. *apozima* (read: *apozema*) *de radicibus* (Arab. مطبوخ الأصول[169]) · Constantinus Africanus, *Viaticum peregrinantis* · trans. Do'eg ha-Edomi, *Sefer Ya'ir Netiv* IV.17: ונאכילהו תרנוגלים טבשאנא עם שולטרי ומשקה השרשים עם שמן שמבוק ועם אישרוב ועם אישנץ עם שמן שקדים ועם מליקראט מבושם. (We administer [the patient] roosters, barley gruel with black nightshade, the roots

167 See entry מָהוּת.

168 See entry זוּז.

169 Cf. Ibn al-Tilmīdh, *Aqrābādhīn*, no. 240 (s.v. *ṭabīkh al-uṣūl*), in: O. Kahl (ed. and trans.), *The Dispensatory of Ibn at-Tilmīḏ*, 255.

decoction with marjoram oil, [absinth wormwood syrup,] almond oil, and fragrant hydromel ...). Hebr. משקה השרשים is not attested in the current dictionaries. Moses ibn Tibbon translates the parallel Arab. term مطبوخ الأصول as בשול השרשים (see entry בִּשּׁוּל for his trans. of Arab. طبيخ الأصول in *Sefer Ṣedat ha-Derakhim* VI.9).

מִשְׁרָה · **decoction**: Arab. مطبوخ (cf. FAQ 245–246) · Ibn al-Jazzār, *Zād al-musāfir wa-qūt al-ḥādir* · trans. Moses ibn Tibbon, *Sefer Ṣedat ha-Derakhim* IV.13: תואר משרה מועיל מרפיון האצטומ׳ והעוות בה והכאב החזק (Composition of a decoction that is good for a weak stomach, for a colic, and for severe pain). Hebr. מִשְׁרָה features in Rabb. literature in the sense of 'infusion; steeping' (cf. JD 858; BM 3419). Ben Yehuda also mentions the term for two attestations, namely Maimonides, *Mishneh Torah: Hilkhot Shekhenim* and Nathan ha-Me'ati, *Sefer ha-Peraqim* (*Pirqei Moshe*) VIII.71 (cf. BMMN 102, ll. 6–8 (corr.); see *Plur.* משרות, next entry).

• *Plur.* **משרות** · **morasses**: Arab. نقايع (cf. FL 326, s.v. نقيعة) · Maimonides, *K. al-Fuṣūl fī al-ṭibb* (*Medical Aphorisms*) · trans. Nathan ha-Me'ati, *Sefer ha-Peraqim* (*Pirqei Moshe*) VIII.71 (cf. BMMN 102, ll. 6–8 (corr.)): המשובח שברוחות מה שינשב מחוף ימים והיותר קרוב אל המשובח שבהם הוא מה שיתנשב מן ההרים. והרע שבהם מה שיתנשב מהיאורים או האגמים או משרות והממוצע שביניהם מה שיתנשב מזולת זה (The best wind is the one that blows from the high sea; the next best is the one that blows from the mountains; the worst is the one that blows from marshes or swamps or morasses. Intermediate between these is the wind that blows from other [directions]). In the sense of 'morasses,' Hebr. מִשְׁרָה, *Plur.* משרות, is a semantic borrowing from Arab. نقايع.

מִשְׁרֶה · **infusion**: Arab. نقوع · Ibn al-Jazzār, *Zād al-musāfir wa-qūt al-ḥādir* · trans. Moses ibn Tibbon, *Sefer Ṣedat ha-Derakhim* V.1: או ישתה מן העוגות המורכבות המועילות לחום הכבד לפי מה שנזכור במה שאחר זה מזה המאמר מן המשקים הקרים אשר להם מן ההקרה כח ינגב ויפתח ויחזק הכבד וישתה המשרות דקות ההרכבה הבטוחות הטובות (He may also take one of the compound pastilles that are beneficial for the heat of the liver, such as I will mention later on in the section on cold drinks that have a cooling power so that they dry, open, and strengthen the liver; he may also take an infusion of fine composition that is safe and good). Hebr. מִשְׁרֶה is not attested in medieval medical literature (cf. BM 3419; EM 1092). Do'eg ha-Edomi translates the parallel Lat. term *sucus* as אשרוב.

מְשָׁרֶת (*Part. Pi'el*) → [שרת].

מִתְחַבֶּרֶת (*Part. Pi'el f.*) → [חבר].

מַתְחִיל (*Part. Hif'il*) → [תחל].

מִתְחַלֵּף (*Part. Hitpa'el*) → [חלף].

מַתִּיךְ (*Part. Hif'il*) → [נתך].

מַתִּיר (*Part. Hif'il*) → [נתר].

מַתְכּוֹנֶת · **recipe**: Arab. صفة · Maimonides, *Maqāla fī al-rabw* (*On Asthma*) · trans. Samuel Benveniste, *Ma'amar 'al ha-Qaṣeret* IV.2 (cf. BMA 2:255, ll. 7–9): ומאלה

המסעדים סומקיא[170] היא בתכלית התועלת וערבת המאכל והיא כרפואה וזה מתכנתה: ישלק בשר הצאן או העוף ויקלה כמו שיקלה שאר המטעמים והתבלין שאזכיר בספר זה (Another dish is that[171] prepared from raisins: it is extremely beneficial and very tasty and is like a remedy. Its recipe is: Boil mutton or fowl that has been roasted in the same way as other foods and spices that I will describe further on). Hebr. מַתְכּוֹנֶת features in the Bible in the sense of 'measurement; relationship' (cf. KB 654), in Rabb. literature in the sense of 'measurement; required amount' (JD 862), and in medieval philosophical literature as 'form; structure' (cf. PESHAT[172]); it is not attested in medieval medical literature. Joshua Shatibi translates Arab. صفة as תואר and Anonymous has טֶפֶס (see entry).

מַתְמִיד (*Part. Hif'il*) → [תמד].

מִתְנַגֵּד (*Part. Hitpa'el*) → [נגד].

מִתְרַחֵב (*Part. Hitpa'el*) → [רחב].

---

170 סומקיא: زبيبية a.

171 'that prepared from raisins': Trans. after a.

172 https://peshat.org/display/peshat_lemmas_00022986 (accessed April 5, 2022).

נֶאֱמָן (*Part. Nifʿal*) → [**אמן**].

נאצור · **fistula**: Arab. ناصور (Gr. κόλπος; cf. UW 357–358) · Ibn al-Jazzār, *Zād al-musāfir wa-qūt al-ḥādir* · trans. Moses ibn Tibbon, *Sefer Ṣedat ha-Derakhim* IV.19: ואם נעשה לו מה שזכרנו ולא סר ממנו החולי אבל שב נאצור והוא מין מפישטולא ידע אז הרופא שלא ירפא עד שיעקר ויחתך (If we give him the mentioned treatment but still [he suffers from hemorrhoids] turning into fistulas, the physician should know that he will not be cured until they will be removed by surgery). Hebr. נאצור is a non-attested calque of Arab. ناصور that is current in medieval Hebr. medical literature. Shem Tov ben Isaac renders the Arab. term as גַּרְגַּתְנִי in his *Sefer ha-Shimmush* XXX.1.17 (cf. BCD 49 (NM 1:84)).

נִבְחָר (*Part. Nifʿal*) → [**בחר**].

[נגד] • *Part. Hitpaʿel* **מִתְנַגֵּד** • **הרפואות המתנגדות למדוים** → **רְפוּאָה**.

נָגוּעַ (*Part. Pass.*) → **נָגַע**.

נָגִיד · **major**: Arab. رئيس · Maimonides, *Maqāla fī al-rabw* (*On Asthma*) · trans. Samuel Benveniste, *Maʿamar ʿal ha-Qaṣeret* V.7 (cf. BMA 2:261, ll. 18–20): ואם השמור הזה חובה בבריאים כל שכן שהוא חובה לידועי החליים הנאמנים וכל שכן למי שאבר מאיבריו הנגידים חלוש בטבע או לפי חלי אשר קרהו (If this [kind] of precaution is indispensable for healthy people, how much more should it be obligatory for chronically ill people and especially for someone who suffers from a weakness of one of the major organs, either inherently or as a result of illness). Hebrew נָגִיד does not feature in a medical context in the current dictionaries. Joshua Shatibi and Anonymous both render Arab. رئيس as ראשי.

נָגַע • **סיד שלא נגע בו מים** → **סִיד**.

• *Part. Pass.* **נָגוּעַ** · **ulcerated**: Arab. متقرّح · Ibn Sīnā, *K. al-Qānūn fī al-ṭibb* · trans. Zeraḥyah Ḥen, *Sefer ha-Qanun* II, fol. 223[b]: כברית ... יושם על הגרב הנגוע (Sulphur: ... [It is useful] when it is put on ulcerated scabies). Hebr. *Part. Pass.* נָגוּעַ does not feature in this sense in the current dictionaries. The term features in the Bible in the sense of ‘touched; afflicted’ (cf. KB 2:668). Nathan ha-Me’ati translates Arab. متقرّح as נגע.

• *Part. Piʿel* **מְנַגֵּעַ** • **הסמים המנגעים** → **סַם**.

• *Part. Puʿal* **מְנֻגָּע** • **הגרב המנוגע** → **גָּרָב**.

• *Hifʿil* **הִגִּיעַ לבגר** • **הגיע לבגר** · **to grow up, reach puberty**: Lat. *venio ad aetatem* (Arab. بلغ) · Constantinus Africanus, *Viaticum peregrinantis* · trans. Do’eg ha-Edomi, *Sefer Ya’ir Netiv* VI.4: אך בהגיעם לבגר אז יולד טבע הזרע שחומם נתרבה ונשלם יותר מקורותם נרחבים ועל כן יניע התולדת לגרש חוץ הטבע שנתרבה ברתיחה בתוך השינה (But when [young boys] reach puberty and the matter of sperm originates in them and becomes increasingly hot and more perfect, their veins become wide and consequently nature moves to expel the accumulated matter by boiling [and expelling] it in their sleep). Hebr. בַּגַר/בֶּגֶר is attested in Rabb. literature and medieval halakhic literature in the sense of 'age of majority (of females after twelve and a half years)' (cf. JD 138; LW 191; BM 460). Moses ibn Tibbon translates Arab. بلغ as הגיע לימי הבגרות (see next entry) and Abraham ben Isaac as הגיע לפרקו (see entry below).

• **הגיע לימי הבגרות** · **to grow up, reach puberty**: Arab. بلغ · Ibn al-Jazzār, *Zād al-musāfir wa-qūt al-ḥādir* · trans. Moses ibn Tibbon, *Sefer Ṣedat ha-Derakhim* VI.4: וכאשר הגיע הנער לימי הבגרות ותתילד בו חמר הזרע ויתחזק חום הגוף ויתרחבו מעברי עורקיהם יתנועע הטבע להוציא החמר כשיתרבה בהם ויוציאהו בחלום[173] (But when boys grow up [i.e., reach puberty] and the matter of sperm originates in them and the heat of their body becomes stronger and the channels of their veins become wide, nature moves to expel that matter when it increases in them, and they expel it in their dream[174]). Hebr. בַּגְרוּת is attested in Rabb. and medieval halakhic literature in the sense of 'a girl who comes of age (after twelve and a half years),' and as a modern term in the sense of 'adulthood; maturity; matriculation exams' (cf. EM 133). Abraham ben Isaac translates Arab. بلغ as הגיע לפרקו (see next entry) and Do'eg ha-Edomi translates the parallel Lat. term *venio ad aetatem* as הגיע לבגר (see previous entry).

• **הגיע לפרקו** · **to grow up, reach puberty**: Arab. بلغ · Ibn al-Jazzār, *Zād al-musāfir wa-qūt al-ḥādir* · trans. Abraham ben Isaac, *Sefer Ṣedah la-Oreḥim* VI.4: וכאשר יגיע הנער לפירקו ותיולד בו מקור הזרע ויתחזק חום יסודות הגוף ויתרחבו שבילי גידיהן (But when a boy grows up (reaches puberty) and the [substance] of sperm originates in them and the heat of his bodily humors increases, and the channels of their veins become wide …). In the sense of 'puberty,' Hebr. פֶּרֶק is attested in Rabb. and medieval liturgical literature (cf. BM 5240). Moses ibn Tibbon translates Arab. بلغ as הגיע לימי הבגרות (see previous entry) and Do'eg ha-Edomi translates the parallel Lat. term *venio ad aetatem* as הגיע לבגר (see entry above).

• *Part. Hif'il* **מַגִּיעַ** • **סבות מגיעות** → **סִבָּה**.

נֶגַע • **נגע המעים** · **[intestinal] abrasion**: Arab. سَحْج · Ibn Sīnā, *K. al-Qānūn fī al-ṭibb* · trans. Nathan ha-Me'ati, *Sefer ha-Qanun* II, fol. 70ᵃ: ביץ ביצים … והמבושל כמות שהוא בחומץ ימנע השלשול ונגע המעיים והאודם שלו ימנע[175] נגעי הכליות וכיס השתן (Eggs: … [Eggs] simply cooked with vinegar prevent diarrhea and [intestinal] abrasion; egg yolk prevents[176] ulcers of the kidneys and urinary bladder). Hebr. נגע המעים is not attested in the current dictionaries, but it also features as *Plur.* נגעי המעים ('intestinal ulcers') in Nathan's *Sefer ha-Peraqim* (*Pirqei Moshe*) VI.83 (cf. BCD 170 (NM 2:65); BMMN 77, l. 8; BMMG no.). For נֶגַע alone in the sense of 'ulcer,' cf. also BCD 170 (NM 1:62) for an attestation from Moses ibn Tibbon, *Sefer Ṣedat ha-Derakhim* VII.14.2 (cf. IJZ 7: 147, l. 28). In his *Sefer ha-Peraqim* (*Pirqei Moshe*) XXI.27, Nathan trans-

173 בחלום: بالا حتلام a.
174 'dream': 'nocturnal emission' a.
175 ימנע: ينفع a.
176 'prevents': 'is useful for' a.

lates Arab. سَحْج as הֶפְשֵׁט (cf. BCD 71 (NM 2:40–41); BMMN 199, l. 6), while Moses ibn Tibbon renders Arab. سحج as חֲמַרְמָרוּת (in his *Sefer Ṣedat ha-Derakhim* VII.29.1 (cf. BCD 104 (NM 1:56); IJZ 7:171, l. 3)) and Arab. سحج الأمعاء as חמרמרות המעיים (in his *Perush Aphorismi shel Apuqraṭ* (*Pirqei Abuqraṭ*) VI.3 (295) (cf. BCD 104 (NM 3:93); BMCH 1:393, l. 12)). Zeraḥyah Ḥen transcribes Arab. سحج as סחג׳ and Anonymous has הפשט המעיים (see also entry הֶפְשֵׁט for Nathan's use of this term in his *Sefer ha-Mezonot*).

• *Plur.* **נגעים** • **הנגעים המוסיפים** · **spreading ulcers**: Arab. القروح الساعية (Gr. νομή, *Plur.* νομαί; cf. UW 436–437) · Ibn Sīnā, *K. al-Qānūn fī al-ṭibb* · trans. Nathan ha-Me'ati, *Sefer ha-Qanun* II, fol. 72ª (Ms Paris, BnF, héb. 1136, fol. 70ª): בלוט ... ימנע מלהגדיל שחין הפה הנקרא קלאע בערבי והנגעים המוסיפים וזה כששורפים אותו (Oak: ... [The application of] burnt oak prevents the growth of aphthae, called QL'ʿ [i.e., *qilāʿ*] in Arab., and spreading ulcers). Hebr. הנגעים המוסיפים is not attested in the current dictionaries. Nathan also translates the Arab. term as הנגעים הפרים (see next entry). Zeraḥyah Ḥen translates Arab. القروح الساعية as הנגעים השורצים (see entry below) and Anonymous has השחינים המתרחבים.

• **הנגעים הפרים** · **spreading ulcers**: Arab. القروح الساعية (Gr. νομή, *Plur.* νομαί; cf. UW 436–437) · Ibn Sīnā, *K. al-Qānūn, fī al-ṭibb* · trans. Nathan ha-Me'ati, *Sefer ha-Qanun* II, fol. 73ª: בול שתן החמור יועיל אל הנגעים[177] הפרים והרטובים ... (Urine: ... The urine of a donkey is useful for spreading, moist ulcers). Hebr. הנגע הפרה, *Plur.* הנגעים הפרים, is not attested in the current dictionaries. Nathan also translates the Arab. term as הנגעים המוסיפים (see previous entry). Zeraḥyah Ḥen translates Arab. القروح الساعية as הנגעים השורצים (see next entry) and Anonymous has השחינים המתרחבים.

• **הנגעים השורצים** · **spreading ulcers**: Arab. القروح الساعية · Ibn Sīnā, *K. al-Qānūn fī al-ṭibb* · trans. Zeraḥyah Ḥen, *Sefer ha-Qanun* II, fol. 216ᵇ: בַּוְל שתן ... שתן החמור ⟨יועיל⟩ לנגעים השורצים והלחים (Urine: ... The urine of a donkey is useful for spreading, moist ulcers). Hebr. הנגע השורץ, *Plur.* הנגעים השורצים, is not attested in the current dictionaries. Nathan ha-Me'ati translates Arab. القروح الساعية as הנגעים הפרים (see previous entry).

[נגר] • *Hifʿil* **הִגִּיר** · **to make [something] flow [copiously]**: Arab. أدرّ · Ibn al-Jazzār, *Zād al-musāfir wa-qūt al-ḥādir* · trans. Moses ibn Tibbon, *Sefer Ṣedat ha-Derakhim* VI.17: עלי פולי כתוש ימית העובר ויגיר דם הנידות (Pounded mint leaves, [used as a vaginal suppository] kill the fetus and make the menstrual blood flow [copiously]). Hebr. [נגר], *Hifʿil* הִגִּיר, is not attested in the current dictionaries for medieval medical literature. *Part. Hifʿil* מַגִּיר features in BCD 187 (NM 4:124–125) in the combinations הסם המגיר הדם, הסם המגיר לזיעה, and הסם המגיר השתן (in attestations from Anonymous, *Sammim Libbiyim*). Abraham ben Isaac translates Arab. أدرّ as הוריד.

177 הנגעים הפרים: הנגעים המתרחבין Ms Paris, BnF, héb. 1136, fol. 70ᵇ.

נִדָּה • *Plur.* **נדות** • **אפיסת דם נידות** → **אֲפִיסָה.**
• **עכוב דם הנדות** → **עִכּוּב**
• **העצר דם הנדות** → **עָצַר¹.**
• **העצר הנדות** → **עָצַר¹.**
• **שופע נידות** → **שֹׁפַע.**

נִדְחָה (*Part. Nifʿal*) → **[דחה].**

[נהג] • *Hifʿil* **הִנְהִיג** · **to treat**: Arab. دبّر · Ibn al-Jazzār, *Zād al-musāfir wa-qūt al-ḥāḍir* · trans. Moses ibn Tibbon, *Sefer Ṣedat ha-Derakhim* IV.16: ואם קרה החולי הזה לנער לא יוכל לשתות הרפואות אשר זכרנו ננהיגהו מחוץ בתחבושות ושמנים וקלוחים ופתילות מרככות (If this illness [i.e., ileus] affects a child, it will not be able to ingest the remedies that I mentioned, but we treat it [with external remedies], such as poultices, oils, clysters, and softening suppositories). Hebr. [נהג], *Hifʿil* הִנְהִיג, does not feature in the sense of 'to treat' in the current dictionaries. The verb features as *Hitpaʿel* הִתְנַהֵג in the sense of 'to be treated' in Moses ibn Tibbon, *Perush Aphorismi shel Apuqraṭ* (*Pirqei Abuqraṭ*) I.1 (19) (cf. BCD 171 (NM 3:151); BMCH 1:323, l. 6). Do'eg ha-Edomi translates the parallel Lat. term *facio* as עשה.

נוֹדִי • **השקוי הנודי** → **שִׁקּוּי.**

נוּסָח · **formula; prescription; recipe**: Arab. نسخة · Ibn al-Jazzār, *Zād al-musāfir wa-qūt al-ḥāḍir* · trans. Moses ibn Tibbon, *Sefer Ṣedat ha-Derakhim* V.11: עוגות כאפר אחרות לפי נסחת בן מאסויה יועילו לכאב הטחול אשר יקרה מן הליחה הרעה והרוח (A recipe for other caper pastilles, formulated by Ibn Māsawayh, that are beneficial for pain in the spleen caused by a malignant humor and wind …). In the sense of 'recipe,' Hebr. נוּסָח features in BM 3578 in later attestations, a.o., from the *Sefer ha-Qanun*.

נוֹסָף (*Part. Nifʿal*) → **[יסף].**

נָזַל • *Part.* **נוֹזֵל** • **המים הנוזלים בעין** → **מַיִם.**

נֵזֶר · **umbel**: Arab. إكليل (Gr. στέφανος; cf. UW 638) · Ibn Sīnā, *K. al-Qānūn fī al-ṭibb* · trans. Anonymous, *Sefer ha-Qanun* II, fol. 69[b]: ג'אושיר … שוקו כמו שוק הכשות ועליו שער כמראה אגבר[178] ועליהו קטן מאד על קצהו נזר דומה לנזר פרח השבת (Opopanax: … Its stem is similar to that of a cucumber; it has dustlike[179] hair; its leaves are very small; its ends have round umbels similar to that of dill). Hebr. נֵזֶר (lit., 'crown') does not feature in this sense in the current dictionaries. Nathan ha-Me'ati translates Arab. إكليل as כִּפָּה (see entry). Zeraḥyah Ḥen transcribes the Arab. term as אכליל (also lit., 'crown'), while in a marginal gloss it features as נֵזֶר as well.

נִחוּר • **נחור הגרון** · **hoarseness**: Arab. بحوحة الصوت · Ibn Sīnā, *K. al-Qānūn fī al-ṭibb* · trans. Nathan ha-Me'ati, *Sefer ha-Qanun* II, fol. 70[a]: ביץ ביצים … והמבושל במים הנקרא נמרשת יועיל מהשעול וממורסת הקרום הנקרא שוצה ומהכליון הנקרא צל בערבי ונחור הגרון מהחום וצרות

---

178 אגבר: الغبار a.
179 'dustlike': Trans. after a.

הנשימה ורקיקת הדם (Eggs: ... [Soft] boiled egg called NMRŠT (i.e, Pers. *nīmbirisht*; cf. VL 1393: 'ovum sorbile, semicoctum;' IG 626) is useful for cough, pleurisy called ŠWṢH [i.e., Arab. *shawṣa*], phthsis called ṢL [i.e., *sill*] in Arab., hoarseness due to temperature, dyspnea, and haemoptysis). In the sense of 'hoarseness,' Hebr. ניחור הגרון features in BCD 173 (NM 3:154–155) in an attestation from Do'eg ha-Edomi, *Sefer Agur* II.40. Zeraḥyah Ḥen translates Arab. بحوحة الصوت as נחירת הקול and Anonymous has נחירות הקול.

נְחִירוּת · **roughness (rawness):** Arab. خشونة · Ibn Zuhr, *K. al-Aghdhiya* · trans. Nathan ha-Me'ati, *Sefer ha-Mezonot*, fol. 5[b]: ואם תשלק עד שתתחמם[180] ולא הגיע הקושי משקיט השעול ההוא מנחירות הריאה (If you boil an egg until it starts[181] to coagulate without becoming hard [and consume it] it alleviates cough hailing from roughness (rawness) of the [membrane] of the lungs). Hebr. נְחִירוּת features in BM 3612 in attestations from the *Sefer ha-Qanun* and from Nathan's *Sefer ha-Peraqim* (*Pirqei Moshe*) VI.41 (cf. BMMN 71, ll. 10–11: והשעול הבטוח הוא אותו שהוא מרוע מזג כלי הנשימה או מנחירות הגרון או מנחירות קנה הריאה; cf. also BMMG no. 1359).

[נחר] • *Hif'il* **הִנְחִיר** · **to make rough (raw):** Arab. خشّن · Ibn Zuhr, *K. al-Aghdhiya* · trans. Nathan ha-Me'ati, *Sefer ha-Mezonot*, fol. 5[b]: ואם תשלק עד שתתחמם[182] ולא הגיע הקושי משקיט השעול ההוא מנחירות הריאה המתחדש מאבק ועשן או מאכילת החומץ וזולתו ממה שינחיר קנה הריאה מהדברים הקובצים והחריפים (If you boil an egg until it starts[183] to coagulate without becoming hard [and consume it] it alleviates cough hailing from roughness (rawness) of the [membrane] of the lungs which is caused by [inhaling] dust or smoke or by drinking vinegar and the like. These astringent, sharp ingredients make the trachea rough (raw)). In the sense of 'to make rough,' Hebr. הִנְחִיר features in BM 3612 in attestations from the *Sefer ha-Qanun* and from Nathan's *Sefer ha-Peraqim* (*Pirqei Moshe*) VII.25 (cf. BMMN 84, l. 20; BMMG no. 1357).

נָחָשׁ • *Plur.* **נחשים** · **intestinal worms:** Arab. حيات · Ibn Zuhr, *K. al-Aghdhiya* · trans. Nathan ha-Me'ati, *Sefer ha-Mezonot*, fol. 3[a]: ואם תאכל החטה נאה כמות שהיא תזיק יותר ותהיה סגולתו להוליד תולעי הבטן הנקראים נחשים (Wheat eaten raw as it is, is more harmful and has the specific property of producing intestinal worms called *neḥashim* [lit., 'snakes']). In the sense of 'intestinal worms,' Hebr. *Plur.* נחשים features as נחשים (בבטן) ('[intestinal] worms') in BCD 173 (NM 266) in an attestation from Nathan's *Sefer ha-Peraqim* (*Pirqei Moshe*) VI.21 (cf. BMMN 68, l. 15).

נָטָה · **to subside:** Lat. *declino* (Arab. انحطاط) · Constantinus Africanus, *Viaticum peregrinantis* · trans. Do'eg ha-Edomi, *Sefer Ya'ir Netiv* V.10: וכאשר יחל החולי לנטות וחדוד הקדחת נכבה אז נסיר האדומה במיץ קושקוטא (When the illness starts to subside and the

---

180 שתתחמם: تختر a.

181 'starts to coagulate': Trans. after a.

182 שתתחמם: تختر a.

183 'starts to coagulate': Trans. after a.

fever has become less acute (ardent), we expel the yellow bile with dodder juice ...). Hebr. נָטָה does not fever in this sense in the current dictionaries. Moses ibn Tibbon translates Arab. انحطاط as יְרִידָה (cf. BCD 120 (NM 3:110) for Ibn Tibbon's use of the term in the sense of 'decline [of a disease]' in his *Perush Aphorismi shel Apuqraṭ* (*Pirqei Abuqraṭ*) II.1 (53) (cf. BMCH 1:335, l. 11)).

נְטִיָּה · paralysis of the facial nerve: Arab. لقوة · al-Rāzī, *K. al-Manṣūrī fī al-ṭibb* · trans. Shem Tov ben Isaac, *Sefer Almansur*, fols. 113^b–114^a: שער בנטיה: כשיתעוררו[184] פני האדם ולא יכול לסגור אחד מעיניו וכשירצה לפחת יראה הנפח יוצא מצד אחד כי אני אומר שיש לו עוות הפה (Chapter on paralysis of the facial nerve: When someone's face is[185] twisted and he cannot close one of his eyes and when he blows [lit., 'wants to blow'] he sees the vapor leave [the mouth] from one side, I say that he suffers from paralysis of the facial nerve). Hebr. נְטִיָּה is not attested in this sense in the current dictionaries. A var. reading נטית הפה features in Shem Tov's *Sefer ha-Shimmush* XXVII and XXX.1.6 (cf. BCD 174 (NM 1:105–106; 4:112)). For the synonymous עוות הפה, see BM 4361 for an attestation from Shabbetai Donnolo, *Sefer Ḥakhmoni*. Gerard de Cremona translates Arab. لقوة as *tortura oris*. See also לקות הפה (entry לָקוּת), העוות שבפנים (entry עִוּוּת), and עקום הפה (entry עִקּוּם).

נְטִילָה · applying fomentations: Arab. تطيل · Ibn al-Jazzār, *Zād al-musāfir wa-qūt al-ḥādir* · trans. Moses ibn Tibbon, *Sefer Ṣedat ha-Derakhim* V.5: ואולם המין השני מן רפואות המים הכרכומים הנה יהיה ברפואות אשר יוציאו המים בזיעה והתכה וזה אמנם יהיה על דרך נטילה ושפיכה (The second kind of remedies for the yellowish fluid [of dropsy] consists of those remedies that expel the fluid through sweating and dissolution. [This should be done by] applying [these remedies] in fomentations and by pouring [the water they have been cooked in] out [over the body]). In the sense of 'applying fomentations,' Hebr. נְטִילָה features in BCD 174 (NM 3:155) in an attestation from Anonymous, *Perush Aphorismi shel Apuqraṭ* (*Pirqei Abuqraṭ*) I.1 (16) (cf. BMCH 1:517, l. 8). Do'eg ha-Edomi translates the parallel Lat. term *suffumigationes* as הקטרות (see entry הַקְטָרָה).

[נטף] • *Hof'al* הֻטַּף • הוטף באף · to be poured (injected) into the nose: Arab. سعط · Ibn Sīnā, *K. al-Qānūn fī al-ṭibb* · trans. Anonymous, *Sefer ha-Qanun* II, fols. 63^b–64^a: בסבאסה ... עם שמן ויאולט יוטף באף לכאב הראש ההוה מרוח עבה בראש ומפלוח הראש (Mace: ... When mixed with violet oil and poured into the nose, [it relieves] the headache caused by dense winds and migraine). Hebr. הוטף באף is not attested in the current dictionaries. Nathan ha-Me'ati translates Arab. سعط as עשה סעוט (see entry עָשָׂה) and Zeraḥyah Ḥen has שם בנחירים.

נִכְאוּת · podagra; gout: Arab. نقرس · Ibn Sīnā, *K. al-Qānūn fī al-ṭibb* · trans. Nathan ha-Me'ati, *Sefer ha-Qanun* II, fols. 66^b–67^a (Ms Paris, BnF, héb. 1136, fol. 66^b): ... אנסאן

184 כשיתעוררו: إذا تعوج a (= כשיתעותו).
185 'is twisted': Trans. after a.

אמרו שדם הוסת ישקיט כאב הנכאות[186]הנקרא נקרס בערבי (Human being: ... Some [physicians] say that menstrual blood is useful for the pain caused by gout, called NQRS [i.e., *niqris*] in Arab.). Hebr. נְכָאוּת, poss. an abbreviated form of נכאות הרגלים (see next entry and this paragraph of Nathan's trans. extant in Ms Paris, BnF, héb. 1136, fol. 66[b]), only features as a modern term in EM 1153.

• **נכאות הרגלים** · **podagra; gout**: Arab. نقرس · Ibn Sīnā, *K. al-Qānūn fī al-ṭibb* · trans. Nathan ha-Me'ati, *Sefer ha-Qanun* II, fol. 94[a]: כשכאש ... עושים ממנו משיחה עם החלב על נכאות הרגלים הנק׳ נקרס בערבי ויועיל (Poppy: ... A plaster of poppy with milk is useful for gout, called NQRS [i.e., *niqris*] in Arab.). Hebr. נכאות הרגלים is not attested in the current dictionaries. It is poss. coined after the biblical נכה רגלים, *Plur.* נכי רגלים ('crippled'); cf. KB 698. It also features in Nathan's trans. extant in Ms Paris, BnF, héb. 1141, fol. 95[a]. However, in Ms Paris, BN héb. 1136, fol. 84[b], Arab. نقرس is merely transcribed as נקרס. The same transcription features throughout Nathan's *Sefer ha-Peraqim* (*Pirqei Moshe*) (cf. BMMG no. 5257).

נִמְלָה • **חולי הנמלה** → חָלִי.

נִמְלָט (*Part. Nif'al*) → [מלט].

נְעִירָה · **shivering fit; rigor**: Arab. نافض (Gr. ῥῖγος; cf. UW 589) · Ibn Sīnā, *K. al-Qānūn fī al-ṭibb* · trans. Nathan ha-Me'ati, *Sefer ha-Qanun* II, fol. 69[b]: בסר ובלח ... אם[187] יסתפקו ממנו הרבה יוליד הנעירה וסמור השער (BSR and BLḤ [i.e., Arab. *busr* and *balaḥ*, 'unripe dates']: ... When one consumes a lot of them, they produce rigor and horripilation). Hebr. נְעִירָה features in BM 3704 in the sense of 'a violent sudden movement;' it is not attested in medieval medical literature. Throughout his *Sefer ha-Peraqim* (*Pirqei Moshe*), Nathan translates Arab. نافض as רתת (cf. BMMG no. 5245), a term already featuring in Do'eg ha-Edomi, *Sefer Agur* IV.46 (cf. BCD 267 (NM 3:223)). Zeraḥyah Ḥen translates Arab. نافض as הקרירות החזק (for קְרִירוּת, as used in his *Sefer ha-Peraqim* (*Pirqei Moshe*) VII.23, cf. BCD 250 (NM 1:185); BMMZ 78, l. 21; BMMG no. 5245) and Anonymous has סְמוּר (which also features in David Caslari, *Sefer Ro'a Mezeg Mitḥallef* VI.4; cf. BCD 192 (NM 2:167)).

• **איברי הנעירה** → אֵבֶר.

נִפּוּץ • **איברי הנפוץ** → אֵבֶר.

נִפְזָר (*Part. Nif'al*) → [פזר].

נֶפַח · **flatulence; inflation; flatus; gas**: Lat. *inflatio* · Constantinus Africanus, *Viaticum peregrinantis* · trans. Do'eg ha-Edomi, *Sefer Ya'ir Netiv* IV.11: הנפח הוא אויר אין מבושל קר וגס נולד שם באסטומכא מהמאכל האין מסודר (Flatulence is crude [lit., 'uncocted'], cold, thick air that originates in the stomach as a result of an irregular diet). In the sense of 'flatulence,' Hebr. נֶפַח features in BCD 177 (NM 4:114) in a later attestation

186 הנכאות: נכאות הרגלים Ms Paris, BnF, héb. 1136, fol. 66[b].

187 אם יסתפקו ממנו: استعمالهما a.

from Nathan ha-Me'ati, *Sefer ha-Qanun* I. Moses ibn Tibbon translates the parallel Arab. term انتفاخ as נֶפַח as well.

נְפִילָה • נפילת תאוה ‧ **loss of appetite**: Arab. سقوط الشهوة ‧ Ibn al-Jazzār, *Zād al-musāfir wa-qūt al-ḥādir* ‧ trans. Moses ibn Tibbon, *Sefer Ṣedat ha-Derakhim* IV.15: ואם היה מה שיצא מן הנגע אשר במעים עב לבן או מוגלא עבה ודם הנה ראוי שנעיין ואם לא יהיה בחולה קדחת ולא צמא ולא חלשה מופלגת ולא נפילת תאוה הנה ראוי לקלחו בזה הקלוח (If the matter that exudes from the intestinal ulcer is thick and white or consists of thick pus and blood, we should examen [the patient]: if there is no fever, thirst, extreme weakness, or loss of appetite, we should apply the following clyster). Hebr. נפילת התאוה features in BCD 178 (NM 2:68) in a later attestation from Nathan ha-Me'ati, *Sefer ha-Peraqim* (*Pirqei Moshe*) VI.90 (cf. BMMN 78, l. 8; BMMG no. 2405). Do'eg ha-Edomi translates the parallel Lat. term *neque appetitus minoratur* as גם לא חסר חפץ המאכל.

נָפַל ‧ **to be put**: Arab. وقع ‧ Ibn Sīnā, *K. al-Qānūn fī al-ṭibb* ‧ trans. Anonymous, *Sefer ha-Qanun* II, fols. 47ª–47ᵇ: באן ... מועיל מן המורסות הקשות כלם ואם יפול באספלנית הנקראת מראהם (B'N [i.e., fruit of the ben oil tree [*Moringa oleifera* Lam.]]: ... When [the fruit] is put in an ointment, called MR'HM [i.e., Arab. *marāhim*], it is useful in all types of hard swellings). In the sense of 'to be put,' Hebr. נָפַל is a non-attested semantic borrowing from Arab. وقع. Nathan ha-Me'ati translates Arab. وقع as עירב and Zeraḥyah Ḥen has נכנס.

• *Hif'il* **הִפִּיל ב- • הפיל ב-** ‧ **to bring about, cause**: Arab. أوقع في ‧ Ibn Sīnā, *K. al-Qānūn fī al-ṭibb* ‧ trans. Anonymous, *Sefer ha-Qanun* II, fol. 54ª: בסר ובלח ... עשייתם הרבה יפילו ברתת ובסמור (BSR and BLḤ [i.e., Arab. *busr* and *balaḥ*, 'unripe dates']: ... Their frequent consumption causes rigor and horripilation). In the sense of 'to bring about, cause,' Hebr. הפיל ב- is a non-attested semantic borrowing from Arab. أوقع في. Nathan ha-Me'ati and Zeraḥyah Ḥen both translate the Arab. term as [ילד], *Hif'il* הוֹלִיד.

נִפְלָא (*Part. Nif'al*) → **[פלא]**.

נֶקֶב ‧ **anus**: Lat. *anus* (Arab. مخرج) ‧ Constantinus Africanus, *Viaticum peregrinantis* ‧ trans. Do'eg ha-Edomi, *Sefer Ya'ir Netiv* IV.15: ואם הוא במעי השפל יאות לטהרו עם קלישטרי בשכונת המעי אל הנקב (If it [i.e., the cause of dysentery] is in the lower intestines, the patient should be treated with clysters because of the proximity of these intestines to the anus). Hebr. נֶקֶב, *Plur.* נקבים, features in Rabb. literature in the sense of 'orifices of the body (anus; urethra);' cf. JD 930, Low LXV. See also NM 5:26 for the Hebr. term בדק נקביו ('to defecate') as used by Zeraḥyah Ḥen for Arab. تغوّط in his *Sefer ha-Peraqim* (*Pirqei Moshe*) XXIV.20 (cf. BMMZ 235, l. 18; BMMG no. 3746). Moses ibn Tibbon translates the parallel Arab. term مخرج as מוֹצָא (see entry) and the Arab. synonym مقعدة as פי הטבעת (see entry פֶּה).

• **הנקב התחתון** ‧ **anus**: Arab. مقعدة (Gr. δακτύλιος; cf. UW 188) ‧ Ibn al-Jazzār, *Zād al-musāfir wa-qūt al-ḥādir* ‧ trans. Abraham ben Isaac, *Sefer Ṣedah la-Oreḥim* VI.12: ואם יהיה הפלגמוני בפי הרחם אז יכאיב השרר והנקב התחתון (If the tumor occurs in the orifice of the uterus, it is followed by pain in the navel and anus). In the sense of 'anus,' Hebr.

הנקה התחתון features in BCD 179 (NM 1:33) in an attestation from Hillel ben Samuel, *Sefer Keritut*. Moses ibn Tibbon translates Arab. مقعدة as פי החלוחלת and פי הטבעת (see entry פֶּה). Do'eg ha-Edomi translates the parallel Lat. term *nates* as עגבות.

[נקה] • *Part. Pu'al* **מְנֻקֶּה** · **seedless**: Arab. منزوع العجم · Ibn al-Jazzār, *Zād al-musāfir wa-qūt al-ḥādir* · trans. Moses ibn Tibbon, *Sefer Ṣedat ha-Derakhim* VI.6: אך יהיה הפלגמוני והניפוח מקור יקח אז צימוקים מנוקים (But if tumor and swelling are caused by cold, he should take seedless raisins ...). Hebr. [נקה], *Part. Pu'al* מְנֻקֶּה, does not feature in this sense in the current dictionaries. Moses ibn Tibbon translates Arab. منزوع العجم as שהוסר זגו.

נִקּוּי · **evacuation**: Arab. استفراغ · Ibn Zuhr, *K. al-Aghdhiya* · trans. Nathan ha-Me'ati, *Sefer ha-Mezonot*, fol. 2b: אמנם הקיץ הוא זמן חם ויבש והעכול בו חלוש והנקוי בו בלתי משובח (But the summer is the hot and dry season in which the digestion is weak and [its] ecacuation is not recommended). Hebr. נִקּוּי is only attested in Rabb. literature in the sense of 'cleansing; clearing from sin' (JD 908; BM 3791). Nathan translates Arab. استفراغ as הרקה throughout his *Sefer ha-Peraqim* (*Pirqei Moshe*) (cf. BMMG no. 3820).

נִקְפָּא (*Part. Nif'al*) → [קפא].

נִרְעָשׁ (*Part. Nif'al*) → [רעש].

נָשׁוּם • **צרות הנשום** → צָרוּת.

נשטרי · **pessary (suppository)**: Lat. *nastare* (var. of *nascale*; cf. DMLBS 2242–2243; ND 708) (Arab. صوفة)· Constantinus Africanus, *Viaticum Viaticum peregrinantis* · trans. Do'eg ha-Edomi, *Sefer Ya'ir Netiv* VI.12: משיחה גם נשטרי (A salve and a pessary (suppository)). Hebr. נשטרי is a non-attested calque of Lat. *nastare*. Moses ibn Tibbon translates Arab. صوفة as צֶמֶר (see entry).

נְשִׁימָה • **כובד הנשימה** → כֹּבֶד.
• **מצוק הנשימה** → מָצוֹק.
• **קצר הנשימה** → קֹצֶר.

[נתך] • *Part. Hif'il* **מַתִּיךְ** • **הסם המתיך** → סַם.

[נתר] • *Part. Nif'al* **נִתָּר** · **having loose bowels; suffering from diarrhea**: Lat. *solutus* · Constantinus Africanus, *Viaticum peregrinantis* · trans. Do'eg ha-Edomi, *Sefer Ya'ir Netiv* V.13: ואם הוא נתר יותר מדאי נתן לו שילי וזרע פאפאויר דרכמ׳ וחצי עם אישרוב רושד או מהדס (If his bowels are too loose, we give him one and a half *dirham* of fleawort and poppy seed with rose juice or myrtle juice). Hebr. [נתר], *Part. Nif'al* נִתָּר, does not feature in this sense in the current dictionaries. Hebr. *Nif'al* נִתַּר in the sense of 'to dissolve' features in BCD 182 (NM 1:173) in an attestation from Zeraḥyah Ḥen, *Sefer ha-Peraqim* (*Pirqei Moshe*) XV.20 (cf. BMMZ 156, l. 1). Moses ibn Tibbon translates the parallel Arab. إن استطلق بطن صاحب العلّة as ואם נתר טבעו.

• *Hif'il* **הִתִּיר** • **התיר הבטן** · **to loosen the bowels, soften the stools, purge, prescribe a purgative**: Lat. *solutio ventris* (Arab. إسهال طبيعته) · Constantinus Africanus, *Viaticum peregrinantis* · trans. Do'eg ha-Edomi, *Sefer Ya'ir Netiv* IV.9: וכן כל הרוצים לשמור הבריאות ואם לא יוכלו להקיא נשתדל להתיר הבטן (Likewise, all those [suffering from indigestion] who want to preserve their health, should be purged in case they cannot vomit). Hebr. התיר הבטן features in BM 3888 in an attestation from Geonic literature. A synonymous term featuring in Abraham Avigdor, *Ha-Ma'amar ha-Teshi'i le-Sefer ha-Mansuri le-Razi* is התיר הטבע (see next entry). For another synonym החליק לטבע, featuring in Zeraḥyah Ḥen, *Sefer ha-Peraqim* (*Pirqei Moshe*) XVII.33, see BCD 101 (NM 1:150); BMMZ 173, l. 3; BMMG no. 4698. Moses ibn Tibbon translates the parallel Arab. term إسهال طبيعته as לשלשל טבעו.

• **התיר הטבע · to loosen the bowels, soften the stools, purge, prescribe a purgative**: Lat. *solvo ventrem* · Gerard de Solo, *Practica super nono Almansoris* · trans. Abraham Avigdor, *Ha-Ma'amar ha-Teshi'i le-Sefer ha-Mansuri le-Razi*, fol. 1b: והתיר הטבע במירבולנש כרכומים והאגסים והתמרידיש והסוכרי הקשה הלבן (One should loosen the bowels (soften the stools) with yellow myrobalans, pear, tamarind, and fine-quality[188] white sugar). Hebr. התיר הטבע is not attested in the current dictionaries. A synonym התיר הבטן features in Do'eg ha-Edomi, *Sefer Ya'ir Netiv* IV.9 (see previous entry).

• *Part. Hif'il* **מַתִּיר • רפואה מתירה/מתרת** → רְפוּאָה.

נִתָּר (*Part. Nif'al*) → [**נתר**].

188 'fine-quality white sugar': סוכר קשה לבן. For סוכר קשה; cf. BCD 186 (NM 4:122).

ס

סֻב • *Plur.* סובין • סובין שבראש · scurf; dandruff; favus: Arab. سعفة (cf. UW 156, s.v. ἀχώρ (cf. LS 298: 'scurf; dandruff') and UW 344, s.v. κηρίον (LS 948: 'honeycomb, *II.* a cutaneous disease; μελικηρίς;' cf. LS 1097, s.v. μελικηρίς: 'a kind of cyst or wen, from its resembling a honeycomb')) · Ibn Sīnā, *K. al-Qānūn fī al-ṭibb* · trans. Zeraḥyah Ḥen, *Sefer ha-Qanun* II, fol. 180[a]: בֵּין ... יועיל מן הקילוף והגרב כשיתנגע ויועיל מן הבתור[189] החלקות ולסובין שבראש (BeYN [i.e., fruit of the ben oil tree [*Moringa oleifera* Lam.]]: ... It is useful for exfoliating and ulcerating scabies, 'milk-like'[190] pimples, and dandruff (favus)). Hebr. סובין שבראש features in BM 3900 in the sense of 'pityr⟨i⟩asis capitis' in an attestation from Shem Tov ben Isaac, *Sefer Almansur*. Nathan ha-Me'ati translates Arab. سعفة as מִסְפַּחַת (see entry). For Hebr. *Plur.* סובין in the sense of 'bran,' see also entry כשך.

סִבָּה • *Plur.* סבות • סבות מגיעות · containing[191] (conjunct) causes: Lat. Sing. *coniuncta* (Gr. συνεκτικόν) · Gerard de Solo, *Practica super nono Almansoris* · trans. Abraham Avigdor, *Ha-Ma'amar ha-Teshi'i le-Sefer ha-Mansuri le-Razi*, fol. 35[b]: עוד ראוי שתדע שאצל הרופאים בהתחדשות הנזילה יש שלשה מינים מהסבות והם מקדימות מתחילות מגיעות והמתחילים הם הדברים החצוניים ... והסבות המגיעות הם הליחות ההם עצמם בהיות בפועל נוזלות מהמוח אל האיברים השפלים (You should also know that according to the physicians a catarrh can have three kinds of causes: antecedent, precedent, and containing. The antecedent causes are external things ... The containing causes are those very humors that actually stream from the brain to the lower organs). Hebr. סבה מגיע, *Plur.* סבות מגיעות, does not feature in the current dictionaries.

• סבות מקדימות · precedent[192] causes: Lat. Sing. *antecedens* (Gr. ἄιτιον προηγούμενον) · Gerard de Solo, *Practica super nono Almansoris* · trans. Abraham Avigdor, *Ha-*

---

189 הבתור החלקות (= البثور اللينة): البثور اللبنية a.

190 ''milk-like' pimples': Trans. after a.

191 'containing (conjunct) causes' (Lat. *coniuncta*): These causes are part of the popular Galenic system of three causes—antecedent, precedent, and containing, cf. P.E. Pormann and N.P. Joosse, 'Commentaries on the Hippocratic *Aphorisms* in the Arabic Tradition: The Example of Melancholy,' in *Epidemics in Context: Greek Commentaries on Hippocrates in the Arabic Tradition*, 233; the containing cause is the cause of the final event, cf. R.J. Hankinson (ed.), *Galen on Antecedent Causes* (Cambridge 1998), 43; the containing cause has also been described as being internal and co-temporal with its effect, cf. K. van't Land, 'Internal, Yet Intrinsic: Conceptions of Bodily Space and Their Relations to Causality in Late Medieval University Medicine,' in *Medicine and Space: Body, Surroundings, and Borders in Antiquity and the Middle Ages*, ed. by P.A. Baker, H. Nijdam, and K. van't Land (Leiden 2011), 105.

192 'precedent causes' (Lat. *antecedens*): 'causes that operate inside the body but are not yet the containing cause of the final event,' cf. Hankinson (ed.), *Galen on Antecedent Causes*, 43; it has also been described as internal and preceding its effect, cf. van't Land, 'Internal, Yet Intrinsic,' 105.

Ma'amar ha-Teshi'i le-Sefer ha-Mansuri le-Razi, fol. 35^{b}: והסבות המקדימות הם הליחות הלבניות או השחורות טרם התחדש מהם ההזלה (The preceding causes are phlegm or black bile before a catarrh originates from them). Hebr. סבה מקדימה, *Plur.* סבות מקדימות, features in KTP 3:84 as a synonym of סבות קודמות as 'vorhergehende Ursachen (Gattungs- und Artmerkmal).'

• **סבות מתחילות** · **antecedent**[193] **(initial) causes:** Lat. Sing. *primitiva* (Gr. *Sing.* ἄιτιον προκαταρκτικόν) · Gerard de Solo, *Practica super nono Almansoris* · trans. Abraham Avigdor, *Ha-Ma'amar ha-Teshi'i le-Sefer ha-Mansuri le-Razi*, fol. 35^{b}: עוד ראוי שתדע שאצל הרופאים בהתחדשות הנזילה יש שלשה מינים מהסבות והם מקדימות מתחילות מגיעות והמתחילים הם הדברים החצוניים (You should also know that according to the physicians, a catarrh can have three kinds of causes: antecedent, precedent, and containing. The antecedent causes are external things). Hebr. סבה מתחילה, *Plur.* סבות מתחילות, does not feature in the current dictionaries.

סָבוּב • *Plur.* **סבובים** · **cycles:** Arab. أدوار · Maimonides, *Maqāla fī al-rabw* (*On Asthma*) · trans. Joshua Shatibi, *Ma'amar 'al ha-Qaṣeret* x.6 (cf. BMA 2:354, ll. 22–25): והכאבים אשר יתחדשו לקצת האברים בסבובים הנה מדרך זאת החפיפה שתעשה בעתות הרוחה שהיא תמנע חידושם ביחוד אם השתמשו בה קודם העונה בשתים או שלש שעות (In the case of pains, which occur to some of the limbs in cycles, one should apply this kind of massage in order to prevent their occurrence, especially when one applies it in the quiet times, two or three hours before the attack). Hebr. סָבוּב, *Plur.* סבובים, does not feature in this sense in the current dictionaries. A synonymous הקפים features in Moses ibn Tibbon, *Perush Aphorismi shel Apuqraṭ* (*Pirqei Abuqraṭ*) IV.59 (196) (cf. BCD 72 (NM 3:69); BMCH 1:370, l. 19). Samuel Benveniste and Anonymous both render Arab. أدوار as תקופות.

סְבִיבָה • *Plur.* **סביבות** · **regarding; with reference to; with respect to:** Lat. *circa* (Arab. في) · Constantinus Africanus, *Viaticum peregrinantis* · trans. Do'eg ha-Edomi, *Sefer Ya'ir Netiv* IV.17: ונתן לו מן האנטידוטום העשוי מצואת הזאב ותקח מצואת זאב ותתן לו לשתות ביין כי זאת הצואה יש לה כח רב סביבות זה החולי (And we administer him [i.e., the patient suffering from a colic] the remedy prepared with the droppings of a wolf. Let him ingest these droppings with wine. Wolf's droppings are a very powerful [remedy] with respect to this illness). In the sense of 'with respect to,' Hebr. סְבִיבָה, *Plur.* סביבות, is a non-attested semantic borrowing from Lat. *circa*. Moses ibn Tibbon translates Arab. في as -בְּ.

---

193 'antecedent (initial) causes' (Lat. *primitiva*): 'causes that are open to inspection, or evident in the sense of the Empiricists,' cf. Hankinson (ed.), *Galen on Antecedent Causes*, 43; it has also been described as external and preceding its effect, cf. van't Land, 'Internal, Yet Intrinsic,' 105; see also Pormann and Joosse, 'Commentaries on the Hippocratic *Aphorisms*,' 233 and NM 2:150–151.

סָבַל · **to apply in a suppository**: Arab. احتمل · Ibn Sīnā, *K. al-Qānūn fī al-ṭibb* · trans. Nathan ha-Me'ati, *Sefer ha-Qanun* II, fols. 68ᵇ–69ᵃ: בורק ... משלשל[194] כשסובלים אותו וכשאוכלים אותו עם סדאב[195] וכמון או תבשיל הסדאב והשבת ישקיט עקיצת המעיים (Borax (sodium borate): ... When one applies it in a suppository, it relaxes the bowels and when one ingests it with rue,[196] cumin, or decoction of rue and dill, it alleviates gripes (colic)). In the sense of 'to apply in a suppository,' Hebr. סָבַל is a non-attested semantic borrowing from Arab. احتمل. Zeraḥyah Ḥen translates Arab. احتمل as סָבַל as well, while Anonymous has הניח למטה. In his *Sefer ha-Peraqim* (*Pirqei Moshe*), Nathan uses both סָבַל and הניח למטה (cf. BCD 171 (NM 2:65–66); BMMG no. 1183). See also next entry.

• **סבל פתילה מלמטה** · **to apply as a suppository**: Arab. احتمل فتيلة · Ibn Sīnā, *K. al-Qānūn fī al-ṭibb* · trans. Nathan ha-Me'ati, *Sefer ha-Qanun* II, fol. 68ᵃ: באן ... שעור שקל מגרגריו ישלשל ליחה לבנה נאה כששותים ממנו בדבש וכן משיחתו וכן אם יסבלו ממנו פתילה מלמטה טבולה בו (B'N [i.e., fruit of the ben oil tree [*Moringa oleifera* Lam.]]: ... One *mithqāl*[197] of its berries when taken with honey, expels the raw phlegm. Similar is the effect of its oil when it is applied in a suppository). Hebr. סבל פתילה מלמטה is not attested in the current dictionaries. Zeraḥyah Ḥen translates Arab. احتمل فتيلة as סבל בפתילה and Anonymous has לקח פתילה ... למטה. See also previous entry.

סֶדֶק • *Plur.* **סדקים** · **fissures**: Arab. شقاق · al-Rāzī, *K. al-Manṣūrī fī al-ṭibb* · trans. Shem Tov ben Isaac, *Sefer Almansur*, fol. 4ᵃ: פ״א בסדקים המתהוים בחדרי הרחם ([Chapter] 81: On fissures occurring in the parts of the uterus). In the sense of 'fissures,' Hebr. סֶדֶק, *Plur.* סדקים, features in MD 293–294. A var. reading סְדִיקָה, *Plur.* סדיקות, features in BCD 184 (NM 4:118 (corr.)) in an attestation from Moses ibn Tibbon, *Sefer Ṣedat ha-Derakhim* VII.30.1 (cf. IJZ 7:171, l. 12). Abraham Avigdor translates the parallel Lat. term *rhagades* as סדקים as well.

סֵדֶר • *Plur.* **סדרים** · **rules; instructions**: Arab. قوانين · Maimonides, *Maqāla fī al-rabw* (*On Asthma*) · trans. Joshua Shatibi, *Ma'amar 'al ha-Qaṣeret* X.1 (cf. BMA 2:353, ll. 10–12): אמנם בענין רפואת המחלות לא יכון לשנות המנהג ולא בשום סבה בשום פנים רק ישגיח השגחה שלימה על מה שביאר לנו גאלינוס בסדריו המועילים (But in the case of the healing of diseases, one should not intend to change the habit in any manner or for any reason. Instead, it should be observed with utmost attention, as Galen explained to us in his helpful instructions). In the sense of 'rules,' Hebr. סֵדֶר, *Plur.* סדרים, features in BCD 184–185 (NM 3:168) in an earlier attestation from Zeraḥyah Ḥen, *Perush Aphorismi shel Apuqraṭ* (*Pirqei Abuqraṭ*) I.1 (16) (cf. BMCH 1:421, l. 23). Samuel Benveniste translates Arab. قوانين as דרכים (see entry דֶּרֶךְ) and Anonymous has עקרים (see entry

---

194 משלשל: add. according to Ms Paris, BnF, héb. 1136, fol. 68ᵃ.
195 סדאב: شراب a.
196 'rue': 'wine' a.
197 Hebr. *sheqel* stands for Arab. *mithqāl*; one *mithqāl* is 4.46 grams; cf. HIM 4–7.

עִקָּר). For *Sing.* סֵדֶר in the sense of 'regimen,' featuring in Do'eg ha-Edomi, *Sefer Ya'ir Netiv* I.22.6, cf. NM 5:137–138; IJZ 1–2:625.

סוּסְיָא (*Aram.*) ‣ **horse (mare)**: Arab. رمكة · Ibn al-Jazzār, *Zād al-musāfir wa-qūt al-ḥādir* · trans. Moses ibn Tibbon, *Sefer Ṣedat ha-Derakhim* V.13: ואם המוגלא עבה מאד נשקה אותו בשול שומר או בשול כרפס או בשול אישנץ וישתה אחר זה ג״כ חלב שנחלב מיד ויהיה החלב מאתון או מסוסיא כי הוא ינקה הנגע נקוי טוב (If the pus is very thick, we administer a decoction of fennel, celery, or absinth wormwood; then [the patient] should also drink fresh milk of a donkey or mare because it cleans the wound properly). Aram. סוּסְיָא is only attested in Rabb. literature (cf. JD 967; DAN 286).

סוֹעֵד (*Part.*) → סָעַד.

סְחִיטָה ‣ **scarification**: Arab. شرط · Ibn al-Jazzār, *Zād al-musāfir wa-qūt al-ḥādir* · trans. Moses ibn Tibbon, *Sefer Ṣedat ha-Derakhim* VI.10: ואם יאריך השפע אחר זאת ההנהגה שים כלי המציצה תחת כל אחד משדדיה וירבה למוץ בלי סחיטה (If the loss [of blood] continues after this regimen, cupping glasses should be placed under each breast, and much blood should be drawn forth without scarification). Hebr. סְחִיטָה is not attested in this sense in the current dictionaries. Do'eg ha-Edomi translates the Lat. parallel term *scarificatio* as כְּרִיתוּת (see entry).

סִיג • סיג הכסף ‣ **silver dross**: Arab. خبث الفضّة (cf. MIG no. 819) · Ibn al-Jazzār, *Zād al-musāfir wa-qūt al-ḥādir* · trans. Moses ibn Tibbon, *Sefer Ṣedat ha-Derakhim* IV.15: ויחבוש פי הטבעת בתחבושת עשויה מנאקרה[198] שרופה וליטרג׳ ובלנקט וסיג הכסף (Put a poultice on the anus made from N'QRH *serufah* [i.e., burnt shells], litharge, ceruse, and silver dross). In the sense of 'silver dross,' Hebr. סיג הכסף features in NM 4:119 (for Arab. خبث الفضة) in a reference to Shem Tov ben Isaac, *Sefer ha-Shimmush* XXIX, list 1 (SHS 1:356–357 (Samekh 6)). Ibn Tibbon also uses סיג הכסף to render Arab. إقليميا الفضّة ('silver cadmia; silver calamine') in his *Sefer Ṣedat ha-Derakhim* I.7.1 (cf. BCD 185 (NM 4:119); IJZ 1–2:450).

סִיד • סיד בלתי מכובה ‣ **unslaked lime; quicklime**: Arab. نورة غير مطفأة · Ibn al-Jazzār, *Zād al-musāfir wa-qūt al-ḥādir* · trans. Moses ibn Tibbon, *Sefer Ṣedat ha-Derakhim* IV.15: תואר עוגות אחרות מארסיניקום ואורופימנט יועילו כמו אשר לפניהם והם חזקות מנוסות ערובם: יקח ארסיניקום ואורופימינט ושמרי חומץ יין מנוגב שרוף ואכסיא וגומא ארביקא מ״א שקל וסיד בלתי מכובה וכאגד שרוף מ״א ב׳ דר׳ אלום לבן דר׳ אופי חצי דר׳ יודקו הסמים וינופו ויולשו ביין אדום ריחני ויעשה עוגות וינגבם בצל וירגילם (A recipe for other pastilles with red and yellow arsenic that are beneficial just like the ones [mentioned] before and that are strong and tested: Take one *sheqel*[199] each of red and yellow arsenic, of dried, burned

198 נאקרה (N'QRH) (صدف a): A non-documented O. Occ. or O. Cat *nacra or *nacre, var. of Mod. Cat. or Mod. Occ. *nacre*, 'white substance with iridescent reflections, which forms the inside of certain sea shells … oyster with pearls' (FEW 19:137). I thank Julia Zwink for this reference.

199 Hebr. *sheqel* stands for Arab. *mithqāl*; one *mithqāl* is 4.46 grams; cf. HIM 4–7.

vinegar sediment, of acacia gum, and of gum Arabic, two *dirhams* each of quicklime and burned papyrus, one *dirham* of white alum, half a *dirham* of opium. Pound the ingredients, sieve them, knead them with fragrant red wine, make pastilles, dry them in the shade, and apply them). In the sense of 'unslaked lime; quicklime,' Hebr. סיד בלתי מכובה is a non-attested calque of Arab. نورة غير مطفأة. Moses ibn Tibbon translates the Arab. synonym نورة لم يصبها ماء as סיד שלא נגע בו מים (see entry below). Do'eg ha-Edomi translates the parallel Lat. term *calx viva* as סיד חי (see next entry).

• **סיד חי · unslaked lime; quicklime**: Lat. *calx viva* · Constantinus Africanus, *Viaticum peregrinantis* · trans. Do'eg ha-Edomi, *Sefer Ya'ir Netiv* IV.15: טרוסיקש ארסניקש סנדראקא שמרי חומץ שרופים אכאסיא גומי דרכמ׳ וחצי סיד חי כאגד שרופה ב׳ דרכמ׳ (Arsenic pastilles: [Take] one and a half *dirham* [each of] orpiment, burnt vinegar sediment, acacia gum; two *dirhams* [each of] quicklime and burned papyrus ...). Hebr. סיד חי features in BCD 185 (NM 1:34) and NM 5:138 in later attestations from Hillel ben Samuel, *Sefer Keritut* and Shem Tov ben Isaac, *Sefer ha-Shimmush* XXIX, list 1 (cf. SHS 1:364–365 (Samekh 21)). Moses ibn Tibbon translates the parallel Arab. term نورة لم يصبها ماء as סיד שלא נגע בו מים (see next entry).

• **סיד שלא נגע בו מים · unslaked lime; quicklime**: Arab. نورة لم يصبها ماء · Ibn al-Jazzār, *Zād al-musāfir wa-qūt al-ḥādir* · trans. Moses ibn Tibbon, *Sefer Ṣedat ha-Derakhim* IV.15: וזה תואר עוגות הארסיניקום ערובם: יקח ארסיניקום ואורופימינט מ״א שקל וסיד שלא נגע בו מים ב׳ שקלים (This is a recipe for arsenic pastilles: Take one *sheqel* each of [red] arsenic and yellow arsenic; two *sheqels* of quicklime ...). In the sense of 'unslaked lime; quicklime,' Hebr. סיד שלא נגע בו מים is a non-attested calque of Arab. نورة لم يصبها ماء. Moses ibn Tibbon translates the Arab. synonym نورة غير مطفأة as סיד בלתי מכובה (see entry above). Do'eg ha-Edomi translates the parallel Lat. *term calx viva* as סיד חי (see previous entry).

סימן → סִמָּן.

סַם • **הסם המרקיק · attenuant drug**: Arab. الدواء الملطّف · Ibn Sīnā, *K. al-Qānūn fī al-ṭibb* · trans. Nathan ha-Me'ati, *Sefer ha-Qanun* II, fol. 56ᵇ: ו⟨הסם⟩ המרקיק הוא סם שמנהגו שיעשה[200] התערוב יותר רקיק בחום ישר כמו בזופא וההאשא והבאבונג (An attenuant drug is a drug that—through its moderate heat—greatly attenuates the humor, [examples of such a drug are:] hyssop, thyme, and camomile). Hebr. הסם המרקיק is not attested in the current dicitionaries. The verb [רקק], *Hif'il* הִרְקִיק, features in BM 6739–6740 in the sense of 'to thin' in an attestation from the *Sefer ha-Qanun*. Zeraḥyah Ḥen translates Arab. الدواء ملطّف as הרפואה המדקדקת (cf. BCD 188 (NM 4:125) for an attestation from Anonymous, *Sammim Libbiyim*) and Anonymous has המדקדק.

• **הסם המתיך · dissolving drug**: Arab. الدواء المحلّل · Ibn Sīnā, *K. al-Qānūn fī al-ṭibb* · trans. Nathan ha-Me'ati, *Sefer ha-Qanun* II, fol. 56ᵇ: ו⟨הסם⟩ המתיך הוא שמנהגו שיפזר התערוב

200 שיעשה: emend. ed. שיש Ms أن يجعل a.

כשמעשן אותו ויוציאנו מן המקום אשר יסתבך בו חלק אחר חלק עד כי בהתמדת אותו הפעל יכלה מה שנשאר ממנו בכח חומו כמו הגנדבא דסתר (A dissolving drug is a drug that—by the intensity of its heat—is capable of dispersing the humor by gradually evaporating and dislodging it through a continuous activity until it eliminates—through its energy—whatever humor is left; [such a drug is] castoreum). Hebr. הסם המתיך features in BCD 190 (NM 4:132) in an attestation from Anonymous, *Sammim Libbiyim*. Zeraḥyah Ḥen translates Arab. الدواء المحلّل as הרפואה המתירה (for רפואה מתירה/מתרת, as used in Do'eg ha-Edomi, *Sefer Ya'ir Netiv* IV.12, see entry רְפוּאָה) and Anonymous has המתיך.

• *Plur.* **סמים • הסמים המנגעים** · **drugs that cause blisters**: Arab. الأدوية المقرحة · Maimonides, *Maqāla fī al-rabw* (*On Asthma*) · trans. Joshua Shatibi, *Ma'amar 'al ha-Qaṣeret* XI.2 (cf. BMA 2:357, ll. 10–12): וכבר זכרו הרופאים ברפואת קצת מיני זה החולי והוא המפורסם אצל כל רופא עשות הסמים המאדמים על הראש אך המנגעים והכוונה בזה מנוע דבר מן הנזילות (The physicians have mentioned as part of the treatment of some types of this disease [i.e., asthma]—and it is well known to every physician—the application of rubefacients, or even drugs that cause blisters, to the head. Their intention with this is the prevention of defluxions). Hebr. הסמים המנגעים is not attested in the current dictionaries. Hebr. *Sing.* הסם המנגע features in BCD 188–189 (NM 4:128) in the sense of 'ulcerative [remedy]' in an attestation from Anonymous, *Sefer ha-Refu'ot ha-Libbiyot*. Samuel Benveniste translates Arab. الأدوية المقرحة as הרפואות המצרבות (see entry רְפוּאָה) and Anonymous has הסמנים המשחינים (see entry סַמָּן).

סְמִירוּת · **shivering**: Arab. اقشعرار (Gr. φρίκη; cf. UW 742) · Maimonides, *Maqāla fī al-rabw* (*On Asthma*) · trans. Anonymous, *Sefer ha-Qaṣeret* V.6 (cf. BMA 2:405, ll. 7–9): או כאב הקולנג או כאב הכליות או כאב הטחול או כאב הכבד או כאב החזה או כאב האברים[201] או שיבוש הגוף או קרירות[202] או סמירות או חמימות (Pain in the colon, intestines, spleen, liver, chest, or joints;[203] indisposition; shivering[204] fit; shivering; or fever). Hebr. סְמִירוּת is not attested in the current dictionaries. A var. reading סמרות features in BCD 192 (NM 1:73) in an attestation from Zeraḥyah Ḥen, *Sefer ha-Peraqim* (*Pirqei Moshe*) XIX.37 (cf. BMMZ 180, l. 21; BMMG no. 4114). Samuel Benveniste translates Arab. اقشعرار as הסתמר and Joshua Shatibi has סִמּוּר (cf. also BMMG no. 4114 for both Zeraḥyah's and Nathan ha-Me'ati's use of סִמּוּר in their *Sefer ha-Peraqim* (*Pirqei Moshe*), as well as BCD 192 (NM 2:167) for an attestation from David Caslari, *Sefer Ro'a Mezeg Mitḥallef* VI.4).

סַמָּן • *Plur.* **סמנים • הסמנים המשחינים** · **drugs that cause blisters**: Arab. الأدوية المقرحة · Maimonides, *Maqāla fī al-rabw* (*On Asthma*) · trans. Anonymous, *Sefer ha-Qaṣeret* XI.2

201 האברים: المفاصل a.
202 קרירות: نافض a.
203 'joints': Trans. after a.
204 'shivering fit': Trans. after a.

וכבר זכרו הרופאים ברפואת מקצת מיני זה החלי והוא המפורסם אצל (cf. BMA 2:425, ll. 10–12): כל רופא כלל הסמנין הנמשחים על הראש המשחינים הכונה ⟨ב⟩זה המנעות הירידות (The physicians have mentioned as part of the treatment of some types of this disease [i.e., asthma]—and it is well known to every physician—the application of drugs that are rubbed on the head, which cause blisters. Their intention with this is the prevention of defluxions). Hebr. הסמנים המשחינים is not attested in the current dictionaries. The verb [שחן], *Part. Hif'il* מַשְׁחִין, features in BM 7027 in the sense of 'ulcerating' in an attestation from Nathan ha-Me'ati, *Sefer ha-Peraqim* (*Pirqei Moshe*) XXIII.46 (cf. BMMN 224, l. 18). Samuel Benveniste translates Arab. الأدوية المقرحة as הרפואות המצרבות (see entry רְפוּאָה) and Joshua Shabiti has הסמים מנגעים (see entry סַם).

סִמָּן · **tattoo(s)**: Arab. وشم · Ibn Sīnā, *K. al-Qānūn fī al-ṭibb* · trans. Zeraḥyah Ḥen, *Sefer ha-Qanun* II, fol. 181ᵇ: בַּלַאדֿר ... היפוי: יתלוש התלול בלע' פּוּרָא ויסיר הבהרת ויעתיק הסימן (Marking nut: ... [Its use in] cosmetics: It removes TLWL [i.e., Arab. *thu'lūl*, 'warts'], in o.l. PWRa'; it also removes *baheret*[205] and tattoos). Hebr. סִמָּן is not attested in this sense in the current dictionaries. Nathan ha-Me'ati translates Arab. وشم as כְּעוּר (see entry) and Anonymous has כֶּתֶם (see entry).

• *Plur.* **סמנים** · I. **spots**: Arab. آثار · Ibn Sīnā, *K. al-Qānūn fī al-ṭibb* · trans. Nathan ha-Me'ati, *Sefer ha-Qanun* II, fol. 91ᵇ (Ms Paris, BnF, héb. 1136, fol. 82ᵇ): ... כברית ואם יערבו אותו בשרף האלון ובערבי בצמג[206] אלבטם יעקר הסמנים אשר על הצפרנים (Sulphur: When mixed with the resin of the turpentine tree, in Arab. ṢMG 'LBṬM [i.e., *ṣumgh al-buṭm*], it removes the spots from the nails). Hebr. *Sing.* סִמָּן is not attested in the sense of 'spot' in the current dictionaries. Zeraḥyah Ḥen translates Arab. آثار as רֹשֶׁם (see entry). The latter term is also used by Nathan in addition to סמנים.

· II. **scars**: Arab. آثار (Gr. οὐλή; cf. UWS 1:813) · Ibn Sīnā, *K. al-Qānūn fī al-ṭibb* · trans. Nathan ha-Me'ati, *Sefer ha-Qanun* II, fol. 73ᵇ: גוז ... אם ישימו הרטוב ממנו על סמני ההכאה יועיל (Walnut: ... If fresh walnut is put on the scars of injuries it is beneficial). Hebr. *Sing.* סִמָּן is not attested in this sense in the current dictionaries. Zeraḥyah Ḥen translates Arab. آثار as סמנים, just like Nathan, and Anonymous has רֹשֶׁם (see entry).

· III. **pimples**: Arab. بثور · Ibn Sīnā, *K. al-Qānūn fī al-ṭibb* · trans. Nathan ha-Me'ati, *Sefer ha-Qanun* II, fol. 71ᵇ: בקלה אלחמקה ... יועיל אל הסמנים אשר בראש אם רוחצים בו מזוג ביין ויסיר קהיית השניים מפני שהוא מחליק העובי (Common purslane: ... It is useful for pimples of the head with it if is washed with [common purslane] mixed

205 '*baheret*': The Hebr. term stands for Arab. *baraṣ*, indicating a skin disease that has two varieties, namely white and black. The white variety is perh. identical with *sclerodermia circumscripta*, while the black variety may be *psoriasis vulgaris* or *ichthyosis vulgaris*. Arab. *baraṣ* stands for Gr. λέπρα; cf. UW 97; see also IJZ 7:108–113, esp. 108, n. 195.

206 בצמג: emend. ed. מגב Ms.

with wine. It removes bluntness of the teeth because it makes their roughness smooth). Hebr. *Sing.* סִמָּן is not attested in this sense in the current dictionaries. In his *Sefer ha-Peraqim* (*Pirqei Moshe*) VI.24, Nathan translates Arab. *Sing.* بثر as צמח (cf. BMMN 68, l. 24; BMMG no. 177) and in XXIII.40 Arab. *Plur.* بثور as בתורים הם צמחים (cf. BMMN 223, l. 18; BMMG no. 179). Zeraḥyah Ḥen transcribes Arab. بثور as בתור and Anonymous has צמחים.

סְנוּן · filtrate: Arab. صفو · Ibn al-Jazzār, *Zād al-musāfir wa-qūt al-ḥāḍir* · trans. Moses ibn Tibbon, *Sefer Ṣedat ha-Derakhim* IV.15: תשליך עליו חצי ליט' מסנון הבשול הקודם (Add to it half a liter[207] of the filtrate of the decoction mentioned before). In the sense of 'filtration' (for Arab. تصفية), the Hebr. term also features in NM 5:140 in an attestation from *Sefer Ṣedat ha-Derakhim* III.6 and in the sense of 'filtrate' (for Lat. *colatura*) in an attestation from R. Isaiah's trans. of Guillaume de Congenis, *Chirurgia* (*Treatise on Surgery*).

סַנְוֵר · night blindness (nyctalopia): Arab. عشا (MMT 253[208]) · al-Rāzī, *K. al-Manṣūrī fī al-ṭibb* · trans. Shem Tov ben Isaac, *Sefer Almansur*, fol. 3ᵇ: כ"ז בסנור המתחדש בעין ([Chapter] 27: On night blindness affecting the eye). Hebr. סַנְוֵר is only attested in the current dictionaries in the general sense of 'blindness' (cf. BM 123–124). See also entries אֹפֶל and לִילִית.

סְנַפִּיר • *Plur.*[1] **סנפירות · incrustation of blood:** Lat. *cortex/crusta* · Gerard de Solo, *Practica super nono Almansoris* · trans. Abraham Avigdor, *Ha-Ma'amar ha-Teshi'i le-Sefer ha-Mansuri le-Razi*, fol. 88ᵇ: שער בנגעים אשר בחוטם. כאשר יהיו בחוטם סנפריות (*סנפירות) ישים בו שעוה ושמן ושומן תרנגולת וישאף ויריח המים החמים פעמים רבות בכל בקר (Chapter on wounds in the nose: If there is an incrustation of blood in the nose, one should put wax, olive oil, and chicken fat in it and repeatedly sniff hot water every morning). Hebr. סְנַפִּיר, *Plur.* סנפירים or סנפירות, does not feature in this sense in the current dictionaries. In the sense of 'dandruff; scurf; eschar; scales' it is attested in BCD 192–193 (NM 1:63; 4:137–138).

• *Plur.*[2] **סנפירים · flakes:** Lat. *cortices* (Arab. صفائح) · Constantinus Africanus, *Viaticum peregrinantis* · trans. Do'eg ha-Edomi, *Sefer Ya'ir Netiv* V.14: וכמו קלפות וסנפירים יתראו בשתן ([Particles] similar to scales and flakes will be visible in the urine). Moses ibn Tibbon translates Arab. صفائح as רקועים ושטחים (see entry רִקּוּעַ).

סָעַד • *Part.* **סוֹעֵד · treating:** Arab. معالجة · Maimonides, *Maqāla fī al-rabw* (*On Asthma*) · trans. Samuel Benveniste, *Ma'amar 'al ha-Qaṣeret* XIII.25 (cf. BMA 2:306, ll. 9–13): אמר ג'אלינוס במאמר ממאמריו הידועים וזה נסחת דבריו אמר: היונים אם נסתפק להם חולי הניחוהו בין הטבע ובינו והוא [כלה] יגרשהו. והביאו טענה לדבריהם שהטבע ממונה ופקיד על

---

207 'liter': Arab. *raṭl*. The weight of a *raṭl* is varying according to region and period; from the twelfth century its general weight in Egypt is 450 grams.

208 The Arab. term can also refer to the opposite of night blindness, i.e., hemeralopia (cf. IJZ 1–2:273, n. 429).

החי בבריאותו וסועד אותו במחלתו ויודע מזג האיברים וישלח לכל אבר הראוי לו מן המסעד אחרי שהכין מקומות למוספי המסעד ולחות מקובלות לגוף (In one of his well-known treatises, Galen said the following: When the Greeks were in doubt about a disease, they left it to nature to expel it. Their argument for this was that nature is in charge of the health of living beings and treats them in the case of disease, and that it knows the temperament of their organs and sends to every individual organ the appropriate kind of nourishment, after first preparing sites for the superfluities of the food and humors appropriate to the body). Hebr. סָעַד, *Part.* סוֹעֵד, does not feature in this sense in the current dictionaries. Joshua Shatibi and Anonymous both render Arab. معالجة as מרפא.

סַעַד · **treatment**: Arab: علاج · Maimonides, *Maqāla fī al-rabw* (*On Asthma*) · trans. Samuel Benveniste, *Ma'amar 'al ha-Qaṣeret* XII.11 (cf. BMA 2:295, ll. 9–11): מבואר הוא שאין הכונה במאמר הזה להשלים כל מה שנזכר ממיני הסעד לחולי זה אבל להזכיר מה שיקל לעשותו. וכבר כתבתי למעלתכם מה שאני חושב שהוא יותר על שאלתכם (It is clear that the intention of this treatise is not to mention all the different kinds of treatment for this disease, but merely to select those medicines which are easily prepared. I have recorded for my Master more of those medicines than you requested). Hebr. סַעַד only features as a modern term in the sense of 'support; help' in EM 1258. In addition to סַעַד, Benveniste translates Arab. *Plur.* علاجات as מסעדים (see entry מִסְעָד). Joshua Shatibi and Anonymous both render Arab. علاج as רפואה.

סעוט • עשה סעוט → עָשָׂה.

סַפַּחַת · **scurf; dandruff; favus**: Arab. سعفة (cf. UW 156, s.v. ἀχώρ (cf. LS 298: 'scurf; dandruff') and UW 344, s.v. κηρίον (LS 948: 'honeycomb, *II.* a cutaneous disease; μελικηρίς;' cf. LS 1097, s.v. μελικηρίς: 'a kind of cyst or wen, from its resembling a honeycomb')) · Ibn Sīnā, *K. al-Qānūn fī al-ṭibb* · trans. Nathan ha-Me'ati, *Sefer ha-Qanun* II, fol. 81b: זרניך ... אם יערבוהו עם חלב ושמן יועיל מהגרב והספחת הרטוב הנקרא סעפה והאגודות[209] (Arsenic: ... Mixed with fat and oil it is useful in scabies, 'moist' scurf (favus), called S'PH [i.e., Arab. *sa'fa*] and putrefaction[210]). Hebr. סַפַּחַת features in the Bible as 'eruption; scab' (BDB 705) and in Rabb. literature as 'rising on the skin; sore' (JD 1012) or 'a scaly skin-disease; pityriasis capitis; psoriasis' (Low LXVII), cf. BM 4155: 'psoriasis' (foll. MD 6069). The term סַפַּחַת features in BCD 194 (NM 4:139) in the sense of 'eczema' (for Arab. قوباء; cf. השחין הדק (s.v. שְׁחִין)) in an attestation from Shem Tov ben Isaac, *Sefer ha-Shimmush* XXVII. A synonym used by Nathan (for Arab. سعفة) in his *Sefer ha-Peraqim* (*Pirqei Moshe*) XXIII.54 is נֶתֶק ('cradle cap,' cf. BCD 182 (NM 2:69); BMMN 225, l. 15). The latter term is also used by Zeraḥyah Ḥen and Anonymous. See also entry מִסְפַּחַת.

---

209 והאגודות: والعفن a.

210 'putrefaction': Trans. after a (عفن). Hebr. אגודות does not feature as a medical term in the current dictionaries; in SHS 1:119–120 (Alef 38) we find it as אגודות בשר with a parallel M. Lat. term *lupia* in the sense of 'epidermal cyst.'

סַפִּירִי • מלח ספירית → מֶלַח.

סַפְלוּל · **long birthwort** [*Aristolochia longa* L.]: Arab. زراوند (cf. MIG no. 321) · *Shinnui ha-Shemot ha-Niqra'im Synonimi*, fol. 77[a]: זדיונכ ה׳ ספלול ה׳ פלפל ארוך ה׳ אריסטולוגיאה ארוכה (ZDYWNYK [read: ZR'WND?, i.e., Arab. *zarāwand*], that is *saflul*, that is *pilpel arokh*, that is 'RYSṬWLWGY'H [i.e., *aristolochia*] *arukkah*). In the sense of 'long birthwort,' Hebr. סַפְלוּל features in EM 1264 as a modern term only.

[ספר] • *Pi'el* **סִפֵּר** · **to prescribe**: Arab. وصف · Ibn al-Jazzār, *Zād al-musāfir wa-qūt al-ḥādir* · trans. Moses ibn Tibbon, *Sefer Ṣedat ha-Derakhim* VI.6: וזאת תאר טיחה ספרה אסחק בן סולימן למורסת הביצים מרוח חמה עבה וכבר נסיתיה (This is the composition of a plaster (salve), which I have tested, prescribed by Isḥāq ibn Sulaymān for a tumor of the testicles caused by a thick, hot flatulence). In the sense of 'to prescribe,' Hebr. *Pi'el* סִפֵּר is a non-attested semantic borrowing from Arab. وصف. Abraham ben Isaac translates Arab. وصف as אָמַר (see entry).

סַפָּר • *Plur.* **ספרים** · **barbers**: Arab. مزيّن, *Plur.* مزيّنون · Maimonides, *Maqāla fī al-rabw* (*On Asthma*) · trans. Samuel Benveniste, *Ma'amar 'al ha-Qaṣeret* XIII.32 (cf. BMA 2:309, ll. 2–3): ואתה רואה דרך בני אדם הבריאים והחולים היאך יסמכו על הספרים להוציא הדם ועל נערים כוחלים[211] לשתות המשלשלים (Nevertheless, you find people, both healthy and sick, who rely on barbers for bloodletting and on young pseudo-oculists[212] for the ingestion of purgatives.) Hebr. סַפָּר features in BM 4190 in attestations from Rabb. literature only (cf. JD 1017). Joshua Shatibi translates Arab. مزيّنون as מקיזים and Anonymous has נסדרים.

[סרך] • *Nif'al* **נִסְרַךְ** · **to get stuck**: Arab. لحج · Ibn al-Jazzār, *Zād al-musāfir wa-qūt al-ḥādir* · trans. Moses ibn Tibbon, *Sefer Ṣedat ha-Derakhim* V.15: והנה תהיה הרקת הדם ג״כ במי שיתילד בכוליתו אבן כשנסרכה במהלך אשר בין הכליות והמקוה (Loss of blood also occurs to someone who gets kidney stones when they get stuck in the passage between the kidneys and urinary bladder). Hebr. *Nif'al* נִסְרַךְ features in BM 4220 in the sense of 'clinging, adhering to' in the context of organs adhering to each other.

סְתִימָה · **obstruction**: Lat. *opilatio* (Arab. سدّة, *Plur.* سدد) · Constantinus Africanus, *Viaticum peregrinantis* · trans. Do'eg ha-Edomi, *Sefer Ya'ir Netiv* V.2: ועוד הסתימה תקרה אל הכבד בשברון האברים האחרים כי אם ישבר היד או הרגל הדם שיהיה רגיל לגדל אותו האבר נשאר בכבד ואז יהיה הכבד נסתם (An obstruction [of the liver] can also occur because of the amputation of [one of] the other organs, for in the case of an amputation of a hand or foot, the blood, which usually nourishes that organ, remains in the liver and consequently the liver suffers from an obstruction). Hebr. סְתִימָה (for Arab. السداد) features in NM 5:141 in a later attestation from Abraham ben Isaac, *Sefer Ṣedah la-Oreḥim* I.23.2 (cf. IJZ 1–2:576), while Arab. *Plur.* سدد is translated by Moses ibn Tibbon

211 כוחלים: كحّالون a.

212 'pseudo-oculists': Trans. after the a (كحّالون), which can mean both 'trained oculists' (cf. WKAS 1:175) or 'pseudo-oculists' (cf. D 2:446).

as סתומים (in his *Sefer Ṣedat ha-Derakhim* I.0.4 (cf. BCD 195 (NM 4:140); IJZ 1–2:441)). Ben Yehuda (BM 4231) explains *Sing.* סָתוּם as having the same meaning as סְתִימָה; i.e., 'closing; filling' (סגירה/מלוי של נקב).

ע

עֹבִי · **roughness**: Arab. خشونة · Ibn Sīnā, *K. al-Qānūn fī al-ṭibb* · trans. Nathan ha-Me'ati, *Sefer ha-Qanun* II, fol. 70r: ביץ ... יועיל מעובי החזה והגרון (Eggs: ... [A soft-boiled egg] is useful for roughness of the chest and pharynx). Hebr. עֹבִי is not attested in this sense in the current dictionaries. In his *Sefer ha-Peraqim* (*Pirqei Moshe*), Nathan translates Arab. خشونة throughout as נחירות (cf. BMMG no. 1359). Anonymous also uses the latter term (נחירות), while Zeraḥyah Ḥen does not have a translation for Arab. خشونة; however, a marginal gloss renders it as גסות.

עָבַר • מה שעבר · **filtrate**: Lat. *colamenta* · Constantinus Africanus, *Viaticum peregrinantis* · trans. Do'eg ha-Edomi, *Sefer Ya'ir Netiv* V.9: כל אלה תבשל בי' ליטרי' מים עד למחצית ותעביר ותוסיף עוד בח' ליטרי' מים ותעביר ותחבר עם מה שעבר תחלה ותשים שם דבש כמו מהכל (Cook all these [ingredients] in ten liters of water until one half remains; sieve this, add eight liters of water, and add this to the first filtrate together with the same quantity of honey). Hebr. עָבַר does not feature in the sense of 'to be filtered' in the current dictionaries. For the active form 'to filter,' Do'eg uses the *Hif'il* conj. הֶעֱבִיר of the same verb (in his *Sefer Ya'ir Netiv* I.17.4; cf. NM 5:143; IJZ 1–2:619).

עֵדוּת · **indication; symptom**: Lat. *significatio* (Arab. علامة) · Constantinus Africanus, *Viaticum peregrinantis* · trans. Do'eg ha-Edomi, *Sefer Ya'ir Netiv* V.16: ואם בכליות גם בעגבות נרגש כמו נשיכת מחט שאינו יכול לסובלו אז יורה עדות נכון בראיית עצם האבן בשתן (If one feels in the kidneys and buttocks as if one is being pricked by a needle and one cannot endure it, then it is a certain indication that the substance of a stone has appeared in the urine). Hebr. עֵדוּת features in NM 5:144 (for Lat. *signum*) in a similar meaning ('prognostic sign') in an attestation from *Sefer Ya'ir Netiv* III.11 (corr.). Moses ibn Tibbon translates Arab. علامة as אות.

עֲדִי · **cosmetics**: Arab. زينة · Ibn Sīnā, *K. al-Qānūn fī al-ṭibb* · trans. Nathan ha-Me'ati, *Sefer ha-Qanun* II, fol. 61b (Ms Paris, BnF, héb. 1136, fol. 63a): אס ... העדי: משיחתו ומיצו ותבשילו יחזק שרשי השער וימנע נפילתו ויאריכנו וישחיר אותו (Myrtle ...: [Its use in] cosmetics: The oil, juice, and decoction [prepared from it] strengthen the roots of the hair and prevent it from falling out and make it grow and darken it). Hebr. עֲדִי features in BM 4335–4336 in the sense of 'ornament.' Zeraḥyah Ḥen translates Arab. زينة as יִפּוּי (see entry) and Anonymous has קִשּׁוּט (see entry).

עֲדִיפָה · **large amount; quantity; abundance**: Lat. *multitudo* (Arab. كثرة) · Constantinus Africanus, *Viaticum peregrinantis* · trans. Do'eg ha-Edomi, *Sefer Ya'ir Netiv* IV.8: והוא נעשה בענינים רבים מהרקה מהשחתת המאכל בתוך האסטומכא ומחלוף עצמו באיכיות נושכות כמחט ומקרירות פי האסטומכא ומהרוח הנופח באסטומכא ומרוב ליחות לחות או מעדיפת המאכל והמשתה (It [i.e., hiccups] is caused by many things: by evacuation [of the stomach]; by corruption of the food in the stomach and its changing into [a substance] with a quality sharp as a needle, by the coldness of the orifice of the stomach, by an inflating wind in the stomach, by a large amount of moistures (moist residues), or by a large quantity of food and drink). Hebr. עֲדִיפָה features in BM 4338 in the sense of 'preference' only. Moses ibn Tibbon translates Arab. كثرة as רבוי.

[עדף] • *Part.* עוֹדֵף • בשר עודף → בָּשָׂר.

עֲדָשָׁה • *Plur.* עדשים · **pimples [in the face]; acne**: Arab. نمش (Gr. ἴονθος; cf. UW 310) · Ibn Sīnā, *K. al-Qānūn fī al-ṭibb* · trans. Nathan ha-Me'ati, *Sefer ha-Qanun* II, fols. 67ª–68ᵇ: באן ... גרגריו יועילו מהעדשים הנקרא' נמש בערבי ומהכתם הנקרא כלף בערבי והבהק וסימני הנגעים (B'N [i.e., fruit of the ben oil tree [*Moringa oleifera* Lam.]]: ... The berries are useful for pimples called NMŠ [i.e., *namash*] in Arab., for freckles called KLP [i.e., *kalaf*] in Arab., for BHQ [i.e., Arab. *bahaq*[213]] and for scars from injuries). Hebr. עֲדָשָׁה, *Plur.* עדשים, features in BM 4350, s.v. *Sing.* עדש, as עדשי הפנים in the sense of 'freckles' (for Arab. كلف); for the same term, see also Moses ibn Tibbon, *Sefer Ṣedat ha-Derakhim* I.0.4 (cf. BCD 197 (NM 4:142); IJZ 1–2:440) and entry כֶּתֶם. Anonymous transcribes Arab. نمش as נמש only.

עובי → עֹבִי.

עוג · **to knead**: Arab. عجن · Ibn Zuhr, *K. al-Aghdhiya* · trans. Nathan ha-Me'ati, *Sefer ha-Mezonot*, fol. 6ª: ומה שיערבו בגבנה הטריה ויעוגו אותה בה ואחר יקלום במרחשת וירגילום בדבש וזה הרע שבמזונות (Some people mix [eggs] with fresh cheese, knead it, then fry it in a pan and [eat] it with honey. This is the worst kind of food). Hebr. עוג features in the sense of 'to bake a [cake]' in the Bible (BDB 728). Ben Yehuda (BM 4351) also quotes the term in an attestation from *Sefer Refu'ot le-Rambam* (ed. M. Grossberg (London 1900)).

עוור → עִוֵּר.

עֲוָוֹת • עוות העצבים · **twisted nerves**: Arab. التواء العصب (Gr. στρέμμα; cf. UW 643) · Ibn Sīnā, *K. al-Qānūn fī al-ṭibb* · trans. Nathan ha-Me'ati, *Sefer ha-Qanun* II, fol. 73ᵇ: ... גוז יועיל מעוות העצבים (Walnut: ... It is beneficial for twisted nerves). Hebr. עוות העצבים is not attested in the current dictionaries. Zeraḥyah Ḥen translates Arab. التواء العصب as לפיתת העצבים (see entry לְפִיתָה) and Anonymous has רצוץ העצבים (see entry רִצּוּץ).
• העוות שבפנים · **paralysis of the facial nerve**: Arab. لقوة · Ibn Sīnā, *K. al-Qānūn fī al-ṭibb* · trans. Zeraḥyah Ḥen, *Sefer ha-Qanun* II, fol. 216ᵇ: בַּלַאדֹר ... יועיל מקרירות העצבים ורפיונם ומן הפלג והעוות שבפנים (Marking nut: ... It is beneficial for cold and laxity of the nerves, for paralysis, and for paralysis of the facial nerve). In the sense of 'paralysis of the facial nerve,' Hebr. העוות שבפנים is not attested in the current dictionaries. Nathan ha-Me'ati translates Arab. لقوة as לקות הפה (see entry לְקוּת). See also עקום הפה (entry עִקּוּם) and נְטִיָּה.

עול • עול ימים · **young**: Arab. صغير · Ibn Zuhr, *K. al-Aghdhiya* · trans. Nathan ha-Me'ati, *Sefer ha-Mezonot*, fol. 6ᵇ: והטוב והמשובח שבהם הוא מה שאינו עול ימים מאד ולא בא בשנים מאד (The best kind of meat [of an animal] is that which is neither very young nor

213 For this skin disease, cf. IJZ 7:108–113, esp. 108, n. 196.

very old). Hebr. עול ימים (lit., 'a suckling of days') features in the current dictionaries in attestations from the Bible (cf. BDB 732) and modern literature (cf. EM 1301).

עומס → עֹמֶס.

עוֹף • לשון עוף → לָשׁוֹן.

עוֹפֶרֶת • **עופרת שחור מימיי** · **tin**: Arab. آنك (KM 1:293–296) · Ibn Sīnā, *K. al-Qānūn fī al-ṭibb* (Ms London, British Library Add. 21.967[214]) · trans. Zeraḥyah Ḥen, *Sefer ha-Qanun* II, fol. 165[b]: אנך הוא עופרת שחור מימיי ('NK [i.e., Arab. *ānuk*.], i.e., Hebr. *'oferet shaḥor meimi* [lit., 'black watery lead']). Hebr. עופרת שחור מימיי is not attested in the current dictionaries.

עוצר → עֹצֶר.

[עור] • *Polel* **עוֹרֵר** • **עורר אסטניסות** · **to cause nausea**: Arab. أغثى · Ibn Zuhr, *K. al-Aghdhiya* · trans. Nathan ha-Me'ati, *Sefer ha-Mezonot*, fol. 3[a]: ולחם הכרסנה והוא אורובי יחדש קיא ורוחות ואינם רבים אך הוא כאלו הוא ינגד עצם האדם כי[215] נעצר ויעורר אסטניסות וחפץ להקיא והוא חם ויבש (Bread from bitter vetch, i.e., [Rom.] 'WRWBY causes vomiting and some flatulence, but not frequently; it is, so to speak, contrary to human nature because it causes[216] distress, nausea, and an urge to vomit; it is hot and dry). In the sense of 'nausea; sickness in the stomach; urge to vomit,' Hebr. אִסְטְנִיסוּת features in BCD 24 (NM 2:30, 10; 4:19), a.o. in an attestation from Nathan's *Sefer ha-Peraqim* (*Pirqei Moshe*) XIII.54 (cf. BMMN 152, l. 18; BMMG no. 3618). Arab. أغثى is also translated as עורר אסטנסות by Nathan in his *Sefer ha-Peraqim* (*Pirqei Moshe*) IX.51, 55 (cf. BMMN 110, l. 15; 111, l. 6; BMMG no. 3616). Shem Tov ben Isaac renders the same Arab. term as גרם אסטניסות in his glossary to the *Sefer Almansur* (cf. BCD 51 (NM 2: 9–10); BMZ 36 (Ḥet 3)).

עִוֵּר • תרנגול עוור → תַּרְנְגוֹל.

עורק → עֹרֶק.

עָזַר · **to heal, cure**: Lat. *medicino* · Constantinus Africanus, *Viaticum peregrinantis* · trans. Do'eg ha-Edomi, *Sefer Ya'ir Netiv* IV.16: וגאלינוס אמר שעזר לעצמו ביין בלבד (Galen said that he cured himself [from ileus caused by crude, cold humors] by drinking wine only). Hebr. עָזַר does not feature in this sense in the current dictionaries. Do'eg uses the same verb in the *Nif'al* conj. נֶעֱזַר for Lat. *curor* ('to be cured') (in his *Sefer Ya'ir Netiv* I.5.1; cf. IJZ 1–2:607); and the noun עֵזֶר for Lat. *cura* in the sense of 'healing; treatment; cure' (in his *Sefer Ya'ir Netiv* I.16.3; cf. IJZ 1–2:617); cf. NM 5:147. Moses ibn Tibbon translates the parallel Arab. term علاج as רפואה.

עַיִן • **עין הבקר** · **plum** [***Prunus domestica* L.**]: Arab. عين البقر (cf. MSh no. 13) · Ibn Sīnā, *K. al-Qānūn fī al-ṭibb* · trans. Nathan ha-Me'ati, *Sefer ha-Qanun* II, fol. 66[a]: אגאץ הוא

---

214 Written in Rome in the earlier part of the fifteenth century by Yeḥiel b. Joab (Margoliouth no. 1026).

215 כי נעצר: فيكرب a.

216 'causes distress': Trans. after a.

עין הבקר והם פרונש והוא שאהלוך (ʾG'Ṣ [i.e., Arab. *ijjāṣ*, 'plum' (esp. *Prunus domestica* L., but in some dialects, esp. in Syria, it is the name of the pear (Arab. *kummathrā*, i.e., *Pyrus communis* L.); cf. IG 59)]; i.e., *ʿein ha-baqar*; i.e., PRWNŠ [i.e., Lat. *prunas*]; i.e., Š'HLWK [i.e., Pers. *shāhlūk*; cf. MSh no. 13; D 717: 'sorte de grande prune blanche']). In the sense of 'plum,' Hebr. עין הבקר is a non-attested calque of Arab. عين البقر.

• **ההתפשטות המתחדש בעין** → **הִתְפַּשְּׁטוּת**.

• **המים הנוזלים בעין** → **מַיִם**.

עיפוץ → **עִפּוּץ**.

עיקור → **עִקּוּר**.

עיקרי → **עִקָּרִי**.

עישוי → **עִשּׁוּי**.

[עכב] • *Part. Puʿal* **מְעֻכָּב** • **יותר מעוכב** · **slower**: Arab. أبطأ · Ibn Sīnā, *K. al-Qānūn fī al-ṭibb* · trans. Nathan ha-Me'ati, *Sefer ha-Qanun* II, fol. 71^b (Ms Paris, BnF, héb. 1136, fol. 71^b): בנדק ... המהות ידוע ועפרירותו הוא יותר מעפרירות האגוזים והוא יותר זן מהאגוזים לפי שהוא יותר ממלא ויותר כבד והפחות השמנינות ויותר מעוכב העכול (Hazelnut: ... What is it (*ha-mahut*)?:[217] It is well-known. It is more earthy than walnuts and more nutritive because it is more compact, heavier, less oily, and slower to digest). Hebr. [עכב], *Part. Puʿal* מְעֻכָּב, features in Rabb. literature in the sense of 'detained; prevented from' (cf. JD 1077; BM 4464–4465). Zeraḥyah Ḥen and Anonymous both translate Arab. أبطأ as יותר מאוחר.

עִכּוּב • **עכוב דם הנדות** · **amenorrhea**: Arab. احتباس الطمث · Ibn al-Jazzār, *Zād al-musāfir wa-qūt al-ḥādir* · trans. Abraham ben Isaac, *Sefer Ṣedah la-Oreḥim* VI.9: שער תשיעי יזכיר עיכוב דם הנידות (Ch. 9: On amenorrhea). Hebrew עכוב דם הנדות is not attested in the current dictionaries. In addition to עכוב דם הנדות, Abraham ben Isaac translates Arab. احتباس الطمث as אפיסת דם נידות (see entry אֲפִיסָה). Moses ibn Tibbon translates the Arab. term as העצר דם הנדות (see entry ¹עָצַר).

[עלה] • *Nifʿal* **נַעֲלָה** · **to be abolished, eliminated, dispelled**: Arab. كان مرتفع · Maimonides, *Maqāla fī al-rabw* (*On Asthma*) · trans. Joshua Shatibi, *Maʾamar ʿal ha-Qaṣeret* XIII.22 (cf. BMA 2:375, ll. 3–5): ואני יודע שאתה תאמר תכלית מה שילקח ממאמרך הוא שנשליך הרפואה ויהיה כל מה שנתעסק ונלאה בזאת המלאכה יהיה דבר בטל. אני אעלה אלו הספקות עם היות שכבר נעלו מכח מאמרי הקודם אכן אישבהו (I know that you could say: The conclusion to be drawn from your words is to abandon medicine, because every effort and attention given to this art is [given] in vain. I will dispel the doubt for you. And if it has already been dispelled by the force of my words so far, I will nevertheless return to the subject [once again]). Hebr. [עלה], *Nifʿal* נַעֲלָה, does not feature in

217 See entry מָהוּת.

this sense in the current dictionaries. In Bibl. Hebr. it features in the sense of 'to be taken up, taken away' (BDB 749); 'to absent oneself from' (KB 2:829); cf. BM 4494: נסתלק. Samuel Benveniste translates Arab. كان مرتفع as יָצָא (see entry) and Anonymous has מוסר.

• *Hifʿil* הֶעֱלָה · **to abolish, eliminate, dispel**: Arab. رفع · Maimonides, *Maqāla fī al-rabw (On Asthma)* · trans. Joshua Shatibi, *Maʾamar ʿal ha-Qaṣeret* XIII.22 (cf. BMA 2:375, ll. 3–5): ואני יודע שאתה תאמר תכלית מה שילקח ממאמרך הוא שנשליך הרפואה ויהיה כל מה שנתעסק ונלאה בזאת המלאכה יהיה דבר בטל. אני אעלה אלו הספקות עם היות שכבר נעלו מכח מאמרי הקודם אכן אישבהו (I know that you could say: The conclusion to be drawn from your words is to abandon medicine, because every effort and attention given to this art is [given] in vain. I will dispel the doubt for you. And if it has already been dispelled by the force of my words so far, I will nevertheless return to the subject [once again]). In the sense of 'to abolish, eliminate, dispel,' Hebr. [עלה], *Hifʿil* הֶעֱלָה, is attested in Rabb. literature only (cf. JD 1081–1082; BM 4498). Samuel Benveniste translates Arab. رفع as הוציא (see entry יָצָא) and Anonymous has הסיר.

עְלוּפִּי • רעב עלופיי → רָעָב.

עָמַד • עמד הגיד · **to have an erection**: Arab. نعظ · Ibn al-Jazzār, *Zād al-musāfir wa-qūt al-ḥāḍir* · trans. Abraham ben Isaac, *Sefer Ṣedah la-Oreḥim* VI.1: ויש שיתאוה ולא יעמוד גידו ולא יוציא זרע (Others have sexual lust but have no erection and do not ejaculate sperm). Hebr. עמד הגיד is not attested in this sense in the current dictionaries. Moses ibn Tibbon translates Arab. نعظ as התקשה (see entry [קשה]) and Doʾeg ha-Edomi translates the parallel Lat. term *erigor* as *Part.* זוקף (see entry זָקַף).

• **כשיעמוד גיד הערוה תדיר** · **priapism**: Arab. الإنعاظ الدائم · Ibn al-Jazzār, *Zād al-musāfir wa-qūt al-ḥāḍir*, trans. Abraham ben Isaac, *Sefer Ṣedah la-Oreḥim* VI.2: השער השיני יזכיר כשיעמוד גיד הערוה תדיר (Chapter 2: On priapism). Hebr. כשיעמוד גיד הערוה תדיר is not attested in the current dictionaries. Moses ibn Tibbon translates Arab. الإنعاظ الدائم as קושי מתמיד (see entry קָשִׁי) and Doʾeg ha-Edomi translates the parallel Lat. term *nimia erectio virgae* as זקיפת האמה ברוב (see entry זְקִיפָה).

• *Hifʿil* הֶעֱמִיד · **to thicken**: Arab. عقّد · Maimonides, *Maqāla fī al-rabw (On Asthma)* · trans. Anonymous, *Sefer ha-Qaṣeret* IV.7 (cf. BMA 2:400, ll. 20–22): ודע שהדברים החמים היבשים ביותר מזיקים בזה החלי ובלבד לזה המזג הנזכר מפני שהן מדבקין מהלחות מה שיש בהן התדשנות ומעמידין ומקפיאין מה שאין בו התדשנות (Know that the hot and dry ingredients are extremely harmful for this disease [i.e., asthma], especially for the temperament that we mentioned because they make the fatty humors sticky and thicken and coagulate those humors that have no fatness). Hebr. [עמד], *Hifʿil* הֶעֱמִיד, is attested in Rabb. literature in the sense of 'to make consistent, curdle' (cf. JD 1086; BM 4552). Samuel Benveniste translates Arab. عقّد as קָשַׁר (see entry) and Joshua Shatibi does not translate the Arab. term.

עֲמִידָה · I. **orthopnea:**[218] Arab. انتصاب (cf. UW 471, s.v. ὀρθόπνοια: نفس الانتصاب) · Maimonides, *Fī tadbīr al-ṣiḥḥa* (*On the Regimen of Health*) · trans. Moses ibn Tibbon, *Hanhagat ha-Beri'ut* IV.22 (cf. BMR 186, ll. 1–3): וכל הנוזלים החמים והקרים לרוב ישפכו לחללי הריאה וימלאו אותם פתאום לרוב הליחה היורדת וחלשת המקבל ויחלש הכח הדוחה מהוציא השעול ההוא ויחנק האדם וימות או יחדשו חולי העמידה שהוא קוצר הנשימה עד שלא יוכל לשכב (All catarrhs, hot and cold, often stream into the cavities of the lungs and fill them all at once because of the abundance of the descending humor and the weakness of the receiving [organ]. The expulsive power is too weak to expel that [humor] through coughing, so that the [patient] suffocates and dies or suffers from the illness of orthopnea, i.e., shortness of breath so that he cannot lie down). Hebr. עֲמִידָה does not feature in this sense in the current dictionaries.

· II. **consistency**: Arab. قوام · Maimonides, *Maqāla fī al-rabw* (*On Asthma*) · trans. Anonymous, *Sefer ha-Qaṣeret* XII.3 (cf. BMA 2:430, ll. 26–29): אחר טוב וקל זכרוהו האחרונים ⟨ראוי⟩ להדרה לסמוך עליו: יוקח הצנובר הגדולים הרב השרף ויבושל עם הפראסיון החדש שיעור חצי הצנובר ומסננין אותו ויעורב באותן המים מהדבש הנקי כמותו ויבושל עד שיהיה בעמדת הדבש ויעשה והוא מנקה כל מה שבחזה ניקוי מופלא (Another beneficial but mild [linctus] mentioned by later [physicians], which my Master should rely upon: Take large pine nuts that contain much resin; cook them with fresh horehound, half the quantity of the nuts; strain this and mix the resulting liquid with a similar amount of pure honey; cook this until it assumes the consistency of the honey; and use this, for it cleanses all that is in the chest in a wonderful way). Hebr. עמדה, read עֲמִידָה, does not feature in this sense in the current dictionaries. Synonymous terms are: ממשות (BCD 151; NM 4:100); מעמד (BCD 155; NM 2:61); עצם (BCD 209; NM 2:72); עצמות (BCD 211; NM 1:178); and תכונה (BCD 294; NM 1:69–70). Samuel Benveniste translates Arab. قوام as מַתְכּוֹנֶת (see entry for Benveniste's use of the same term for Arab. صفة ('recipe')).

• **עמידת הגיד** · **[penile] erection** Arab. إنعاظ · Ibn al-Jazzār, *Zād al-musāfir wa-qūt al-ḥāḍir* · trans. Abraham ben Isaac, *Sefer Ṣedah la-Oreḥim* VI.1: ויש מקצת אנשים שיתחזק בו זה הרוח ויתמעט רטיבותו ואז יהיה עמידת הגיד בלשון ישמעאל אנעאט[219] ולא יוציא זרע כלל (Some men who have a strong flatulency but only little moisture, may have an erection [called] in Arab. 'N°Ṭ [i.e., *in'āẓ*] but not an ejaculation of sperm). Hebr. עמידת הגיד is not attested in the current dictionaries. Moses ibn Tibbon translates Arab. إنعاظ as קִשׁי (cf. BCD 251–252 for an attestation, a.o., from Ibn Tibbon, *Perush Aphorismi shel Apuqraṭ* (*Pirqei Abuqraṭ*) VI.30 (322) (cf. NM 3:211); BMCH 1:399, l. 3) and Do'eg ha-Edomi translates the parallel Lat. term *erigo* as זְקִיפָה (see entry).

---

218 I.e., discomfort in breathing that is brought on or aggravated by lying flat (cf. BMA 1:2, n. 5).
219 אנעאט: emend. ed. אנטעאט Ms.

עֹמֶס · **tenesmus**: Lat. *pondus tenesmon* · Constantinus Africanus, *Viaticum peregrinantis* · trans. Do'eg ha-Edomi, *Sefer Ya'ir Netiv* IV.15: אחר זה טוב אל דישנטריא דיאריאה ולעומס טנסמון ולנגעי המעים והפשטתם ולחזק האסטומכא (Another [pastille] that is good for dysentery, diarrhea, tenesmus, ulcers, abrasion (excoriation) of the intestines, and for strengthening the stomach). Hebr. עֹמֶס does not feature in this sense in the current dictionaries. A synonym from the same Hebr. root עמס used by Do'eg is מַעֲמָס (see entry).

עֵנָב • *Plur.* ענבים • **עצירת הענבים** → עֲצִירָה[1].

עִסָּה • **מלח העסה** → מֶלַח.

עִסּוּי → עִשּׁוּי.

עִפּוּץ · **astringency**: Arab. قبض · Maimonides, *Maqāla fī al-rabw* (*On Asthma*) · trans. Anonymous, *Sefer ha-Qaṣeret* XI.1 (cf. BMA 2:425, ll. 7–9): ועל כל פנים יש לנו בחיזוק כל אבר עם השבתו למזגו הטבעי שנשים בסמניו מה שיש בו עיפוץ לכל אבר לפיהו (To strengthen any organ and to restore its natural temperament, it is unavoidable that we use astringent drugs [in accordance with what is appropriate to each organ]). Hebr. עִפּוּץ features in the current dictionaries in the sense of 'tanning' (cf. BM 4614: עבוד העור על ידי עפצים). Joshua Shatibi renders Arab. قبض as קביצות (cf. BCD 236 (NM 2:78) for an attestation from Nathan ha-Me'ati, *Sefer ha-Peraqim* (*Pirqei Moshe*) IX.71 (cf. BMMN 113, l. 10; BMMG no. 3990)) and Samuel Benveniste has חֲבִישׁוּת (see entry).

עַפְעַף • *Plur.* עפעפים • **השער המתהפך בעפעפים** → שֵׂעָר.

[עפץ] • *Part. Hif'il* **מַעֲפִיץ** · **astringent**: Arab. مقبّض · Ibn al-Jazzār, *Zād al-musāfir wa-qūt al-ḥāḍir* · trans. Abraham ben Isaac, *Sefer Ṣedah la-Oreḥim*, VI.10: ואם בכל זאת יזוב דמה אז נעשה לה הרפואות המעפיצות (If the loss of blood continues nevertheless, we treat her with astringent remedies). Hebr. עפץ is only attested in the current dictionaries in the *Pu'al* conj. in the sense of 'to be made with gallnut' (BM 4619). Moses ibn Tibbon translates Arab. مقبّض as קָבֵץ, *Part.* קובץ (cf. BCD 237 for attestations (for Arab. قابض) from the *Sefer ha-Peraqim* (*Pirqei Moshe*) by both Zeraḥyah Ḥen (VIII.63; cf. NM 1:183, corr. 2:198; BMMZ 96, l. 10) and Nathan ha-Me'ati (IX.37; cf. NM 2:81; BMMN 107, l. 26; 108, l. 2); cf. also BMMG no. 3993).

עָפָר • *Plur.* **עפרים** · **powders**: Arab. ذرورات · Maimonides, *Maqāla fī al-rabw* (*On Asthma*) · trans. Joshua Shatibi, *Ma'amar 'al ha-Qaṣeret* XIII.6 (cf. BMA 2:364, ll. 20–21): ואמנם מה שיחזק המוח בזה החולי הנה אבן זהר זכר שהוא מצא העפרים יותר טובים מן הרטיות (As for [drugs] that strengthen the brain in this disease [i.e., asthma], Ibn Zuhr has remarked that he found powders better for this than ointments). Hebr. עָפָר, *Plur.* עפרים, does not feature in this sense in the current dictionaries. In addition to עפרים, Joshua Shatibi translates Arab. ذرورات as עפרים נפזרים (see next entry). Samuel Benveniste and Anonymous both render Arab. ذرورات as אבקים.

• **עפרים נפזרים** · **powders**: Arab. ذرورات · Maimonides, *Maqāla fī al-rabw* (*On Asthma*) · trans. Joshua Shatibi, *Ma'amar 'al ha-Qaṣeret* XI.2 (cf. BMA 2:357, ll. 14–15): וכן כבר זכרו הרופאים עפרים נפזרים ורטיות מחזקות המח בזאת המחלה אך כלם חמים ואין טוב לו

מה שיחמם חמום חזק (The physicians have also mentioned powders and liniments that strengthen the brain in this disease [i.e., asthma]. However, all these have a warming effect, and for you anything that has a strong warming effect is not good). Hebr. עפר נפזר, *Plur.* עפרים נפזרים, does not feature in the current dictionaries. In addition to עפרים נפזרים, Joshua Shatibi translates Arab. ذرورات only as עפרים (see previous entry). Samuel Benveniste translates Arab. ذرورات as אבקים and Anonymous renders Arab. ذرورات وأطلية ('powders and liniments') as תחבושות ומשיחות.

עָצָב • *Plur.* **עצבים** • **לפיתת העצבים** → לְפִיתָה.

• **עוות העצבים** → עַוּוּת.

• **רצוץ העצבים** → רִצּוּץ.

עִצּוּר · I. **dysentery**: Arab. سحج (cf. SN 1:111 (265), s.v. إسهال وهو سحج: 'dysenteria rheumatica') · Ibn al-Jazzār, *Zād al-musāfir wa-qūt al-ḥāḍir* · trans. Moses ibn Tibbon, *Sefer Ṣedat ha-Derakhim* IV.15: ואולם אותות העצור הכולל העוות הוא המשברים והצער ויציאת הדם מעורב בליחה כרכומית (In general, the symptoms of dysentery are colic, i.e., [Hebr.] *mishbarim*, pain, loss of blood mixed with yellow bile). Hebr. עִצּוּר features in BCD 207 as 'constipation' (NM 2:179) and 'cramps; pressure' (NM 1:64). For the use of the term in the sense of 'extract' (s.v. עצור העופרת for Arab. عصارة الرصاص ('lead extract')) and 'contraction,' cf. NM 5:153. In the sense of 'squeezing; contraction' (סחיטה/התכוצות) it also features in BM 4641. In addition to עִצּוּר, Ibn Tibbon uses the term חֲמַרְמְרוּת (see entry) to refer to 'dysentery;' cf. also BCD 104 (NM 1:56) for חֲמַרְמְרוּת with the meaning of '[intestinal] abrasion' (in his *Sefer Ṣedat ha-Derakhim* VII.29.1; cf. IJZ 7:171, l. 5). The common Arab. term for 'dysentery' is اختلاف دم (cf. SN 1:110 (264); BCD 58 (NM 3:53)). This term is rendered in medieval Hebr. medical literature as דם שותת (cf. ibid.); הגרת הדם (cf. BCD 62 (NM 1:138)); הזלת הדם (cf. BCD 64 (NM 3:62)); הזלת דם הבטן (cf. BCD 65 (NM 3:62)); עירוב הדם (cf. BCD 214 (NM 3:184)), שלשול (ה)דם (cf. BCD 276 (NM 3:228)); שלשול עם דם (cf. BCD 276 (NM 3:229–230)) and שנוי דם (cf. BCD 280 (NM 3:233)). In addition to these Hebr. terms, we find the Rom. loan word פונץ (*pons*, cf. entry). Do'eg ha-Edomi transcribes the parallel Lat. term *disenteria* as דישנטריא.

· II. **tenesmus**: Arab. زحير (Gr. τεινεσμός; cf. UW 669) · Ibn al-Jazzār, *Zād al-musāfir wa-qūt al-ḥāḍir* · trans. Moses ibn Tibbon, *Sefer Ṣedat ha-Derakhim* IV.15: תאר אבק חברתיו לעצורים והנגעים המתילדים במעים ממרה כרכומית חדה ולמי שיש בו שלשול הדם בכאבים ועצור ועוות (A recipe for a powder that I composed for those suffering from dysentery and intestinal ulcers originating from sharp yellow bile, and for those suffering from bloody diarrhea with pains, tenesmus, and colic). Do'eg ha-Edomi translates the parallel Lat. term *pondus* as מַעֲמָס or עֹמֶס (see entries). Synonymous terms for 'tenesmus' featuring in medieval medical literature are עִסּוּי (cf BCD 205 (NM 3:177)); עִצּוּם (cf. BCD 207 (NM 4:152)); and שלשול מעיים (cf. BCD 277 (NM 3:229)).

‣ III. **narrowing; narrowness; obstruction**: Lat. *strictio* (Arab. سدّة) · Constantinus Africanus, *Viaticum peregrinantis* · trans. Do'eg ha-Edomi, *Sefer Ya'ir Netiv* V.20: עצור הדרך מאשר יוצא השתן מהמקוה יקרה בסתימת האבן ואפיסת הדם או הליחות הגסות או הבלוי או מאיזה דבר שנולד שם כמו ורוגא או בשר עודף (An obstruction in the passage through which the urine passes from the bladder occurs when it is blocked by a stone or by a blood clot or by coarse humors or by pus or by whatever grows there, such as a tumor or fleshy excrescence). Moses ibn Tibbon translates Arab. سدّة as צרות.

עֲצִירָה¹ ‣ **juice**: Arab. عصارة · Maimonides, *Maqāla fī al-rabw* (*On Asthma*) · trans. Joshua Shatibi, *Ma'amar 'al ha-Qaṣeret* IX.7 (cf. BMA 2:348, l. 22): אחרת עצירת הסלק חצי ליטרא שמן טוב ב׳ אוקיות יחמם זה ויתחקן בו (Another [enema]: [Take] half a liter of beet juice and two ounces of fine olive oil, heat this, and use it as an enema). In the sense of 'juice,' Hebr. עֲצִירָה is a non-attested noun coined from the verb עָצַר meaning 'to press, squeeze' (cf. BM 4661). Samuel Benveniste translates the Arab. term as עסיס and Anonymous has מים.

• **עצירת הענבים** ‣ **must from grapes**: Arab. عصير العنب · Ibn Zuhr, *K. al-Aghdhiya* · trans. Nathan ha-Me'ati, *Sefer ha-Mezonot*, fol. 14[a]: אמנם עצירת הענבים הם שרש ליינות המבושלות ולמיני החומץ והוא חם רטוב אם ישתה מיד שיעצר מנפח הבטן ויחדש קרקורים בו (Must from grapes is the basis for wines made from boiling (fermenting) [the must] and for the [different] kinds of vinegar. It [i.e., the must] is hot and moist; when it is drunk immediately after [the grapes have] been pressed it causes flatulency and rumblings in the stomach).

עֲצִירָה² • **עצירת השתן** ‣ **urinary retention**: Arab. احتباس البول · Ibn al-Jazzār, *Zād al-musāfir wa-qūt al-ḥāḍir* · trans. Moses ibn Tibbon, *Sefer Ṣedat ha-Derakhim* V.20: השער הכ׳ בעצירת השתן: יציאת השתן יגיעהו הנזק אם בסבת הכליות ואם בסבת המקוה ויקרה הבחורים לבד בכליות לחום מזגם ויקרה לנערים מרוע הנהגתם (Ch. 20: On urinary retention: Peeing problems can be caused either by the kidneys or by the bladder. They are caused by the kidneys especially in young people because of their hot temperament and in young children because of their bad regimen). Hebr. עצירת השתן features in BM 4642 in later attestations, a.o., from Meir Aldabi, *Shevilei Emunah*. Do'eg ha-Edomi transcribes the parallel Lat. term *stranguria* as אשטרנגוריאה.

עֲצִירוּת ‣ **constipation**: Arab. عقل Ibn Sīnā, *K. al-Qānūn fī al-ṭibb* · trans. Nathan ha-Me'ati, *Sefer ha-Qanun* II, fol. 70[b]: בדנגאן ... ואין אל הבדנגאן ערך אל העצירות ולא אל השלשול אבל אם יבשלוהו בשמן זית ישלשל ובחומץ יעצור (Eggplant: ... Eggplant has nothing to do with constipation or relaxation of the bowels, but when it is cooked in olive oil, it relaxes the bowels, and when cooked with vinegar, it causes constipation). In the sense of 'constipation,' Hebr. עֲצִירוּת is attested in EM 1356 in an attestation from the *Sefer Ḥasidim* and in BM 4643 in a later attestation from the *Moreh Darkhei ha-Refu'ah*, a Hebrew trans. of the *Enchridium medicum* (Zhitomir 1869). Anonymous has עֲצִירָה (just like Bonfos (for Lat. *constipatio*) in his trans. of *On the Treatment of Small Children*, attributed to al-Rāzī, cf. BCD 207 (NM 2:72)).

עָצָל • *Plur.* **עצלים** • **רצוץ העצלים** → **רצוץ**.

עַצְלָה · **fatigue**: Arab. إعياء · Ibn Sīnā, *K. al-Qānūn fī al-ṭibb* · trans. Nathan ha-Me'ati, *Sefer ha-Qanun* II, fol. 74ᵃ: גואשיר ... אמרו קצתם שהוא רע אל העצבים ויראה לי שיהיה זה אל העצב הבריא אבל לא המרוטב והוא מועיל לגיד הנשה ושותים מיצו כמו כן ויועיל ממנו ויסיר העצלה ויועיל ממכאובי הפרקים כולם ולנכאות הרגלים כשעושים ממנו תחבשת (Opopanax: ... Some [physicians] state that it is bad for the nerves. It seems to me that this might be [true] for healthy nerves but not for moist [temperament of the] nerves. It is useful for sciatica. Drinking its juice is good for removing fatigue. Its plaster is useful for all kinds of pains of the joints and gout). In the sense of 'fatigue,' Hebr. עַצְלָה features in BCD 208 (NM 4:154) in an attestation from Anonymous, *Sammim Libbiyim*.[220] Zeraḥyah Ḥen translates Arab. إعياء as עיפות and Anonymous has יגיעה. The latter term also features throughout Nathan's *Sefer ha-Peraqim* (*Pirqei Moshe*) (cf. BMMG no. 3599).

עֶצֶם • *Plur.* **עצמות** • **העצמות מלמטה מן הצואר על החזה** · **collarbones**: Arab. ترقوة · Ibn al-Jazzār, *Zād al-musāfir wa-qūt al-ḥāḍir* · trans. Moses ibn Tibbon, *Sefer Ṣedat ha-Derakhim* V.1: ואם יתחבר בכבד איד וירבה ולא יהיה לו מעבר יוצא ממנו ולא ירגיש בעליו בכבדות לבד אבל ימצא משיכה ג"כ ובעל הסתום ימצא כאב במה שבין העצמות מלמטה מן הצואר על החזה הנק' אורוגוש ובין הכבד (If many vapors collect in the liver but do not have a way out, the patient will not only feel heaviness but also tension, and the patient suffering from an obstruction [in the liver] will feel pain in the region between the collarbones called 'WRWGWŠ [read: 'WRWGNLŠ; i.e., Rom. *organals*/*orguenals*][221] and the liver). Hebr. *Sing.* העצם מלמטה מן הצואר על החזה does not feature in the current dictionaries. A synonym used by Moses ibn Tibbon in *Sefer Ṣedat ha-Derakhim* III.12 is Rom. אורגנא (cf. NM 5:170, s.v. צמידי הראש). In his *Sefer ha-Peraqim* (*Pirqei Moshe*) VI.55, 57; VII.54; XII.27; XV.62, Nathan ha-Me'ati transcribes the Arab. term as תרקוה (cf. BMMN 73, ll. 12, 20; 89, ll. 7, 9; 142, ll. 15–16; 164, l. 5), while Zeraḥyah Ḥen translates it as קטולא (XII.27; XV.62; cf. BMMZ 140, ll. 1, 3; 162, l. 15) or קטיולה (VI.55, 57; VII.54; cf. BMMZ 67, l. 21; 68, l. 4; 83, l. 21) (cf. also BMMG no. 453). Do'eg ha-Edomi translates the parallel Lat. term *furculas* as צמידי הראש (see NM 5:170 for an attestation from *Sefer Ya'ir Netiv* III.12).

עָצַר¹ · 1. **to suffer from tenesmus**: Arab. تزحّر · Ibn al-Jazzār, *Zād al-musāfir wa-qūt al-ḥāḍir* · trans. Moses ibn Tibbon, *Sefer Ṣedat ha-Derakhim* IV.20: אלו החלאים אשר יקרו

220 So far, I have encountered Hebr. עַצְלָה in this sense in no other medical text than these two trans. of works by Ibn Sīnā. This might indicate that both trans. were done by Nathan ha-Me'ati and therefore the anonymous translator of the *Sammim Libbiyim* is indeed Nathan. To be certain, however, one would need further definite proof.

221 Cf. SHS 1:196 (Waw 3): ורידי הצואר ב"ה אודאג' וב"ל אורגונאלש ([Hebr.] WRYDY HṢW'R, Arab. 'WD'Ǧ, o.l. 'WRGWN'LŠ); i.e., jugular veins.

בפי הטבעת ר״ל הטחורים והמורסות והנגעים והסדיקות יכאב מהם פי הטבעת ויעצור החולה בעבור זה ומקוה אל המרגוע ממה שימצא מן הכאב (Those illnesses that affect the anus—i.e., hemorrhoids, tumors, ulcers, and fissures—cause pain to the anus and as a result the patient suffers from tenesmus and hopes to find relief from the pain). Hebr. עָצַר features in the sense of 'to cause constipation' in BM 4660 (עצר את הבטן) and as *Part. Pass.* עָצוּר in the sense of 'suffering from constipation' in NM 5:154 in an attestation from Do'eg ha-Edomi, *Sefer Ya'ir Netiv* III.7 (see also the Hebr. term עצור הבטן ('he who has constipated bowels') in BCD 211–212 (NM 3:179), as it features in Ibn Tibbon's *Perush Aphorismi shel Apuqraṭ* (*Pirqei Abuqraṭ*) III.25 (131) (cf. BMCH 1:355, l. 19)). Hebr. עָצַר also features in medieval medical literature (cf. BCD 211) in the sense of 'to be astringent' (NM 1:178–179; see also *Part.* עוֹצֵר ('astringent; styptic') in BCD 211 (NM 2:180; 3:181–182); NM 5:154), 'to bind (tightly)' (NM 1:35), and 'to be difficult' (NM 1:178).

‣ **II. to contract**: Lat. *constringo* (Arab. انضمّ) · Constantinus Africanus, *Viaticum peregrinantis* · trans. Do'eg ha-Edomi, *Sefer Ya'ir Netiv* VI.16: ובעת החורף אשר קרירות האויר יעצור דרכי הרחם ([Difficult childbirth also happens] in the winter season because the cold contracts the passages of the uterus). Hebr. עָצַר does not feature in this sense in the current dictionaries. For the noun עִצּוּר in the sense of 'contraction,' cf. NM 5:153 for an attestation from *Sefer Ya'ir Netiv* III.11. Moses ibn Tibbon translates the parallel Arab. term انضمّ as סתם and Abraham ben Isaac has עבה וצמק.

• **עצר הבטן** ‣ **to cause constipation**: Arab. عقل البطن · Ibn Zuhr, *K. al-Aghdhiya* · trans. Nathan ha-Me'ati, *Sefer ha-Mezonot*, fol. 3[a]: ולחם אורז והוא ריש חם ויבש קשה מאוחר העכול יהיה ממנו ליחה עבה ויוליד סתום בקרבים ובשאר הגוף ועוצר הבטן (Bread from rice, i.e., [Rom.] RYŠ, is hot and dry and hard, it is slow to digest, produces thick humors and blockages in the intestines and the rest of the body, and causes constipation). Hebr. עצר הבטן features in BM 4660 in the sense of 'to close the openings [of the body]' (סתם את הנקבים) in an attestation from Maimonides, *Millot Higgayon*; cf. also *Part. Pass.* עצור הבטן ('he who has constipated bowels') in BCD 211–212 (NM 3:179) for an attestation from Moses ibn Tibbon, *Perush Aphorismi shel Apuqraṭ* (*Pirqei Abuqraṭ*) III.25 (131) (cf. BMCH 1:355, l. 19).

• *Inf. Nif'al* **הֵעָצֵר** • **העצר דם הנדות** ‣ **amenorrhea**: Arab. احتباس الطمث · Ibn al-Jazzār, *Zād al-musāfir wa-qūt al-ḥādir* · trans. Moses ibn Tibbon, *Sefer Ṣedat ha-Derakhim* VI.9: שער ט' בהעצר דם הנדות (Ch. 9: On amenorrhea). Hebrew העצר דם הנדות is not attested in the current dictionaries. A var. used by Ibn Tibbon is העצר הנדות (see next entry). Abraham ben Isaac translates Arab. احتباس الطمث as עכוב דם הנדות (see entry עִכּוּב). For yet another var. העצר הפרחים, featuring in *Sefer ha-Refu'ot le-Ḥakham Qosṭa'ntin*, see entry below.

• **העצר הנדות** ‣ **amenorrhea**: Arab. احتباس الطمث · Ibn al-Jazzār, *Zād al-musāfir wa-qūt al-ḥādir* · trans. Moses ibn Tibbon, *Sefer Ṣedat ha-Derakhim* VI.9: העצר הנדות יהיה

על שני פנים (Amenorrhea occurs in two ways). Hebrew העצר הנדות is not attested in the current dictionaries. A var. used by Ibn Tibbon is העצר דם הנדות (see previous entry). Abraham ben Isaac translates Arab. احتباس الطمث as אפיסת דם נידות (see entry אֲפִיסָה) and Do'eg ha-Edomi translates the parallel Lat. term *ablatio* as העדרה. For yet another var. העצר הפרחים, featuring in *Sefer ha-Refu'ot le-Ḥakham Qosṭa'ntin*, see next entry.

• **העצר הפרחים** · **amenorrhea**: *Sefer ha-Refu'ot le-Ḥakham Qosṭa'ntin*, fol. 212[a]: בהעצר הפרחים: אמר פלאטיאריש: דרך הנשים להוציא בטבעם דם בכל חדש בזמן קבוע ולפיפך נעצר דמם בטבע כשהן מעוברות וכשהן זקנות (On amenorrhea: Says Platearius: It is in the nature of women to have a menstruation every month at a fixed time. For this reason, they do not have a menstruation anymore when they are pregnant and when they are old). Hebrew העצר הפרחים is not attested in the current dictionaries. For vars. העצר דם הנדות and העצר הנדות, featuring in Moses ibn Tibbon, *Sefer Ṣedat ha-Derakhim* VI.9, see entries above.

עָצַר[2] · **to press out**: Arab. عصر · i. Maimonides, *Maqāla fī al-rabw* (*On Asthma*) · trans. Joshua Shatibi, *Ma'amar 'al ha-Qaṣeret* XII.3 (cf. BMA 2:362, ll. 17–18): אחר חזק זכרהו גאלינוס: ילקח בצל אל ענצל ותעצר וישים עם הנעצר בכמותו מדבש ויתעבה משקה ילקח ממנו שיעור אוקיא קודם המאכל וכן אחריו (Another strong [linctus] mentioned by Galen: Take squill, press it out, add to the juice a similar amount of honey, thicken it until it becomes a syrup, and take one ounce of it before and after meals). In the sense of 'to press, squeeze,' Hebr. עָצַר features in BM 4661 and EM 1359. For other meanings in a medical context, cf. BCD 211. Samuel Benveniste translates Arab. عصر as שָׁחַט (see entry) and Anonymous has יָצָא, *Part. Hif'il* מוֹצִיא (see entry).

· ii. Ibn Zuhr, *K. al-Aghdhiya* · trans. Nathan ha-Me'ati, *Sefer ha-Mezonot*, fol. 14[a]: אמנם עצירת הענבים הם שרש ליינות המבושלות ולמיני החומץ והוא חם רטוב אם ישתה מיד שיעצר מנפח הבטן ויחדש קרקורים בו (Must from grapes is the basis for wines made from boiling (fermenting) [the must] and for the [different] kinds of vinegar. It [i.e., the must] is hot and moist; when it is drunk immediately after [the grapes have] been pressed, it causes flatulency and rumblings in the stomach).

עֹצֶר • **עוצר ההריון** · **difficulty in conception**: Arab. عسر الحبل · Ibn Sīnā, *K. al-Qānūn fī al-ṭibb* · trans. Nathan ha-Me'ati, *Sefer ha-Qanun* II, fol. 80[a]: הליון ... תבשיל עקרו ישלשל השתן ויועיל מעצירותו ויוסיף בטפת הזרע ותאות המשגל ויועיל לעוצר ההריון (Asparagus: ... A decoction of its root is diuretic. It increases the quantity of semen and also improves libido. It is also useful for difficulty in conception). In the sense of 'difficulty,' Hebr. עֹצֶר features in different combinations in BCD 212 (עוצר הבטן ('constipation'); עוצר הלידה ('difficult labor'); עוצר הניפוש ('dyspnea'); עוצר השתן ('dysuria')). Anonymous has קושי ההריון.

עָקֵב • **העורק אשר אצל העקב לצד פנימי** → עֹרֶק.

עָקוּם • עקום הפה · **paralysis of the facial nerve; facial paresis**: Lat. *tortura oris* (Arab. لقوة) · Gerard de Solo, *Practica super nono Almansoris* · trans. Abraham Avigdor, *Ha-Ma'amar ha-Teshi'i le-Sefer ha-Mansuri le-Razi*, fol. 35b: שער ט' דֵי טוֹרטוּרַא אוֹרִיש: ראוי שתדע בבאור הרובריקא כי עקום הפה הוא חולי כליי מפסיד תמונת הפנים וצורתם (Chapter 9: DeY ṬWoRṬWuRa' 'WoRiYŠ [i.e., *De tortura oris*]: Regarding the explanation of the heading you should know that paralysis of the facial nerve is an[222] illness that impedes the functioning of an organ and corrupts (distorts) the form and shape of the face). In the sense of 'paralysis of the facial nerve,' Hebr. עקום הפה features in BCD 212 (NM 4:158–159) in an attestation from Moses ibn Tibbon, *Sefer Ṣedat ha-Derakhim* I.23.3 (cf. IJZ 1–2:477). See also לקות הפה (entry לָקוּת), נְטִיָּה, and העוות שבפנים (entry עִוּוּת).

עִקּוּר · **infertility**: *Sefer ha-Refu'ot le-Ḥakham Qoṣṭa'ntin*, fol. 216b: בעקור: אמר פלאטיאריש: עיקור שאין האשה יכולה לקבל הריון בא ברוב סבות (On infertility: Says Platearius: Infertility, i.e., that a woman cannot become pregnant, happens for many reasons). In the sense of 'infertility,' Hebr. עִקּוּר features in BM 4673 in an attestation from Nachmanides' commentary on Ex 23:28.

עֲקִיצָה • עקיצת המעיים · **gripes; colic**: Arab. مغص (Gr. στρόφος; cf. UW 644) · Ibn Sīnā, *K. al-Qānūn fī al-ṭibb* · trans. Nathan ha-Me'ati, *Sefer ha-Qanun* II, fols. 68b–69a: בורק ... משלשל[223] כשסובלים אותו וכשאוכלים אותו עם סדאב[224] וכמון או תבשיל הסדאב והשבת ישקיט עקיצת המעיים (Borax (sodium borate): ... When one applies it in a suppository, it relaxes the bowels and when one ingests it with rue,[225] cumin, or a decoction of rue and dill, it alleviates gripes (colic)). Hebr. עקיצת המעיים is not attested in the current dictionaries. For the term עֲקִיצָה on its own in the sense of 'gripes; colic,' cf. BCD 212–213 (NM 3:182) for an attestation from Zeraḥyah Ḥen, *Perush Aphorismi shel Apuqraṭ* (*Pirqei Abuqraṭ*) V.41 (261) (cf. BMCH 1:480, l. 18). In his *Sefer ha-Peraqim* (*Pirqei Moshe*) XII.7 (cf. BMMN 139, l. 16), Nathan renders the Arab. var. مغس as כאב מעים (cf. BCD 123 (NM 2:52–53)). Zeraḥyah translates Arab. مغص as פונטורא (i.e., Lat. *punctura*) and Anonymous has חבלי הבטן (see entry חֵבֶל). For other synonyms, see entries חִיל and חִתּוּךְ.

עִקָּר • *Plur.* עקרים · **rules; instructions**: Arab. قوانين · Maimonides, *Maqāla fī al-rabw* (*On Asthma*) · trans. Anonymous, *Sefer ha-Qaṣeret* X.1 (cf. BMA 2:421, ll. 11–13): ואמנם בענין רפואת החלאים לא יכוון לשנות מנהג בשום פנים ולא בשום סבה אלא נושאין פניה [מנהג] שאת גמור כפי מה שבאר לנו גאלינוס בעקריו המועילים (But in the case of the healing of diseases, one should not intend to change the habit in any manner or for any reason.

222 'an illness that impedes the functioning of an organ' (חולי כליי): See entry חֳלִי.

223 משלשל: add. according to Ms Paris, BnF, héb. 1136, fol. 68a.

224 סדאב: شراب a.

225 'rue': 'wine' a.

Instead, it should be observed with utmost attention, as Galen explained to us in his helpful instructions). In the sense of 'rules,' Hebr. עִקָּר, *Plur.* עקרים, does not feature in the current dictionaries. Samuel Benveniste translates Arab. قوانين as דרכים (see entry דֶּרֶךְ) and Joshua Shatibi has סדרים (see entry סֵדֶר).

עִקָּרִי • החום העקרי → חֹם.

• החמימות העיקרי → חֲמִימוּת.

עָרֹב · **insects; vermin**: Arab. هوامّ · Ibn Sīnā, *K. al-Qānūn fī al-ṭibb* · trans. Zeraḥyah Ḥen, *Sefer ha-Qanun* II, fols. 260ᵇ–261ᵃ: מֶנְטְרַשְׁטְרֵי[226] ... כשישתהו ויחבשנו בו יועיל מנשיכת הערוב (Mint: ... When a person drinks [its extract] and puts it [on the spot of the sting or bite] it is good for insect (vermin) bites). Hebr. עָרֹב is a Biblical term of uncertain meaning, variously interpreted as: 'vermin in general; pests; noxious insects,' or 'a particular type of fly, esp. a horse-fly' (cf. KB 2:879). Nathan ha-Me'ati translates Arab. هوامّ as שרצים.

עָרֵב · **I. low (re: fire)**: Lat. *suavis* (Arab. ليّن) · Constantinus Africanus, *Viaticum peregrinantis* · trans. Do'eg ha-Edomi, *Sefer Ya'ir Netiv* V.2: כל אלה תבשל בח' ליטרי' מים עד השליש ותעביר ואחר תקבל מנא כ' דרכמ' קשיא פישטולא י' דרכמ' ואלה תעביר ותשים שם ב' ליטרי' סוקרי ותבשל באש ערב עד העשותו אישרוב (Cook all these [ingredients] in eight liters of water until one third is left; sieve it, take 20 *dirhams* of manna and ten *dirhams* of purging cassia [*Cassia fistula* L.]. Put this through a sieve and add two pounds [Lat. *libra*] of sugar and cook it on a low fire until it turns into a syrup). Hebr. עָרֵב is not attested in this sense in the current dictionaries. Moses ibn Tibbon translates the parallel Arab. term ليّن as רפה.

· **II. softening; mitigating**: Lat. *mitigans* (Arab. ملطّف; i.e, 'thinning; diluting') · Constantinus Africanus, *Viaticum peregrinantis* · trans. Do'eg ha-Edomi, *Sefer Ya'ir Netiv* V.10: העזר זה ההדרוקן יאות להרפא בדברים ערבים ומקררים האדומה (Its cure: This [kind of] jaundice should be treated with ingredients that mitigate and cool [the heat of] the yellow bile). Hebr. עָרֵב is not attested in this sense in the current dictionaries.

עֶרְוָה • גב הערוה → גַּב.

• גיד הערוה → גִּיד.

עָרְלָה • ערלת הגרון · **uvula**: Arab. لهاة · al-Rāzī, *K. al-Manṣūrī fī al-ṭibb* · trans. Shem Tov ben Isaac, *Sefer Almansur*, fol. 3ᵇ: מ"ד בנפילת ערלת הגרון ([Chapter] 44: On prolapse of the uvula). Hebrew ערלת הגרון features in BM 4734 in attestations from Nathan ben Yeḥiel, *Sefer ha-Arukh* and Zedekiah ben Abraham Anav, *Shibbolei ha-Leqet*. A var. reading ערלת הגרגרת features on fol. 122ᵃ. Abraham Avigdor renders the parallel Lat. term *uvula* as אונקלי הוא אל להאה.

---

226 פֿנדַנג': מֶנְטְרַשְׁטְרֵי Ms¹.

עֹרֶק • העורק אשר על הכף בין האצבע הקטן ושכנו · **salvatella vein**: Arab. أسيلم · Ibn al-Jazzār, *Zād al-musāfir wa-qūt al-ḥādir* · trans. Moses ibn Tibbon, *Sefer Ṣedat ha-Derakhim* v.1: וכשיהיה בכבד סתום והיה הסתום ההוא מליחה חמה ר״ל מפני דם עב או מרה כרכומית ... הנה ראוי שנצוה החולה להקיז הגיד התחתון מן הצד הימני או להקיז העורק אשר על הכף בין האצבע הקטן ושכנו (If there is an obstruction in the liver and that obstruction is caused by a hot humor, i.e., thick blood or yellow bile ... we should order the patient to be bled from the basilic vein on the right side or from the salvatella vein). Hebr. העורק אשר על הכף בין האצבע הקטן ושכנו does not feature in the current dictionaries. A var. used by Ibn Tibbon in his *Sefer Ṣedat ha-Derakhim* III.7 is העורק אשר בין האצבע הקטן וחברו הנקרא אסילם (cf. NM 5:146). Do'eg ha-Edomi translates the parallel Lat. term *vena que est inter pollicem et indicem* as המקור שהוא בין הגודל והאצבע (see entry מָקוֹר).

• **העורק אשר אצל העקב לצד פנימי** · **the saphenous vein**: Arab. الصافان (lit., 'both saphenous veins') · Ibn al-Jazzār, *Zād al-musāfir wa-qūt al-ḥādir* · trans. Moses ibn Tibbon, *Sefer Ṣedat ha-Derakhim* v.2: אם היה מתילד הסתום בכבד מפני הפסק דם הנדות נצוה החולה להקיז העורק אשר אצל העקב לצד פנימי הנקרא צפאן הנקרא צפאן משני הרגלים ולהכנס במרחץ (If the obstruction of the liver originates from the cessation of the menstrual blood, we order the patient to be bled from the saphenous vein called [in Arabic] ṢP'N [read Ṣ'PN; i.e., *ṣāfin*] from both legs and to go to the bathhouse). Hebr. העורק אשר אצל העקב לצד פנימי is not attested in the current dictionaries. A var. reading by Ibn Tibbon in his *Sefer Ṣedat ha-Derakhim* III.8 is העורק אשר אצל העקב (cf. NM 5:146). Cf. also the definition of the Arab. term صافن in Nathan ha-Me'ati's glossary to the *Sefer ha-Qanun*: צאפן הוא העורק שמקיזים בו על הקרסול לצד פנים (Ṣ'PN ([small] saphenous vein): This is the vein, on the inner side of the ankle, which is bled) (cf. NM 2:118, 155–156 (Ṣade 2)). Do'eg ha-Edomi translates the parallel Lat. term *ambas venas in cruribus* as שני המקורות הירכים.

• **עורק הראש** · **cephalic vein**: Lat. *cephalica* · Gerard de Solo, *Practica super nono Almansoris* · trans. Abraham Avigdor, *Ha-Ma'amar ha-Teshi'i le-Sefer ha-Mansuri le-Razi*, fol. 1b: הקיז הקיפאל הוא עורק הראש אשר בזרוע מן הצד אשר בכאב יותר ([In the case of headache,] bleed the cephalic vein, which is in the arm that is on the same side as that part [of the head] in which the pain is worse). Hebr. עורק הראש is not attested in the current dictionaries. For the synonymous גיד הראש, cf. BCD 45 for attestations from Shem Tov ben Isaac, *Sefer ha-Shimmush* XXX.2.95 (cf. NM 1:82) and Moses ibn Tibbon, *Sefer Ṣedat ha-Derakhim* I.1.3 (cf. NM 4:31–32; IJZ 1–2:443).

עַרְקָא (*Aram.*) · **leech**: Arab. علق · al-Rāzī, *K. al-Manṣūrī fī al-ṭibb* · trans. Shem Tov ben Isaac, *Sefer Almansur*, fol. 3b: כשיהיה האדם מוצא מציצה בגרונו ורקיקת דם רקיק צריך לסבור כי כבר בלע ערקא (When a person has the sensation of sucking in his throat and he gives up thin blood, he should consider [the possibility] that he has swallowed a leech). Aram. עַרְקָא (cf. SDA 854) is not attested in medieval Hebr. medical literature. Abraham Avigdor translates the parallel Lat. term *sanguisuca* as עלוקה.

עֶרֶשׂ • השתין בערשו → הִשְׁתִּין.

עֵשֶׂב • עשב השוטה · **common purslane** [*Portulaca oleracea* L.]: Arab. *baqla al-ḥamqā'* (lit., 'the stupid vegetable', or perh. 'the insipid herb')[227] · Ibn Sīnā, *K. al-Qānūn fī al-ṭibb* · trans. Nathan ha-Me'ati, *Sefer ha-Qanun* II, fol. 71ᵇ: בקלה אלחמקה כלומר עשב שוטה ובערבי רקלסי (BQLH 'LḤMQH [i.e., Arab. *baqla al-ḥamqā'*]; i.e., [Hebr.] *'esev ha-shoṭeh*; Arab. RQLSY [read: RYGLH; i.e., *rijla*[228]). Hebr. עשב השוטה features in NM 5:157 in an attestation from [*Synonima*], Ms Vatican, Biblioteca Apostolica, ebr. 550, fol. 126ᵃ.

עָשָׂה • עשה סעוט · **to drip (inject) a medicine into the nose**: Arab. سعط · Ibn Sīnā, *K. al-Qānūn fī al-ṭibb* · trans. Nathan ha-Me'ati, *Sefer ha-Qanun* II, fols. 72ᵃ–72ᵇ: בסבאסה ... עושים ממנו סעוט עם שמן בנפסג לכאב הראש הנולד מרוחות גסות בראש (Mace: ... When mixed with violet oil and dripped into the nose, it relieves the headache caused by dense winds in the head). Hebr. עשה סעוט is not attested in the current dictionaries. The term סעוט is actually a loan word from Arab. سعوط 'errhine; sternutatory;' cf. FAQ 265–266. In his *Sefer ha-Peraqim* (*Pirqei Moshe*) XV.58, Nathan translates Arab. سعط as [עטש], *Pi'el* עִטֵּשׁ (cf. BMMN 163, l. 17; BMMG no. 2389). Zeraḥyah Ḥen translates the Arab. term as שם בנחירים and Anonymous has הטיף באף.

• עשה קנקן · **to apply an enema**: Arab. حقن · Ibn Sīnā, *K. al-Qānūn fī al-ṭibb* · trans. Nathan ha-Me'ati, *Sefer ha-Qanun* II, fol. 71ᵇ (Ms Paris, BnF, héb. 1136, fol. 69ᵇ): בקלה אלחמקה ... עושין ממנו קנקן[229] לנגעי המעיים והשלשול המררי (Common purslane: ... When one makes an enema with it [and applies it], it is useful for intestinal abrasions and bilious diarrhea). Hebr. קַנְקַן does not feature in this sense in the current dictionaries. In his *Sefer ha-Peraqim* (*Pirqei Moshe*), Nathan translates the Arab. verb حقن throughout as עשה חוקן and the noun حقنة as חוקן (cf. BMMG nos. 1019, 1021). Zeraḥyah Ḥen translates Arab. حقن as O. Occ./O. Cat. קירישטיר (i.e., *cristeri, crestiri, cresteri* or *cristiri*; cf. SHS 1:421–422 (Pe 36)) and Anonymous has חוקן, just like Nathan in his *Sefer ha-Peraqim* (*Pirqei Moshe*).

עִשּׁוּי (i.e., **עִסּוּי**) · **1. evacuation; extraction**: Lat. *extractio* · Constantinus Africanus, *Viaticum peregrinantis* · trans. Do'eg ha-Edomi, *Sefer Ya'ir Netiv* IV.14: אם הוא מהטבע המקובץ שם יאות לטהר הליחות עם רפואות מטהרות בעשוי (If [the lack of power] results from [humors] that have accumulated there [i.e., in the stomach] these humors should be cleansed with remedies that cleanse through evacuation). In the sense of 'evacuation; extraction,' Hebr. עִסּוּי features in BCD 205 (NM 4:149) in a later attestation from Nathan ha-Me'ati, *Sefer ha-Qanun* I. Moses ibn Tibbon translates the parallel Arab. term عصر as סחיטה.

---

227 Cf. Tanḥum Yerushalmi, *Al-Murshid al-kafi*, ed. and trans. by H. Shy (Jerusalem 2005), 190–191: חלק: לגלוגות מין רגילה הנקרא 'פרפחין' ... הידוע לרופאים בשמו 'אלבקלה אלחמקא' בשל הסתעפותו הרבה והתפשטות ענפיו.

228 Arab. *rijla* (رجلة), a synonym of *baqla al-ḥamqā*; cf. IG 751.

229 קנקן: חקנה הנקר' קנקן Ms Paris, BnF, héb. 1136, fol. 69ᵇ.

‣ II. **tenesmus** Lat. *extractio* (Arab. التزّحر) · Constantinus Africanus, *Viaticum peregrinantis* · trans. Do'eg ha-Edomi, *Sefer Ya'ir Netiv* IV.20: אם כן יאות לעין מאין יולד ואם הוא מעשוי יכאב כאב רב ויאות שהחולה ישב במים שנתבשלו בם דברים עוצרים (For this reason, one should pay attention to the cause [lit., origin] of [the rectal prolapse]: If it is caused by tenesmus, it is very painful and the patient should sit in waters in which astringent ingredients have been cooked ...). In the sense of 'tenesmus,' Hebr. עִסּוּי features in BCD 205 (NM 3:177) in a later attestation from Nathan ha-Me'ati, *Pirqei Abuqraṭ* VII.27. For synonymous terms, see entry עִצּוּר above. Moses ibn Tibbon translates Arab. التزّحر as עצר.

‣ III. **labor pains**: Lat. *expressio* (Arab. طلق) · Constantinus Africanus, *Viaticum peregrinantis* · trans. Do'eg ha-Edomi, *Sefer Ya'ir Netiv* VI.14 ופעמים תצא ברב העישוי בשעת הלידה (Sometimes [the uterus] suffers from a prolapse because of severe labor pains). Hebr. עִסּוּי does not feature in this sense in the current dictionaries. Moses ibn Tibbon translates Arab. طلق as הַמְלָטָה (see entry; he also translates the Arab. term as הַתָּרָה (see entry) in *Sefer Ṣedat ha-Derakhim* V.16) and Abraham ben Isaac has הלידה בקושי.

עֲשִׂיָּה · **application**: Arab. استعمال · Ibn al-Jazzār, *Zād al-musāfir wa-qūt al-ḥāḍir* · trans. Moses ibn Tibbon, *Sefer Ṣedat ha-Derakhim* IV.10: וכאשר נקינו האצטו' מהליחה ההיא הרעה נשתדל לתקן מזגה אשר קרה לה מפני רוע הליחה ההיא ונחזק כחה בעשיית דברים אשר יחזקו גרמה ויתקנו מזגה ויסירו הקבסא (Once we cleansed the stomach from that bad humor, we try to improve its temperament caused by that bad humor and to increase its strength by the application of ingredients that strengthen its substance and improve its temperament and take away the indigestion). In the sense of 'application,' Hebr. עֲשִׂיָּה is a non-attested semantic borrowing from Arab. استعمال. In the sense of 'consumption; intake,' it features in Nathan ha-Me'ati, *Sefer ha-Peraqim* (*Pirqei Moshe*) III.91 (cf. BCD 216 (NM 2:74); BMMN 53, l. 2; BMMG no. 3569). For the verb עָשָׂה in the sense of 'to apply [medicines],' see BCD 215 (NM 1:65) for an attestation from *Sefer Ṣedat ha-Derakhim* VII.9.3 (cf. IJZ 7:139, l. 2).

פ

[פגג] • *Piʿel* ‣ **to make [something] crude**: Arab. فجّج · Maimonides, *Maqāla fī al-rabw* (*On Asthma*) · trans. Joshua Shatibi, *Maʾamar ʿal ha-Qaṣeret* VII.3 (cf. BMA 2:343, ll. 10–11): אכן מים כבר ידעו רוב האנשים כי שתותו על המאכל יפגגוהו ויכנס בין האצטומכה והמאכל ויצוף למעלה וירע עכולו (Regarding water, most people know that, if one drinks it with a meal, it [keeps] the food crude because it forms a barrier between it and the stomach so that the food floats and is poorly digested). Hebr. [פגג], *Piʿel* פִּגֵּג, does not feature in this sense in the current dictionaries. It is poss. coined analogous to Arab. فجّج, but cf. the meaning of the noun פַּג ('unripe fig;' BM 4809). Ben Yehuda (ibid.) refers to a verb פגג only featuring in the *Piʿel* conj. in the sense of 'to thicken, coagulate, clot.' Samuel Benveniste translates Arab. فجّج as [פגג], *Hifʿil* הֵפֵג (see next entry) and Anonymous renders Arab. فجّج as *Piʿel* פִּגֵּג, just like Joshua Shatibi.

• *Hifʿil* הֵפֵג ‣ **to make [something] crude**: Arab. فجّج Maimonides, *Maqāla fī al-rabw* (*On Asthma*) · trans. Samuel Benveniste, *Maʾamar ʿal ha-Qaṣeret* VII.3 (cf. BMA 2:266, ll. 12–13): אבל המים כבר נודע לרוב בני אדם כי שתותם על המאכל יפיגוה ויבדילו בין האסטומכה ובין המאכל ויצוף ויפסד העכול (Regarding water, most people know that, if one drinks it with a meal, it [keeps] the food crude because it forms a barrier between it and the stomach so that the food floats and is poorly digested). Hebr. [פגג], *Hifʿil* הֵפֵג, does not feature in this sense in the current dictionaries. Joshua Shatibi and Anonymous both render Arab. فجّج as [פגג], *Piʿel* פִּגֵּג (see previous entry).

פֶּה • **לקות הפה** → לָקוּת.

• **עקום הפה** → עִקּוּם.

• **פי החלוחלת** ‣ **anus**: Arab. مقعدة · Ibn al-Jazzār, *Zād al-musāfir wa-qūt al-ḥādir* · trans. Moses ibn Tibbon, *Sefer Ṣedat ha-Derakhim* IV.20: ואלו הסמים הקובצים כלם כשיעשו אחר שהכניסו פי הטבעת ברירים הדבקים המבושלים או באבק יחזקו פי החלוחלת וימנעו יציאתה בע"ה (All these astringent remedies, when their viscous boiled mucilages have been inserted into the anus or they have been [pulverized and strewn upon it,] strengthen it and prevent its prolapse, God willing). Hebr. פי החלוחלת does not feature in the current dictionaries. The term חלוחלת alone features as חַלְחֹלֶת in JD 466 (cf. Low LI) in the sense of 'mesentery' and in BM 1568 as 'rectum.' Moses ibn Tibbon also translates Arab. مقعدة as פי הטבעת (see next entry) and the Arab. synonym مخرج as מוֹצָא (see entry), both in his *Sefer Ṣedat ha-Derakhim* IV.15.

• **פי הטבעת** ‣ **anus**: Arab. مقعدة · Ibn al-Jazzār, *Zād al-musāfir wa-qūt al-ḥādir* · trans. Moses ibn Tibbon, *Sefer Ṣedat ha-Derakhim* IV.15: ואם קרה לו עצור הוא הנקרא בער' זחיר הנה ראוי שיתרחץ מי שהיה בו החולי הזה בדברים קובצים אשר יחזקו פי הטבעת (If he is affected by tenesmus, which is called in Arab. ZḤYR [i.e., *zuḥair*], he should wash himself with astringent ingredients that strengthen the anus). Hebr. פי הטבעת features in BM 1845 (s.v. טבעת) and 4834 in attestations from Rabb. literature only (cf. JD 519, s.v. טבעת). In addition to פי הטבעת, Ibn Tibbon translates Arab. مقعدة as פי

החלוחלת (see previous entry) and the Arab. synonym مخرج as מוֹצָא (see entry). Do'eg ha-Edomi translates the parallel Lat. term *anus* as נֶקֶב (see entry) and Abraham ben Isaac renders مقعدة as הנקב התחתון in his *Sefer Ṣedah la-Oreḥim* VI.12 (see also entry נֶקֶב).

• **בליטת פי הטבעת → בְּלִיטָה.**

• **יציאת פי הטבעת → יְצִיאָה.**

פּוֹלֵט (*Part.*) → **פָּלַט.**

פּוּנְץ · **dysentery**: Arab. سحج · Maimonides, *Maqāla fī al-rabw* (*On Asthma*) · trans. Samuel Benveniste, *Ma'amar 'al ha-Qaṣeret* XIII.10 (cf. BMA 2:300, ll. 5–7): וכמה פעמים ראיתי מי שהשקה משלשל חזק למי שלא יצטרך אפילו למשלשל קל ויצא ממנו דם רב מלמטה עד שהיו לו פונץ עצומים והבריא אחרי כן (I have seen several times how someone administered a strong purgative to a person who did not even need a weak purgative. [As a result,] this person lost much blood from below, which [condition] lasted [for several days, and] he suffered from severe dysentery; yet he recovered afterwards). Hebr. פונץ is a widely spread non-attested loan word from O. Cat. *pons* ('dysentery'), stemming from Lat. *pondus*; cf. SHS 1:157 (Gimel 17). Thus it features, a.o., in Moses ibn Tibbon, *Perush Aphorismi shel Apuqraṭ* (*Pirqei Abuqraṭ*) VII.27 (379) (BMCH 1:410, l. 1), in Jacob ibn Tibbon, *Hanhagat ha-Beri'ut le-Abu 'Ali ben Zuhr* (cf. RSA 161), and in the *Sefer ha-Refu'ot le-Ḥakham Qosṭa'ntin* (see חולי הזחיר (entry חֳלִי)). Anonymous renders Arab. سحج as שחנות and Joshua Shatibi translates Arab. انسحج سحجا as התנגעו מעיו. For other Hebrew terms for 'dysentery,' see entry **עִצּוּר.**

פּוּרְנִי (*Aram.*) · **brick oven fuelled with wood, similar to glass-making furnaces**: Arab. فرن (NA 681–682) · Ibn Zuhr, *K. al-Aghdhiya* · trans. Nathan ha-Me'ati, *Sefer ha-Mezonot*, fol. 2b: והמשובח שבכל מיניו מה שישלים אפייתו בתנור ואחריו מה שיאפה בפורני (The best kind [of bread] is that which is properly baked in a domed clay oven, followed by that which is baked in a brick oven). Aram. פּוּרְנִי features in BCD 219 (NM 4:162–163) in an attestation from Shem Tov ben Isaac, *Sefer ha-Shimmush* XXVII.

[פזר] • *Part. Nif'al* **נִפְזָר** • **עפרים נפזרים → עָפָר.**

[פטר] • *Part. Hif'il* **מַפְטִיר** • **להיות מפטיר** · **taking for dessert**: Arab. التنقّل · Maimonides, *Maqāla fī al-rabw* (*On Asthma*) · trans. Samuel Benveniste, *Ma'amar 'al ha-Qaṣeret* III.8 (cf. BMA 2:253, ll. 1–4): ויתמיד[230] להיות מפטיר בפסטק ושקדים וכל שכן המרים מעורבים עם המתוקים עד שילמד אכלם מפני שהם רפואה גדולה לחולי זה ומדקקים הליחה פותחים כל הסתומים מנקים הריאה עוזרים לרוק שימהו במחשבתך (And for dessert, one[231] should take pistachio nuts and almonds, especially the bitter [nuts], which one may mix with sweet [nuts] until one becomes accustomed to eating them. For [this] is an excellent remedy for this disease, because it thins the humors, opens all the obstructions,

---

230 ויתמיד: ويعتمد a.

231 'one should take': Trans. after a.

cleans the lungs, and helps expectoration; keep it in mind). In the sense of 'to take for dessert,' Hebr. [פטר], *Part. Hif'il* מַפְטִיר, features in mPes x.8 as: אין מפטירין אחר הפסח אפיקומן (After the Passover meal, they may not finish with dessert); cf. JD 104, s.v. אפיקומן; BM 4900. Joshua Shatibi translates Arab. التنقّل as אכול אחר האכילה and Anonymous has אפיקימון (see entry אֲפִיקוֹמָן).

[פלא] • *Part. Nif'al* • **נִפְלָא** • **השבכה הנפלאת** → **שְׂבָכָה.**

פְּלוּחַ • **פלוח הראש** · **migraine**: Arab. شقيقة · Ibn Zuhr, *K. al-Aghdhiya* · trans. Nathan ha-Me'ati, *Sefer ha-Mezonot*, fol. 4[a]: ואמנם אפרוחיהם הם יותר רבי הלחות מותרי מאד ולהם סגולה לחדש כאיבי ראש הידועים בפלוח הראש והוא מיקרניא[232] (However, young [pigeons] have a very large quantity of residual moisture and are known to produce a headache that is known as migraine, i.e., [Lat./Rom.] MYQRNY'). In the sense of 'migraine,' Hebr. פלוח הראש features in BM 4940–4941, a.o., in attestations from the *Sefer ha-Qanun* and from Nathan's *Sefer ha-Peraqim* (*Pirqei Moshe*) VI.35: בעלי פלוח הראש הנקר' מיקראניא (cf. BMMN 70, l. 7; BMMG no. 2711). Shem Tov ben Isaac translates Arab. شقيقة as Aram. צלחתא in his *Sefer ha-Shimmush* XXX.1.3 (cf. BCD 229 (NM 1:111)).

פְּלוּשׁ • *Plur.* **פלושים** · **passages; channels**: Arab. منافذ · Maimonides, *Maqāla fī al-rabw* (*On Asthma*) · trans. Anonymous, *Sefer ha-Qaṣeret* II.1 (cf. BMA 2:393, ll. 20–21): שהכונה שיהיו הגידים כולם והפילושים פתוחי השביל נקיים מהאוטם והצוק עד שירוצו בהם הרוחות והלחות ונדחים מהם היתרונות (One's intention should be that all the veins and passages are open and clean and free from obstruction and constriction so that the pneumas and humors stream through them [freely] and the superfluities are expelled). Hebr. פְּלוּשׁ features in BM 4941 in attestations from medieval literature in the sense of 'hollowness,' and in EM 1430 in the sense of 'opening; open passage.' Samuel Benveniste translates Arab. منافذ as נקבים and Joshua Shatibi has מעברים.

פָּלַט • *Part.* **פּוֹלֵט** • **הכח הפולטת** → **כֹּחַ.**

פְּנִימִי • **העורק אשר אצל העקב לצד פנימי** → **עֹרֶק.**

פעולה → **פְּעֻלָּה.**

פְּעֻלָּה • *Plur.* **פעולות** · **[healing] effects**: Arab. أفعال · Ibn Sīnā, *K. al-Qānūn fī al-ṭibb* · trans. Zeraḥyah Ḥen, *Sefer ha-Qanun* II, fol. 239[b]: מַרְזוּנְגוֹשׁ הטבע חם ויבש הפעולות והסגולות דק ומתיר פותח בכח (Marjoram: Its nature: It is hot and dry. Its healing effects and specific properties: It thins, dissolves, and opens with force). Hebrew פְּעֻלָּה, *Plur.* פעולות, does not feature in this sense in the current dictionaries. Nathan ha-Me'ati translates Arab. أفعال as מפעלים (see entry מִפְעָל).

פְּקוֹקֶלֶת • *Plur.* **פקוקליות** · **buttocks; lower back**: Arab. قطاة (cf. VL 3:470: 'nates et locus inter coxas') · al-Rāzī, *K. al-Manṣūrī fī al-ṭibb* · trans. Shem Tov ben Isaac, *Sefer Almansur*, fol. 139[a]: שער בשחין הפקוקליות: כשתארך השכיבה פרקדן לפעמים יכהה מקום הקוליות וישחין שחין רע (Chapter on swelling of the lower back: If a person lies too

232 מיקרניא: emend. ed. מיקדניא Ms.

long on his back, the area between the thigh bones becomes pale (dark) and then develops a bad swelling ...). Hebr. פְּקוֹקֶלֶת only features in the current dictionaries in the *Plur.* פקוקלות as a Rabb. term in the sense of 'ramication of sinews [in the loins]' (JD 1208) or 'ramification of veins, of fleshy parts' (cf. LW 4:94: '... die sich verzweigenden Fleischteile oder Adern'); cf. Aram. פקוקלה, *Det.* פקוקלתה (SD 443: 'ramification of sinews'). Abraham Avigdor translates the parallel Lat. term *ulceres lumborum et renum* (extant in Ms Munich, Bayerische Staatsbibliothek, Cod. hebr. 296, fol. 177[a], as part of the header שער די אולששיריבוש לומבורום ויל רינום) as התנגע קצה השדרה ('swelling of the lower spine').

[פרד] • *Inf. Nif'al* הִפָּרֵד • **הפרד הדבוק** · **dissolution of continuity; separation of connected parts**: Arab. تفرّق الاتّصال · Maimonides, *Maqāla fī al-rabw* (*On Asthma*) · trans. Samuel Benveniste, *Ma'amar 'al ha-Qaṣeret* v.1 (cf. BMA 2:259, ll. 8–10): ועקר הדבר בכל זה להשמר מן השבעה המביאה למתיחת הבטן ביותר ממה שבטבע כי כל אבר שימתח ישתבשו פעלותיו בהכרח כי ההמתח הוא ממיני הפרד הדבוק (The main principle in this entire matter is to avoid satiation, which causes unnatural distension of the stomach, because when any organ is distended, its functions are necessarily impaired. For distension is a kind of separation of connected parts (dissolution of continuity)). Hebr. הפרד הדבוק is not attested in the current dictionaries. Joshua Shatibi translates Arab. تفرّق الاتّصال as פרוק החבור (see entry פֵּרוּק) and Anonymous has הפרדות החיבור (see entry הִפָּרְדוּת).

פָּרָה • *Part. m. Plur.* פֹּרִים • **הנגעים הפרים** → **נֶגַע**.

פֵּרוּד • **פרוד החבור** · **dissolution of continuity; separation of connected parts**: Arab. انحلال الفرد · Ibn al-Jazzār, *Zād al-musāfir wa-qūt al-ḥāḍir* · trans. Moses ibn Tibbon, *Sefer Ṣedat ha-Derakhim* v.4: הנה יתחדש הרקת דם מן הכבד מפני סבות רבות ויהיו מיני הדם המורק מתחלפים כי מהם מין מפרוד החבור ר"ל שיקרה בגרם הכבד נגע או יפתח בו עורק (There are many causes for the evacuation of blood from the liver, while the kinds of blood that is evacuated vary; one kind hails from the dissolution of continuity; i.e., that an ulcer occurs in the substance of the liver or that a vein bursts). Hebr. פרוד החבור is not attested in the current dictionaries. Do'eg ha-Edomi translates the parallel Lat. term *separatio iuncture* as הפרדת החבור (see entry הַפְרָדָה).

פֵּרוּק • **פרוק החבור** · **dissolution of continuity; separation of connected parts**: Arab. تفرّق الاتّصال · Maimonides, *Maqāla fī al-rabw* (*On Asthma*) · trans. Joshua Shatibi, *Ma'amar 'al ha-Qaṣeret* v.1 (cf. BMA 2:335, ll. 9–10): ועיקר הדבר בזה שישמר מן השובע המזיק המושך האצטו' לפי שכל אבר ימשך יתבטלו פעולותיו בהכרח לפי שההמשך ממיני פרוק החבור (The main principle in this matter is to avoid harmful satiation that causes distension of the stomach, because when any organ is distended, its functions are necessarily impaired. For distension is a kind of separation of connected parts (dissolution of continuity)). Hebr. פרוק החבור features as פירוק חבור in BCD 223 (NM 2:75) in an attestation from Nathan ha-Me'ati, *Sefer ha-Peraqim* XXV.21 (cf. BMMN 247, ll. 2, 4, 7; BMMG no. 3828). Samuel Benveniste translates Arab. تفرّق الاتّصال as הפרד הדבוק (see entry [פרד]) and Anonymous has הפרדות החיבור (see entry הִפָּרְדוּת).

פֶּרַח • *Plur.* **פרחים** • **הֲעצר הפרחים** → עָצַר[1].
פַּרְסִי • **האש הפרסי** → אֵשׁ.
פֶּרֶק • **הגיע לפרקו** → נָגַע.
• *Plur.* **פרקים** • **אבון הפרקים** → אִבּוּן.
• **התאבנות הפרקים** → הִתְאַבְּנוּת.

[פרר] • *Piʿel* **פֵּרֵר** • **to grind**: Arab. حكّ · Maimonides, *Maqāla fī al-rabw* (*On Asthma*) · trans. Anonymous, *Sefer ha-Qaṣeret* XII.9 (cf. BMA 2:435, ll. 1–3): נוסח מעשה הסמנין המשלשלין כלם שנסו אותם בקיאי הרופאים במערב וראינום עין בעין ונתרבה נסיונו בנוסח עשיית המשלשל הוא מה שאזכור לך: האגאריקון מפררין אותו על הכברה עד שיכבר (Description of the preparation of all the purgatives, which the skillful physicians in the Maghreb have tested repeatedly in my presence. The description of the preparation of [such a] purgative is as follows: Agaric should be ground over a sieve until it is sifted). Hebr. [פרר], *Piʿel* פֵּרֵר, is attested in Rabb. literature in the sense of 'to crumble' (cf. JD 1241; BM 5242). Samuel Benveniste translates Arab. حكّ as חיכך and Joshua Shatibi has גרד.

פָּשַׁט • *Inf.* **פְּשׁוֹט** • **making glad: gladdening**: Arab. بَسط · Maimonides, *Maqāla fī al-rabw* (*On Asthma*) · trans. Joshua Shatibi, *Maʾamar ʿal ha-Qaṣeret* VII.2 (cf. BMA 2:341, ll. 15–17): ולפי שנאסר הרב והמעט ממנו בין הישמעאלים עשו הרופאים תחבולה במה שיהיה בקצת תמורת היין והוא משקה הדבש המתובל שהוא היה במקום היין ברוב סגולותיו הטובות זולתי בפשט הנפש והסרת המותר העשני מן הרוחות (But since the consumption of both a large and a small quantity of [wine] is forbidden under Islam, the physicians have taken pains to find a beverage that can replace it to a certain degree. This beverage is that consisting of honey seasoned with spices, for it can substitute for most of the excellent qualities of wine, except for the gladdening of the soul and the removal of the turbid, gaseous superfluity from the pneumas …). In the sense of 'gladdening,' Hebr. פְּשׁוֹט is a non-attested semantic borrowing from Arab. بَسط. Samuel Benveniste translates the Arab. term as שמח and Anonymous has שימוח.

• *Part. Hifʿil* **מַפְשִׁיט** • **abrasing; excoriating**: Lat. *excorians* · Constantinus Africanus, *Viaticum peregrinantis* · trans. Doʾeg ha-Edomi, *Sefer Yaʾir Netiv* IV.15: וזה סובל החולה כאשר האדומה המחודדת עוברת במעי ונוקבת ומפשטת או מנגעת בחדודה (The patient suffers from this [illness] when the sharp yellow bile passes through the intestines, has a biting effect on them, and excoriates them or causes ulcers because of its sharpness). In the sense of 'to abrade,' Hebr. *Hifʿil* הִפְשִׁיט features in BCD 225 (NM 2:75) in a later attestation from Nathan ha-Meʾati, *Sefer ha-Peraqim* (*Pirqei Moshe*) VI.90 (cf. BMMN 78, l. 7; BMMG no. 2325). Moses ibn Tibbon translates the parallel Arab. term سحج as חמרמר; cf. BCD 104 (NM 3:93) for חֲמַרְמַר as an intrans. verb in the sense of 'to be abraded' in an attestation from Ibn Tibbon's *Perush Aphorismi shel Apuqraṭ* (*Pirqei Abuqraṭ*) IV.24 (161) (cf. BMCH 1:363, l. 2).

• *Inf. Hitpaʿel* **הִתְפַּשֵּׁט** • **rejoicing**: Arab. انبساط · Maimonides, *Maqāla fī al-rabw* (*On Asthma*) · trans. Joshua Shatibi, *Maʾamar ʿal ha-Qaṣeret* VIII.2 (cf. BMA 2:345, ll. 14–

15): והשמחה והששון יעשו הפך זה כלו להתפשט הנפש ותנועת הדם לחוץ הגוף ויראו פעולות האברים על השלמות (But joy and pleasure have an effect opposite to all these things because of the rejoicing of the soul and the movement of the blood and pneuma to the outside of the body so that the functions of the organs seem to be at their very best). In the sense of 'rejoicing,' Hebr. הִתְפַּשֵּׁט is a non-attested semantic borrowing from Arab. انبساط. Samuel Benveniste translates Arab. انبساط as הַרְחָבָה (see entry) and Anonymous has הִתְפַּשְּׁטוּת (see entry).

פְּשִׁיאוּת · **fineness; thinness**: Lat. *subtilitas* (Arab. رقّة) · Constantinus Africanus, *Viaticum peregrinantis* · trans. Do'eg ha-Edomi, *Sefer Ya'ir Netiv* v.12: אם הכאב ואפיסת הכליות יהיו מחבור רע יאות לעיין אם הוא מחום אז נעשה חום הזרע ופשיטותו והשחתת השומן אשר בכליות ויהיה השתן אדום או מכורכם (If the pain and weakness of the kidneys are caused by a bad temperament, one should look whether it is caused by heat; for then the sperm will be hot and thin and the fat in the kidneys will be corrupted and the urine will be red or like saffron). Hebr. פְּשִׁיאוּת does not feature in this sense in the current dictionaries. Moses ibn Tibbon translates the parallel Arab. term رقّة as דקות.

פִּתּוּחַ · **deobstruent quality [of a drug]**: Arab. تفتيح (cf. UW 229, s.v. ἐκφρακτικός: 'Obstruktionen beseitigend') · Ibn Sīnā, *K. al-Qānūn fī al-ṭibb* · trans. Nathan ha-Me'ati, *Sefer ha-Qanun* II, fol. 69b: בטיך ... והאבטיח אשר אינו מבושל הוא בטבע הקשואים ובו פתוח איך שיהיה (Melon: ... Unripe melons are similar to cucumbers in nature and deobstruent quality, anyhow). Hebrew פִּתּוּחַ does not feature in this sense in the current dictionaries. Zeraḥyah Ḥen translates Arab. تفتيح as פִּתּוּחַ, just like Nathan, but also as פְּתִיחָה (see next entry).

פְּתִיחָה · **deobstruent quality [of a drug]**: Arab. تفتيح (cf. UW 229, s.v. ἐκφρακτικός: 'Obstruktionen beseitigend') · Ibn Sīnā, *K. al-Qānūn fī al-ṭibb* · trans. Zeraḥyah Ḥen, *Sefer ha-Qanun* II, fol. 216b: חַבָּה אלכַצְ'רָה ... ויש בו פתיחה טובה ובישול וחלקות וימשוך מן העומק ואל הרבה מן החליים[233] יעמוד במקום המצטכי (Turpentine: ... It is a good deobstruent and has laxative and maturative [properties]. It extracts [superfluous matters] from the depth [of the body] and often[234] its actions are similar to mastic). Hebrew פְּתִיחָה does not feature in this sense in the current dictionaries. In addition to פְּתִיחָה, Zeraḥyah translates Arab. تفتيح as פִּתּוּחַ, just like Nathan ha-Me'ati (see previous entry). Anonymous has פְּתִיחָה, just like Zeraḥyah.

פְּתִילָה • סבל פתילה מלמטה → סָבַל.

233 החליים: الأوقات a.

234 'often': Trans. after a.

צ

צֵאָה · **dung; droppings:** Arab. روث · Ibn Sīnā, *K. al-Qānūn fī al-ṭibb* · trans. Nathan ha-Me'ati, *Sefer ha-Qanun* II, fol. 112ᵇ: ענבר המהות הענבר כפי מה שאני חושב מעין נובע בים ומה שאמרו שהוא מקצף הים או מצאת בהמה רחוק בעיני (Ambergris: What is it (*ha-mahut*)?:[235] In my opinion [the source] of ambergris is a spring in the sea. The opinion of some that it is the sea foam or droppings of an animal is unlikely in my eyes). Hebrew צֵאָה features in BCD 227 (NM 3:191) in the sense of 'emptying; excrement; voiding' (for Arab. براز), a.o., in an attestation from Zeraḥyah Ḥen, *Perush Aphorismi shel Apuqraṭ* (*Pirqei Abuqraṭ*) IV.83 (220) (cf. BMCH 1:472, l. 4). Here, Zeraḥyah translates Arab. روث as רעי and Anonymous has צואה.

צֶבַע • *Plur.* **צבעים** • **רוג׳ה של צבעים** → **רוג׳ה**.

צַד • **בעלת הצד** → **בַּעֲלָה**.

• **העורק אשר אצל העקב לצד פנימי** → **עֹרֶק**.

צַוָּאר • **צואר המקוה** · **neck of the bladder (cervix; collum vesicae):** Lat. *collum vesicae* (Arab. عنق المثانة) · Constantinus Africanus, *Viaticum peregrinantis* · trans. Do'eg ha-Edomi, *Sefer Ya'ir Netiv* V.16: והאבן נולדת לבחורים בכליות ולנערים במקוה אשר צוארה קצר בהם ומונעת לצאת הטבע ועל כן נולדת שם האבן (Adults develop stones in the kidneys and children [develop stones] in the bladder because they have a narrow neck of the bladder which prevents the matter (urine) to pass. As a result, stones develop in it). Hebr. צואר המקוה is attested in BM 5412 in a later attestation from Meir Aldabi, *Shevilei Emunah*. Moses ibn Tibbon has the same Hebr. term for the parallel Arab. term عنق المثانة.

• **העצמות מלמטה מן הצואר על החזה** → **עֶצֶם**.

צוּרָה · **I. species; kind:** Lat. *species* (Arab. صنف) · Constantinus Africanus, *Viaticum peregrinantis* · trans. Do'eg ha-Edomi, *Sefer Ya'ir Netiv* IV.14: וזאת הצורה מליאנטריא אין לה בתחלה אוקשירימיא[236] (In the beginning of this kind of lienteria, [one does not suffer] from acidic eructation). In the sense of 'species,' Hebr. צוּרָה features in PESHAT[237] in a later attestation from Shem Tov ben Joseph Falaquera, *De'ot ha-Philosophim*. Moses ibn Tibbon translates the parallel Arab. term صنف as מין.

· **II. appearance; looks:** Lat. *figura* (Arab. سحنة;[238] Gr. ἕξις) · Constantinus Africanus, *Viaticum peregrinantis* · trans. Do'eg ha-Edomi, *Sefer Ya'ir Netiv* VI.9: ושבה צורתה למתכונתה (Her appearance became normal again). Hebr. צוּרָה features in the sense of 'external form; perceived by the senses' in later attestations from

---

235 See entry מְהוּת.

236 אוקשירימיא: *oxiregmia* L جشاء حامض a.

237 https://peshat.org/display/peshat_lemmas_00003613 (accessed April 9, 2022).

238 The faulty سخنة in BIJS 132, l. 551, should be corrected as سحنة.

medieval philosophical literature (cf. PESHAT[239]). Moses ibn Tibbon translates the parallel Arab. term سحنة as תֹּאַר (see entry) and Abraham ben Isaac has תוכן הבריאות.

צִיּוּר · **imagination:** Lat. *imaginatio* (Arab. تخيّل) · Constantinus Africanus, *Viaticum peregrinantis* · trans. Do'eg ha-Edomi, *Sefer Ya'ir Netiv* VI.4: ולפעמים יראה אשה ויחשוק אותה והנפש בתוך שנתו מציירת אותה אצלו כאלו היה שם ומשם יחול הגיעול ההוא כי ציור הנפש אינו כי אם חבור הגוף (Sometimes a man sees a woman and longs for her. When he is asleep, the soul imagines her near to him as if he was with (had intercourse with) her and this causes the nocturnal pollution, for the imagination of the soul is nothing else but a temperament of the body). In the sense of 'imagination,' Hebr. צִיּוּר features in medieval philosophical literature, cf. KT 3:241–243. Moses ibn Tibbon and Abraham ben Isaac both translate Arab. تخيّل as דמיון.

צְלִיל • **צליל באוזן** · **tinnitus:** Arab. دويّ (Gr. ἦχος; cf. UW 288) · Ibn Sīnā, *K. al-Qānūn fī al-ṭibb* · trans. Nathan ha-Me'ati, *Sefer ha-Qanun* II, fols. 67[b]–68[a]: באן ... יפסיק רעיפת דם הנחירים ויקבצהו[240] והוא נאות לכאב האוזן ואל הצליל אשר בה ויותר עם שמן אווזות (B'N [i.e., fruit of the ben oil tree [*Moringa oleifera* Lam.]]: ... It stops nosebleeds because[241] of its astringency. It is good for earache and tinnitus, especially with duck fat). Hebr. צליל באוזן features as צליל באזנים in BM 5493 in an attestation from Nathan ben Jo'el Falaquera, *Sefer Ṣori ha-Guf*.[242] A var. reading צְלִילָה is attested in Moses ibn Tibbon, *Sefer Sedat ha-Derakhim* II.8.4 (cf. BCD 229 (NM 4:172); IJZ 1–2:495). Other synonyms featuring in medieval Hebr. medical literature are הברה, הברה באזנים, and הברת השמע (cf. NM 5:57), as well as צלצול (האזנים) (in Do'eg ha-Edomi, *Sefer Ya'ir Netiv* II.8.0–1; cf. NM 5:168; IJZ 1–2:639)). Zeraḥyah Ḥen translates Arab. دويّ as הקול הנשמע באוזן (see entry קול) and Anonymous has צלצול באוזן.

[צלל] • *Pi'el* **צִלֵּל** · **to filter, strain:** Arab. صفّى · Maimonides, *Maqāla fī al-rabw* (*On Asthma*) · trans. Samuel Benveniste, *Ma'amar 'al ha-Qaṣeret* IX.1 (cf. BMA 2:271, ll. 4–6): וכבר שבח אבו מרון בן זהר להרפות בזה אמר: ימרס מן התמר אינדי עשרה זוזים במה שיכסהו מן המים החמים וישרה בו ריברברי רצוץ שלשה רביעי זוז כ״ד שעות וצללהו באוקיה משקה קלפת האתרוג (Abu Marwan ibn Zuhr has recommended softening [the stools] with the following [drug]: Macerate ten *zuzim* of Indian tamarind in sufficient warm water to cover them, and then soak three-quarters of a *dirham* of ground Chinese rhubarb for twenty-four hours and strain this into one ounce of lemon peel juice). Hebr. צלל is not attested in the *Pi'el* conj. in the current dictionaries. It features in the *Qal* conj. in NM 5:167 in the sense of 'to clarify, clear, purify, filter' in an attestation from Abra-

239 https://peshat.org/display/peshat_lemmas_00003613 (accessed April 9, 2022).

240 ויקבצהו: بقبضه a.

241 'because of its astringency': Trans. after a.

242 See G. Bos and R. Fontaine, 'Medico-Philosophical Controversies in Nathan b. Jo'el Falaquera's *Sefer Ṣori ha-Guf*,' *The Jewish Quarterly Review* 90, nos. 1–2 (1999): 27–60.

ham ben Isaac, *Sefer Ṣedah la-Oreḥim* I.14.3 (cf. IJZ 1–2:561). Joshua Shatibi translates Arab. صفّى as *Pi'el* זִכֵּךְ (see entry [זכך]) and Anonymous has *Pi'el* סִנֵּן.

צֶלַע • *Plur.* **צלעות** • **hypochondrium**: Lat. *hypochondria* (Arab. شراسيف; Gr. ὑποχόνδριον; cf. UW 715) · Constantinus Africanus, *Viaticum peregrinantis* · trans. Do'eg ha-Edomi, *Sefer Ya'ir Netiv* V.9: אשירוף מאשקינגט זה טוב לסתימת הכבד ולטחול ולרוח הצלעות הם אפוקנדריא (A syrup of camel grass that is good for obstruction of the liver and spleen and for wind in the hypochondrium, i.e., [Lat.] 'PWQNDRY' ...). As an anatomical term, Hebr. צֶלַע, *Plur.* צלעות, only features in the current dictionaries in the sense of 'ribs.' Instead of צלעות, which features regularly in the *Sefer Ya'ir Netiv*, Do'eg uses the more precise term תחת הצלעים in his *Sefer Agur* IV.64 (cf. BCD 293 (NM 3:242–243)). For var. readings תחת החלצי(י)ם, תחת הטבור, and תחת הכסלים, cf. BCD 292–293 (NM 1:93 (corr. 4:229), 149; 3:242–243)). Moses ibn Tibbon translates Arab. شراسيف as צלעות as well.

• **כאב צדי הצלעות** → כְּאֵב.

צִמּוּק • **digestion**: Arab. هضم · Ibn al-Jazzār, *Zād al-musāfir wa-qūt al-ḥāḍir* · trans. Moses ibn Tibbon, *Sefer Ṣedat ha-Derakhim* IV.11: וכשיהיה לאחד הקיא מבלתי שלקח מזון רב או מאכל רע הנה הוא מהמבואר כי הסבה בזה ליחות רעות עוקצות פי האצטו' והנה ימצא אות זה בקיא עצמו שאם היה ממרה כרכומית או חם יתבאר רושם זה בצמוק המאכל (If a person needs to vomit while he did not take food in a large quantity or of a bad quality, it is clear that it is caused by bad humors that bite the cardia of the stomach. An indication for this can be found in the vomit itself; when it consists of yellow bile and it is hot, it means that the food is digested). Hebr. צִמּוּק does not feature in this sense in the current dictionaries. Do'eg ha-Edomi translates the parallel Lat. term *digestio* as בשול.

צִמּוּקִיָּה • **a compound dish consisting of raisins, meat, and other ingredients**: Arab. زبيبية (cf. NTT 131–132) · Maimonides, *Maqāla fī al-rabw* (*On Asthma*) · trans. Anonymous, *Sefer ha-Qaṣeret* IV.2 (cf. BMA 2:399, ll. 7–9): ומזה צמוקיה היא בתכלית התועלת ועריבת הטעם והיא כרפואה וטופסה: שולקין בשר הצאן או העוף וקולין אותו כמו שקולין כל התבשילין בתבלין שאזכרם אחר כן (Another dish is that prepared from raisins; it is extremely beneficial and very tasty and is like a remedy. Its recipe is: Boil mutton or fowl and roast it in the same way as other foods [and] spices that I will describe further on)(corr.). Hebr. צִמּוּקִיָּה, coined after Arab. زبيبية, is not attested in the current dictionaries. Samuel Benveniste translates the Arab. term as סומקיה and Joshua Shatibi has מטעם הצמוקים.

צֶמַח • *Plur.* **צמחים** • **abcesses**: Lat. *apostemata* (Arab. أورام) · Constantinus Africanus, *Viaticum peregrinantis* · trans. Do'eg ha-Edomi, *Sefer Ya'ir Netiv* V.13: הצמחים הם אפושטמש ונולדים בכליות מהליחות היורדות בהם ועל כן הכאב נרגש בעגבות והקושי בקחדת (Abscesses, i.e., 'PWŠṬMŠ [i.e., Lat. *apostemas*] occur in the kidneys from humors descending into them. For this reason, the patient will feel pain and hardness in the buttocks and he will suffer from fever). In the sense of 'abscess,' Hebr. *Sing.* צֶמַח

features in BCD 231 (NM 1:36–37) in a later attestation from Hillel ben Samuel, *Sefer Keritut*. Moses ibn Tibbon translates Arab. أورام as מורסות.

צֶמֶר · **vaginal suppository (pessary)**: Arab. صوفة (lit., 'wool') (Gr. πέσσος; cf. the definition in Paul of Aegina, *Epitomes iatrikes biblia hepta* III.61 (cf. PAE 1:276, l. 17): πέσσος δέ ἐστιν ἔριον διεξασμένον (a pessary consists of carded wool)) · Ibn al-Jazzār, *Zād al-musāfir wa-qūt al-ḥādir* · trans. Abraham ben Isaac, *Sefer Ṣedah la-Oreḥim* VI.12: ונעשה מהם תחבושת ונניח מבחוץ ויכניס ממנו מעט ברחם בצמר (We should also make a salve from [the mentioned ingredients] and smear it on the outside [of the uterus] and apply some of it internally in the form of a pessary). Hebr. צֶמֶר does not feature in this sense in the current dictionaries. Moses ibn Tibbon translates Arab. صوفة as מוֹךְ (see entry).

צִנּוּן · **paralysis; hemiplegia**: Arab. فالج (Gr. ἀπόπληξις; cf. UW 123–124) · Ibn Sīnā, *K. al-Qānūn fī al-ṭibb* · trans. Nathan ha-Me'ati, *Sefer ha-Qanun* II, fols. 73ᵇ–74ᵃ: גנדבא דסתר ... יועיל אל העצב ויועיל אל הרעישה והקיווץ הרטוב ומהתנועה אשר בלי חפץ הנקרא כזאז הנולדת בעד רוטבה ומהבטול הנקרא כדר והצנון הנקרא פלאג (GNDB' DSTR [i.e., Arab. *jandubādastar* ('castoreum')[243]]: ... It is beneficial for the nerves, and also for tremors, 'humid' spasms, shivers called KZ'Z [i.e., Arab. *kuzāz*] that are caused by moisture, numbness called KDR [i.e., Arab. *khadar*], and paralysis called PL'G [i.e., Arab. *fālij*]). Hebr. צִנּוּן features in EM 1537 in the sense of 'cooling' only. Zeraḥyah Ḥen translates Arab. فالج as פלג and Anonymous transcribes the Arab. term as פאלג׳. The latter term and vars. פאלג, פלאג, פלג׳ also feature in Nathan's *Sefer ha-Peraqim* (*Pirqei Moshe*) (cf. BMMG no. 3942).

צף • צף החרדל · **mustard foam**: Lat. *spuma sinapi* · Constantinus Africanus, *Viaticum peregrinantis* · trans. Do'eg ha-Edomi, *Sefer Ya'ir Netiv* IV.17: ויאכל פרדיץ מבושלים עם זרעונים ואניט ותרנגלי יונים גם תרנגלים ישנים מלאים אניט כמון רודא שלגימא מנטא שמן שישמני ונתן לו צף[244] חרדל כתוש עם שמן שקדים ועם חומץ אשקיליטיק (He should eat partridges cooked with chickpeas, dill, young doves; likewise old roosters filled with dill, cumin, rue, salt, mint, sesame oil. We also give him mustard foam pounded with almond oil and squill vinegar). Hebr. צף features in the sense of 'froth' in the combined term צף הים ('sea froth') in NM 5:171 in an attestation from Do'eg ha-Edomi, *Sefer Ya'ir Netiv* I.1.7 (cf. IJZ 1–2:603). Note, that the learned copyist of Ms Moscow, Russian State Library, Guenzburg 1481, fol. 102ᵇ, has replaced the uncommon term צף with the regular term קצף.

צֶמֶד · **glue**: Arab. غراء · Ibn Sīnā, *K. al-Qānūn fī al-ṭibb* · trans. Nathan ha-Me'ati, *Sefer ha-Qanun* II, fol. 76ᵇ (Ms Paris, BnF, héb. 1136, fol. 73ᵃ): גרא הטבע חם ויבש בראשונה

---

243 'castoreum': I.e., a medicament often defined as testicles of a water animal; in fact, it is an excretion derived from the scent glands of the Eurasian beaver [*Castor fiber* Linnaeus, 1758]; cf. MIG no. 183.

244 צף: קצף Ms Moscow, Russian State Library, Guenzburg 1481, fol. 102ᵇ.

והצפד העשוי מהדג הנקרא גרא בערבי והוא פחות החום אבל הוא פחות יבש (Glue: Its nature is hot and dry in the first degree; the glue made from fish called GR' [i.e., *ghirā'* [*al-samak*]] in Arab. is less hot but [also] less dry). In the sense of 'glue,' Hebr. צֶפֶד is not attested in medieval medical literature. In his *Sefer ha-Peraqim* (*Pirqei Moshe*) IX.123, Nathan translates Arab. غراء as דבק (cf. BMMN 121, l. 13; BMMG no. 3657).

צְפַרְדֵּעַ · (lit., 'frog'); swelling, inflammation beneath the tongue (ranula): Arab. غدّة · al-Rāzī, *K. al-Manṣūrī fī al-ṭibb* · trans. Shem Tov ben Isaac, *Sefer Almansur*, fol. 122^b: שער בצפרדע אשר תחת הלשון (Chapter on swelling beneath the tongue (ranula)). In the sense of 'swelling beneath the tongue,' Hebr. צְפַרְדֵּעַ features in BM 5607 in attestations from the *Sefer ha-Qanun*: צפרדע הוא דומה לגדד תחת הלשון ('ranula is similar to a GDD [i.e., Arab. *ghudda*, Plur. *ghudad* ('gland')] beneath the tongue'), and Nathan ben Jo'el Falaquera, *Sefer Ṣori ha-Guf*. The same Arab. term is rendered by Shem Tov as צמח מתחת הלשון in his *Sefer ha-Shimmush* XXIX, list 1 (see NM 5:169; SHS 1:441 (Ṣade 27)). Abraham Avigdor translates the parallel Lat. term *nodus* as אֲגֻדָּה (see entry).

צִפֹּרֶן • מורסת הצפורן → מֻרְסָה.

• *Dual* **צפרנים • צפרני הרפואות · onycha (*unguis odorati*):** Arab. أظفار الطيب (cf. IG 610) · Ibn Sīnā, *K. al-Qānūn fī al-ṭibb* · trans. Zeraḥyah Ḥen, *Sefer ha-Qanun* II, fol. 170^b: אַטְפַר אלטֵיב צפרני הרפואות ('aṬəPaR 'LṬeYB; [i.e., Hebr.] *ṣippornei ha-refu'ut*). Hebr. צפרני הרפואות is a non-attested loan translation hailing from reading Arab. الطيب ('fragrancy') as الطبّ ('medicine').

[צרב] • *Part. Pi'el* **מְצָרֵב • הרפואות המצרבות → רְפוּאָה.**

צָרוּת • צרות החזה · angina pectoris: Arab. ضيق الصدر · Ibn al-Jazzār, *Zād al-musāfir wa-qūt al-ḥādir* · trans. Moses ibn Tibbon, *Sefer Ṣedat ha-Derakhim* VI.12: ואם לא ימהרו לרפואת מורסת הרחם בהנהגה טובה והרפואה הנאותה תגדל ותתעקם[245] וימשך אחר העקום[246] כאב באצטו' ונפח במה שלמטה מן החלצים וצרות החזה עם רפיון וחולשה (If the tumor in the uterus is not healed quickly with the right regimen and treatment, it will become worse and more serious and it will be followed by pain in the stomach, swelling under the epigastrium, angina pectoris, languor, and weakness). Hebr. צרות החזה is not attested in the current dictionaries. Abraham ben Isaac translates Arab. ضيق الصدر as דוחק בחזה (see entry דֹּחַק).

• **צרות הנשום · breathing difficulty; shortness of breath; asthma:** Arab. ربو · al-Rāzī, *K. al-Manṣūrī fī al-ṭibb* · trans. Shem Tov ben Isaac, *Sefer Almansur*, fol. 3^b: נ"ג בצרות[247] הנשום ([Chapter] 53: On breathing difficulty). Hebr. צרות הנשום is not attested in the current dictionaries. A var. reading צרות הנשימה features in Moses ibn Tibbon, *Sefer Ṣedat ha-Derakhim* III.6 (cf. NM 5:172). Abraham Avigdor translates the parallel Latin term *asma* as התיצבות הנשימה.

---

245 ותתעקם (= ?ותתעצם): وتفاقم a.

246 העקום (= ?העצום): تفاقمه a.

247 בצרות: emend. ed. בצרת Ms.

ק

קֳבָה · **vagina**: Arab. قبل (Gr. αἰδοῖον; cf. UW 77–79) · Ibn al-Jazzār, *Zād al-musāfir wa-qūt al-ḥāḍir* · trans. Moses ibn Tibbon, *Sefer Ṣedat ha-Derakhim* VI.12: ואם היה התחדש המורסא בקודם מן הרחם ימשך אחר זה כאב בקבה חזק עם אדמימות השתן (If the tumor occurs in the front part of the uterus, it is followed by a heavy pain in the vagina with redness of the urine). In the sense of 'vagina,' Hebr. קֳבָה features in BM 5670–5671 in attestations from *The Alphabet of Ben Sira*, ed. Eisenstein.[248] Ben Yehuda (ibid.) mentions a var. reading קיבה, which actually features instead of קֳבָה in the *The Alphabet of Ben Sira*, ed. Yassif.[249] Ben Yehuda adds that קיבה is a var. of נקבה, a term also featuring in ed. Yassif.[250] See also Low LXXV, s.v. קבה: 'a euphemism for genitalia; cf. קיבה;' CD 7:170, s.v. קֹבָה* (featuring in Num 25:8): 'female genitals or breast (unless from קֵבָה stomach);' EM 1556, s.v. קֳבָה: 'uterus; female genitals' (cf. BM 5670: מלה מסופקה). Abraham ben Isaac renders Arab. قبل as אלקבל הנק׳ בלע׳ קופמא ([Arab.] *al-qubl* (*qubul*), called in o.l. QWPM'[251]).

קִבּוּץ · I. **firmness**: Arab. تلزز · Maimonides, *Maqāla fī al-rabw* (*On Asthma*) · trans. Anonymous, *Sefer ha-Qaṣeret* X.4 (cf. BMA 2:422, ll. 9–11): אולם ראוי שינהיג יציקת המים החמין ביותר עד עוד מעט שתתאדם עור הראש שזה מחמם מוח הראש חום אמצעי ייטבו בו פעולותיו ויחסרו יתרונותיו ממנו ומקנה עור הראש קיבוץ וחוזק עד שלא יפעל לסבה מועטת שתפגשנו (One should accustom oneself to pour water [over the head] that is so hot that the skin of the head almost turns red, because this warms the brain with a balanced heat so that its activities improve and its superfluities are reduced. It also makes the skin of the head firmer and stronger so that it is not affected [anymore] by the slightest cause). As a medical term, Hebr. קבוץ features in BCD 235 in the sense of 'astringency' (NM 1:66, 182); 'collection (accumulation [of residues])' (NM 2:168); 'density' (NM 2:78); 'flexion' (NM 4:177); and in NM 5:173 as 'coagulation.' Samuel Benveniste translates Arab. تلزز as דִּבּוּק (see entry) and Joshua Shatibi has קְבִיצָה (see entry).

· II. **constipative quality; constipation**: Arab. قبض · Ibn Sīnā, *K. al-Qānūn fī al-ṭibb* · trans. Nathan ha-Me'ati, *Sefer ha-Qanun* II, fol. 70a: ביץ ביצים ... יש בו קבוץ וקל וחומר באודם הצלוי ממנו והלובן שלו ישקיט כל הכאבים הנושנים וזה בדבוק אשר בו (Eggs: ... They are constipative, especially the fried yolk. The egg white relieves all chronic pains due to its agglutination). Zeraḥyah Ḥen translates Arab. قبض as דבוק and Anonymous has קביצות.

248 J.D. Eisenstein (ed.), *Oṣar Midrashim* (New York 1915), 1:43.

249 E. Yassif (ed.), *Sippurei Ben Sira bi-Yemei ha-Benayyim: The Tales of Ben Sira in the Middle Ages* (Jerusalem 1984), 198, l. 6 (בקיביהם); 199, l. 18 (בקיבתה).

250 Yassif (ed.), *Sippurei Ben Sira*, 198, l. 16 (בנקבתן).

251 QWPM': Poss. O. Fr. *con* [*de*] *fame* ('vagina of a woman') (for *con* < Lat. *cunnus*; cf. FEW 2:1540–1541). I thank Sandra Hajek for this explanation.

קְבִיצָה · I. **firmness:** Arab. تلزّز · Maimonides, *Maqāla fī al-rabw* (*On Asthma*) · trans. Joshua Shatibi, *Ma'amar 'al ha-Qaṣeret* x.4 (BMA 2:354, ll. 7–10): ואמנם ראוי שירגיל המים חזקי החום עד שכמעט יאדימו עור הראש כי זה יחמם המוח חימום שוה ויטיב בו פעולותיו וימעיט מותריו ממנו ויקנה עור הראש קביצה וכח עד שלא יקבל רושם מסבה מעוטה תפגשנו (One should accustom oneself to water that is so hot that the skin of the head almost turns red, because this warms the brain with a balanced heat so that its activities improve and its superfluities are reduced. It also makes the skin of the head firmer and stronger so that it is not affected [anymore] by the slightest cause). As a medical term, Hebr. קְבִיצָה features in the sense of 'astringency' in BCD 236 (NM 1:183) in an attestation from Zeraḥyah Ḥen, *Sefer ha-Peraqim* (*Pirqei Moshe*) XIII.45 (cf. BMMZ 149, l. 16; BMMG no. 3990). Samuel Benveniste translates Arab. تلزّز as דִּבּוּק (see entry) and Anonymous has קִבּוּץ (see entry).

· II. **fistful:** Arab. قبضة · Maimonides, *Maqāla fī al-rabw* (*On Asthma*) · trans. Joshua Shatibi, *Ma'amar 'al ha-Qaṣeret* XII.7 (cf. BMA 2:365, ll. 21–23): ויותר חזק מזה שבת ופודנאג׳ וקנטריון מכל אחד קביצה ירתח הכל במים ויצרף אליו שמן זית טוב ב׳ אוקיות ודבש ב׳ אוקיות כיאר שנבר אוקיא יתחקן בו והוא פושר (A stronger enema is: [Take] a fistful each of dill, mint, and centaury; cook all these in water and add to it two ounces of fine olive oil and the sweet, honeylike pulp of Indian laburnum and use it as an enema when it is lukewarm). Hebr. קְבִיצָה does not feature in this sense in the current dictionaries. Samuel Benveniste translates Arab. قبضة as מלא קמצו and Anonymous has מלא כף.

קַבָּלָה · **taking [a medicine]:** Lat. *acceptio* (Arab. شرب) · Constantinus Africanus, *Viaticum peregrinantis* · trans. Do'eg ha-Edomi, *Sefer Ya'ir Netiv* V.12: ואמר גיאלינוס על איפיטימא כאב הכליות נעזור מאד לתועלת בתנועת נחת ובמעצור משפעת המאכלים ומקבלת הדברים השוברים ([In his commentary on the book *Epidemics*,] Galen said that a very efficient therapy for kidney pain is to do moderate exercise, to abstain from large quantities of food, and to take diuretics). In the sense of 'taking a medicine,' Hebr. קַבָּלָה is a non-attested semantic borrowing from Lat. *acceptio*. For Do'eg's use of [קבל], *Pi'el* קִבֵּל, in the sense of 'to take' (for Lat. *accipio* in *Sefer Ya'ir Netiv* III.1), cf. NM 5:173–174. Moses ibn Tibbon translates the parallel Arab. term شرب as שתיה.

[קבץ] • *Pi'el.* קִבֵּץ · **to coagulate, congeal:** Arab. جمّد · Ibn al-Jazzār, *Zād al-musāfir wa-qūt al-ḥāḍir* · trans. Moses ibn Tibbon, *Sefer Ṣedat ha-Derakhim* IV.1: כי כל הדברים אשר יקררו יחזקו התאוה והדברים החמים יחסרו ממנה וישקיטוה. ואמנם זה מפני כי הדברים הקרים יקבצו הדם אשר בעורקים אשר בגלדי האצטומ׳ עד שימעט חמרו ויקטן שעורו ויוסיף בתאוה ויעוררנה כאשר תהיה נעדרת (All cooling things strengthen the appetite and all heating things reduce and satisfy the appetite. The reason is, that cooling things congeal the blood that is in the veins in the layers (coats) of the stomach so that its substance and quantity is diminished, for the appetite is whetted when there is less blood). In the sense of 'to coagulate,' Hebr. *Qal* קָבַץ features in NM 5:174 for Lat. *coagulo* (Arab. جمع) in an earlier attestation from Do'eg ha-Edomi, *Sefer Ya'ir Netiv* I.25.1 (cf. IJZ 1–

2:631). Here, Do'eg translates the parallel Lat. term *aduno et coagulo* as מאסף ומקבץ (see entry [אסף]).

• *Part. Pu'al* מְקֻבָּץ · **coagulated**: Lat. *coagulatus* (Arab. جامد) · Constantinus Africanus, *Viaticum peregrinantis* · trans. Do'eg ha-Edomi, *Sefer Ya'ir Netiv* v.15: טרוסיקש אלה מן גיאלינוס מטהרים הדם המקובץ משברון מקורות הכבד והכליות והוא נזול ברוח המקוה (These pastilles compounded by Galen dissolve the blood that has coagulated because of a burst vessel in the liver or kidneys and that has flown into the hollow part of the urinary bladder). Hebr. [קבץ], *Part. Pu'al* מְקֻבָּץ, does not feature in this sense in the current dictionaries. For *Pi'el.* קִבֵּץ in the sense of 'to coagulate, congeal,' see previous entry. Moses ibn Tibbon translates the parallel Arab. term جامد as קרוש; cf. BCD 57 (NM 3:52–53), s.v. דם קרוש ('blood clots'), in a later attestation from Nathan ha-Me'ati, *Pirqei Abuqraṭ* IV.69.

[קדם] • *Part. Hif'il* מַקְדִּים • סבות מקדימות → סִבָּה.

• *Part. Hof'al* מֻקְדָּם · **principal**: Lat. *principalis* (Arab. رئيس) · Constantinus Africanus, *Viaticum peregrinantis* · trans. Do'eg ha-Edomi, *Sefer Ya'ir Netiv* VI.1: כי הבצים נותנים חום רב ועצמה וכח לגוף והם סבות להעמיד התולדות ועל כן אמר גיאלינוס כי הם מן האברים המוקדמים (Since the testicles give the body much heat and strength, which are the cause of permanent (continuous) reproduction, Galen said that they rank among the principal organs). Hebr. [קדם], *Part. Hof'al* מֻקְדָּם, does not feature in this sense in the current dictionaries. Moses ibn Tibbon translates the parallel Arab. term رئيس as ראשי and Abraham ben Isaac has מיוחס. Other synonyms are: מושל (cf. BCD 15 (NM 1:76), s.v. האבר המושל); and שרי (cf. BCD 285 (NM 1:193)).

קֵהוּת · **bluntness [of teeth]**: Arab. ضَرَس (Gr. αἱμωδία; cf. UW 83) · Ibn Sīnā, *K. al-Qānūn fī al-ṭibb* · trans. Zeraḥyah Ḥen, *Sefer ha-Qanun* II, fol. 187ª: בַּקְלָה חַמְקָה ... תועיל ללבתור שבראש לרחוץ אותו בה מזוגה עם יין ויסיר קהות השנים בחלקותו לגסות (Common purslane: ... It is useful for pimples of the head if it is washed with it, mixed with wine. It removes bluntness[252] of the teeth because it makes their roughness smooth). In the sense of 'bluntness,' Hebr. קֵהוּת features as a modern term in BM 5006 and EM 1571. Nathan ha-Me'ati translates Arab. ضَرَس as קְהִיָּה (see next entry) and Anonymous has הקיון (read קהיון?).

252 Note, that Ibn Sīnā, *The Canon of Medicine* (*al-Qānūn fī'l-ṭibb*) (*The Law of Natural Healing*), trans. L. Bakhtiar (Chicago 2015), 2:906, faultily reads ضِرس ('molars') instead of ضَرَس ('bluntness'): '[Common purslane]: Pimples on the head washed with common purslane, particularly, when mixed with wine. Common purslane may remove molars if they are rubbed with it.' This should be corrected as: 'It is useful for pimples on the head when washed with it, mixed with wine. Common purslane may remove bluntness of the teeth if they are rubbed with it.' The same mistake already occurs in the trans. published in 1998 by the Department of Islamic Studies, Hamdard University, New Delhi, India.

קְהִיָּה · **bluntness [of teeth]**: Arab. ضَرَس (Gr. αἱμωδία; cf. UW 83) · Ibn Sīnā, *K. al-Qānūn fī al-ṭibb* · trans. Nathan ha-Me'ati, *Sefer ha-Qanun* II, fol. 71[b]: יועיל ... בקלה אלחמקה אל הסמנים אשר בראש אם רוחצים בו מזוג ביין ויסיר קהיית השניים מפני שהוא מחליק העובי (Common purslane: ... It is useful for pimples of the head if it is washed with it, mixed with wine. It removes bluntness[253] of the teeth because it makes their roughness smooth). Hebr. קְהִיָּה, coined from the root קהה (cf. KB 3:1078), is mentioned as a modern term and var. of קהיון in EM 1571 without attestations. Zeraḥyah Ḥen translates Arab. ضَرَس as קְהוּת (see previous entry) and Anonymous has הקיון (read קהיון?).

קוֹל • **הקול הנשמע באוזן** · **tinnitus**: Arab. دويّ (Gr. ἦχος; cf. UW 288) · Ibn Sīnā, *K. al-Qānūn fī al-ṭibb* · trans. Zeraḥyah Ḥen, *Sefer ha-Qanun* II, fol. 180[a]: בֵּין ... ייפסיק הגרת דם הנחירים בקיבוצו ויהיה נאות לכאב האוזן והקול הנשמע בה כל שכן עם שומן האווז (BeYN [i.e., fruit of the ben oil tree [*Moringa oleifera* Lam.]]: ... It stops nosebleeds because of its astringency. It is good for earache and tinnitus, especially with duck fat). Hebr. הקול הנשמע באוזן is not attested in the current dictionaries. Nathan ha-Me'ati translates Arab. دويّ as צליל באוזן (see entry צְלִיל). Synonyms featuring in medieval medical literature are צְלִילָה (cf. BCD 229 (NM 4:172)) and צלצול (האזנים) (NM 5:168), as well as הברה, הברה באזנים, and הברת השמע (cf. NM 5:57).

• *Plur.* **קולות** · **intestinal rumblings (borborygmus)**: Arab. قرقرة, *Plur.* قراقر · Ibn Sīnā, *K. al-Qānūn fī al-ṭibb* · trans. Zeraḥyah Ḥen, *Sefer ha-Qanun* II, fol. 183[b]: בֹּסֶר ובלח ... מנפח וכל שכן כשישתה מיד מים ובהיותו מתוק יחדש קולות יותר ויחדשו הסתימות בקרבים (BoSeR and BLḤ [i.e., Arab. *busr* and *balaḥ*, 'unripe dates']: ... They are flatulent, particularly when one drinks water immediately [after their consumption]. Sweet dates especially produce intestinal rumblings; they also produce obstructions in the intestines). Hebr. קוֹל, *Plur.* קולות, is not attested in this sense in the current dictionaries. In his *Sefer ha-Peraqim* (*Pirqei Moshe*) VII.55, Zeraḥyah translates Arab. *Sing.* قرقرة as רַעַם (cf. BCD 264 (NM 1:187–188); BMMZ 84, l. 1; BMMG no. 4080). The latter term recurs in the same paragraph on 'unripe dates' in Nathan ha-Me'ati, *Sefer ha-Qanun* II.

קוצר → קֹצֶר.

[קטר] • *Part. Pu'al* **מְקֻטָּר** · **fumigated**: Arab. مبخّر · Ibn al-Jazzār, *Zād al-musāfir wa-qūt al-ḥāḍir* · trans. Abraham ben Isaac, *Sefer Ṣedah la-Oreḥim* VI.1: כתוש כל הסמים ותן בכלי מצופה[254] מבפנים מקוטר באקסיללואה הוא עץ אלואי ותן בשעור קטן קודם אכילה ולאחר

253 Note, that Ibn Sīnā, *Canon of Medicine*, trans. L. Bakhtiar, 2:906, faultily reads ضِرْس ('molars') instead of ضَرَس ('bluntness'): '[Common purslane]: Pimples on the head washed with common purslane, particularly, when mixed with wine. Common purslane may remove molars if they are rubbed with it.' This should be corrected as: 'It is useful for pimples on the head when washed with it, mixed with wine. Common purslane may remove bluntness of the teeth if they are rubbed with it.' The same mistake already occurs in the trans. published in 1998 by the Department of Islamic Studies, Hamdard University, New Delhi, India.

254 מצופה: أملس a.

אכילה יועיל (Pound all these ingredients, fumigate them with ʾQSYLLWʾH [i.e., Lat. *agallocha*; i.e., *Aquilaria malaccensis* Lam. (syn. *A. agallocha* Roxb.)]; i.e., agarwood, and put [the substance] in a vessel covered[255] [with a smooth layer] on the inside. Give [the patient] a small dosis before and after dinner; it will be beneficial). Hebr. [קטר], *Part. Puʿal* מְקֻטָּר, is not attested in medieval medical literature. In the *Hifʿil* conj. (הִקְטִיר), the verb features in NM 5:175 (for Lat. *fumigo*) in an attestation from Do'eg ha-Edomi, *Sefer Ya'ir Netiv* II.14.5 (cf. IJZ 1–2:643). Moses ibn Tibbon translates Arab. مبخّر as מעושן.

קְטֹרֶת · **fumigant**: Arab. بخور · Maimonides, *Maqāla fī al-rabw* (*On Asthma*) · trans. Samuel Benveniste, *Maʾamar ʿal ha-Qaṣeret* XI.4 (cf. BMA 2:284, ll. 21–22): ומרפואות החלי הזה חקנות יחקן בהם בזמן המשמרה למשוך הליחה להפך העבר וקטרת להריח לחזק המוח וליבש מה שיש בו מן הליחות ולמנוע דליפתם (One can also treat this disease with enemas, which should be administered during the attack in order to attract the [superfluous] humor in the opposite direction, or with a fumigant, which should be inhaled to strengthen the brain and to dry any moisture it contains in order to prevent its streaming down). In the sense of 'fumigant,' Hebr. קְטֹרֶת is not attested in medieval Hebr. medical literature. In the sense of 'soot' (Arab. دخان), it features in Shem Tov ben Isaac's glossary to the *Sefer Almansur* (cf. BCD 242 (NM 2:18); BMZ 28 (Dalet 7)). Joshua Shatibi and Anonymous both render Arab. بخور as קְטֹרֶת as well.

קִיא • קיא ושלשול יחד · **(lit., vomiting and diarrhea at the same time); cholera**: Arab. هيضة · al-Rāzī, *K. al-Manṣūrī fī al-ṭibb* · trans. Shem Tov ben Isaac, *Sefer Almansur*, fol. 125ª: שער בקיא והשלשול יחד הנקרא בלשונם אלהיצה: כשיתחדש באדם חבלים וצירים ויקיצה ויתחדש עמהם או אחריהם קיא ושלשול צריך להשקותו מים חמים פעמים רבות תוכפות (On cholera called in [Arab.] ʾLHYṢH [i.e., *al-haiḍa*]: When a person suffers from pains and sleeplessness and from vomiting and diarrhea at the same time or later on, one should let him drink hot water time and again). Hebr. קיא ושלשול יחד does not feature in this sense in the current dictionaries. A var. reading שלשול וקיא features in Shem Tov ben Isaac, *Sefer ha-Shimmush* XXVII (cf. BCD 277 (NM 4:206)). Synonyms featuring in medieval medical literature are: הרקת הירוקה מלמעלה ומלמטה (cf. BCD 73 (NM 3:73)) and כאב הקיבה (BCD 123 (NM 3:113)).

קִיבּוּץ → קִבּוּץ.

קִימָה · **orthopnea**:[256] Arab. انتصاب (cf. UW 471, s.v. ὀρθόπνοια: نفس الانتصاب) · Maimonides, *Maqāla fī al-rabw* (*On Asthma*) · trans. Joshua Shatibi, *Maʾamar ʿal ha-Qaṣeret* N.2 (cf. BMA 2:320, ll. 1–4): וכבר ידעתי בעדות ברורה ובמה שסדרה אלי המעלה הנשאה שסבת זה החולי נזילה נגרת מן המוח בעתים ידועות ועל הרוב בסתיו והקימה והמצוקה

255 'covered [with a smooth layer]': Trans. after a.

256 I.e., discomfort in breathing that is brought on or aggravated by lying flat (cf. BMA 1:2, n. 5).

לא יסורו ימים בלילותיהם כפי אורך העונה וקצרותה עד שתעמד הנזילה ותתבשל מה שנגר אל הריאה עד שתתנקה (I know from what I have witnessed [with my own eyes] and from what [my Master] has described to me, that the cause of this illness is a defluxion that descends from the brain at certain times [of the year], but mostly in winter. [And I know] that the orthopnea and distress do not cease through the night for days on end, according to the length or brevity of the attack, until the defluxion decreases and until that [fluid] that has reached the lungs has been cocted so that the latter have become clean). Hebr. קִימָה does not feature in this sense in the current dictionaries. Samuel Benveniste translates Arab. انتصاب as זְקִיפָה (see entry) and Anonymous has הִתְיַצְּבוּת (see entry).

קַל • קל וחומר · **especially**: Arab. لا سيما · Ibn Sīnā, *K. al-Qānūn fī al-ṭibb* · trans. Nathan ha-Me'ati, *Sefer ha-Qanun* II, fols. 71ª–71ᵇ: באדרוג׳ ... כשמטיפים ממיצו יועיל מרעיפת הנחירים קל וחומר בחומץ יין וכאפור (Sweet basil: ... When one drips its juice into the nose it is useful for nosebleeds, especially with wine vinegar and camphor). Hebr. קל וחומר is not attested in this sense in the current dictionaries. The Arab. synonym خصوصا is translated by Nathan as יוֹתֵר (see entry). Zeraḥyah Ḥen translates both Arab. لا سيما and the synonymous خصوصا as כל שכן (see entry כֹּל). Anonymous has כל שכן, just like Zeraḥyah.

קִלּוּף · **exfoliating scabies**: Arab. جرب متقشّر · Ibn Sīnā, *K. al-Qānūn fī al-ṭibb* · trans. Nathan ha-Me'ati, *Sefer ha-Qanun* II, fol. 68ª: באן ... כשמערבין אותו באספלנית הנקרא מרהם בערבי עם חומץ יועיל מהקלוף והגרב המנוגע ויועיל מהסמנים[257] הרפים והמספחת הנקרא סעפה[258] בערבי (B'N [i.e., fruit of the ben oil tree [*Moringa oleifera* Lam.]]: When it is mixed with vinegar in an ointment, called MRHM [i.e., *marham*] in Arab., it is useful for exfoliating and ulcerating scabies, 'milk-like'[259] pimples, and favus, called S'PH [i.e., *sa'fah*] in Arab.). Hebr. קִלּוּף is not attested in this sense in the current dictionaries. Zeraḥyah Ḥen translates Arab. جرب متقشّر as קִלּוּף as well and Anonymous has התקלפות.

[קלח] • *Pi'el* קִלֵּחַ · **to apply a clyster**: Arab. حقن · Ibn al-Jazzār, *Zād al-musāfir wa-qūt al-ḥāḍir* · trans. Moses ibn Tibbon, *Sefer Ṣedat ha-Derakhim* IV.15: ואם היה מה שיצא מן הנגע אשר במעים עב לבן או מוגלא עבה ודם הנה ראוי שנעיין ואם לא יהיה בחולה קדחת ולא צמא ולא חלשה מופלגת ולא נפילת תאוה הנה ראוי לקלחו בזה הקלוח (If the matter that exudes from the intestinal ulcer is thick and white or consists of thick pus and blood, we should examine [the patient]: If there is no fever, thirst, extreme weakness, or loss of appetite, we should apply the following clyster). Hebr. [קלח], *Pi'el* קִלֵּחַ, features in the sense of 'to apply a clyster' in BM 5945 in a later attestation from Meir Aldabi,

257 מהסמנים הרפים (= البثور اللينة): البثور اللبنية a.
258 סעפה: emend. ed. סחפה Ms سعفة a.
259 ''milk-like' pimples': Trans. after a.

Shevilei Emunah. Hebr. *Part. Pi'el* מְקַלֵּחַ, *Plur.* מקלחים, features in BCD 243 (NM 4:104) in the sense of 'clysters' in an attestation from Moses ibn Tibbon, *Sefer Ṣedat ha-Derakhim* I.23.4 (cf. IJZ 1–2:477). Do'eg ha-Edomi translates/transcribes the parallel Lat.-Rom. term *facio clistere* as עשה קלישטרי.

קֶלַח • *Plur.* **קלחים** · **shoots:** Arab. عساليج · Maimonides, *Maqāla fī al-rabw* (*On Asthma*) · trans. Anonymous, *Sefer ha-Qaṣeret* IV.4 (cf. BMA 2:400, ll. 1–3): וכשלוקחין הקלחים של שומר כשיגדלו ויאריכו וקולפין אותן וחותכין לבותן ויבושל בהן כפי מה שזכרנו יהיה תבשיל טוב מסייע להריק הלחות (And if one takes the shoots of fennel, once they have grown large and peels them and cuts their hearts and cooks them with it, as we have described, it is a dish beneficial and helpful for expectoration). Hebr. *Sing.* קֶלַח features in the current dictionaries in the sense of 'tube; stem; stalk' (cf. JD 1374; BM 5946–5947) and is used by Anonymous also in this sense (for Arab. قضبان) in *Sefer ha-Qaṣeret* VII.2 (see entry קָנֶה). Samuel Benveniste translates Arab. عساليج as לולבים (see entry לוּלָב) and Joshua Shatibi has שריגים.

קָלִי • **רפואת הקלי** → רְפוּאָה.

• **שתיתת קלי קמח השעורים** → שְׁתִיתָה.

[קלל] *Hif'il* הֵקֵל • **הקל הבטן** · **to open (empty) the bowels:** Arab. سهّل البطن (cf. D 1:696) · Ibn al-Jazzār, *Zād al-musāfir wa-qūt al-ḥādir* · trans. Moses ibn Tibbon, *Sefer Ṣedat ha-Derakhim* IV.17: אם הריק הקלוח הזה והקל בו הבטן ושקטו הכאבים ונתכו הרוחות טוב (If this clyster has an evacuating effect and has relieved the bowels and the pains have subsided and the winds have been dissolved, it is well). In the sense of 'to open (empty) the bowels,' Hebr. הקל הבטן is a non-attested semantic borrowing from Arab. سهّل البطن.

קְלִפָּה · **membrane; lining:** Lat. *cortex* (Arab. قشر) · Constantinus Africanus, *Viaticum peregrinantis* · trans. Do'eg ha-Edomi, *Sefer Ya'ir Netiv* V.18: אחר: קלפת קורקבן מתרנגולת הפנימית (Another [remedy]: The inner lining of the gizzard of a chicken). Hebr. קְלִפָּה does not feature in this sense in the current dictionaries. For the different meanings in a medical context of both *Sing.* קְלִפָּה and *Plur.* קלפות in medieval literature, see BCD 244 and NM 5:176. Moses ibn Tibbon translates Arab. قشر as קְלִפָּה as well.

Plur. **קלפות** • **קלפות יבשות** · **eschar:** Arab. خشكرشة (Gr. ἐσχάρα; cf. UW 270) · Ibn Sīnā, *K. al-Qānūn fī al-ṭibb* · trans. Nathan ha-Me'ati, *Sefer ha-Qanun* II, fol. 94[r]: כשכש ... עלי המקרין יועילו מן הנגעים המטונפים ואוכלים הבשר הנוסף וזה בתמרוק והוא חותך הקלפות היבשות ובער' חשכריישה (Poppy: ... The leaves of horned [poppy] are useful for dirty ulcers. They erode the excessive flesh due to their detergence and remove eschars, in Arab. ḤŠKRYŠH [i.e., *khashkarīsha*]). Hebr. קלפה יבשה, *Plur.* קלפות יבשות, is not attested in the current dictionaries. In his *Sefer ha-Peraqim* (*Pirqei Moshe*) XV.9, Nathan renders Arab. خشكرشة as הכשכרישה הוא הצרבת (cf. BCD 233 (NM 2:77–78); BMMN 155, l. 18). For קליפות on its own and also in the sense of 'eschar,' cf. BCD 244 (NM 1:112–113) for an attestation from Shem Tov ben Isaac, *Sefer ha-Shimmush* XXX.1.52.

קֶמַח · **powder**: Arab. سفوف · Ibn al-Jazzār, *Zād al-musāfir wa-qūt al-ḥādir* · trans. Abraham ben Isaac, *Sefer Ṣedah la-Oreḥim* VI.9: וזה מעשה קמח הנק׳ בלשון ישמעאל ספוף[260] מאשר חבר יצחק בן עמראן לנשים שלא יראו נדות מן הבחרות (Prescription for a powder composed by Isḥāq ibn ʿImrān for young women who do not menstruate). In the sense of 'powder,' Hebr. קֶמַח features in NM 5:176 in another attestation from Abraham ben Isaac, *Sefer Ṣedah la-Oreḥim* I.23.11 (cf. IJZ 1–2:579). Moses ibn Tibbon translates Arab. سفوف as אָבָק (as already in *Sefer Ṣedat ha-Derakhim* I.23.11, cf. BCD 15 (NM 4:11); IJZ 1–2:480). The same term is used by Do'eg ha-Edomi to render the parallel Lat. term *pulvis*.

• **שתיתת קלי קמח השעורים** → **שְׁתִיתָה**.

קָנֶה · **stalk**: Arab. قضبان · Maimonides, *Maqāla fī al-rabw* (*On Asthma*) · trans. Joshua Shatibi, *Ma'amar ʿal ha-Qaṣeret* VII.2 (cf. BMA 2:341, ll. 23–25): וכשיוסר הקצף ישליך בו חצי אוקי׳ לשון השור וקנה נענע ומן התבלין כפי השנים והמזג וכפי עניני האברים (And when there is no froth left, add to it [i.e., the remedy] half an ounce of borage, [three] stalks of cultivated mint, and spices according to the age [of the patient], his temperament, and the condition of his organs). Hebr. קָנֶה is attested in the Bible in the sense of 'stalk; reed' or 'water-plant; reed' (BDB 889) and in Rabb. literature in the sense of 'calamus; reed; anything resembling a reed' (JD 1388–1389); cf. EM 1616. For קָנֶה as an anatomical term, see BCD 245 (NM 4:184) and NM 5:177. Samuel Benveniste translates Arab. قضبان as בדים and Anonymous has קֶלַח (see entry).

קַנְקַן • **עשה קנקן** → **עָשָׂה**.

[קפא] • *Part. Nifʿal* **נִקְפָּא** · **suffering from lethargy**: Lat. *patior subeth* (Arab. سبات) · Gerard de Solo, *Practica super nono Almansoris* · trans. Abraham Avigdor, *Ha-Ma'amar ha-Teshiʿi le-Sefer ha-Mansuri le-Razi*, fol. 27^b: כאשר יהיה האדם מושלך כישן ולא יתנועע אלא שעיניו פתוחות ולא יניע העפעפים הנה הוא נקפא (If a person is lying down as if he is asleep and he does not move himself nor his eyelids while his eyes are open, he suffers from lethargy). Hebr. [קפא], *Part. Nifʿal* נִקְפָּא, does not feature in this sense in the current dictionaries.

קְפִיאָה · **catalepsy**: Lat. *congelatio* (Arab. جمود) · Gerard de Solo, *Practica super nono Almansoris* · trans. Abraham Avigdor, *Ha-Ma'amar ha-Teshiʿi le-Sefer ha-Mansuri le-Razi*, fol. 27^a: ראוי שתדע בבאור הרובריקאה שהקפיאה היא רוע מזג קר יבש עם חומר או בלתי חומר בחלק האחרון מהמוח ובסבת הרוע מזג ההוא ישובו הרוחות הנפשיות עבות ובלתי מתנועעות ולא יוכלו להתפשט לחוץ אל כליהם ולזה לא ירגיש ולא יתנועע (You should know as an explanation of the [term *congelatio* in the] RWBRYQ'H [i.e., *rubrica* ('heading'), i.e., *De congelatione*] that catalepsy is a bad, cold, [and] dry temperament with or without [superfluous] matter in the posterior part of the brain. Because of the bad temperament, the psychical pneumas become thick and immobile; they cannot

---

260 ספוף: emend. ed. ספקס Mss.

spread out to their organs and as a result, [the patient] does not sense nor move). In the sense of 'catalepsy,' Hebr. קְפִיאָה features (for Arab. جمود) in BCD 247 (NM 2:83) in an attestation from Nathan ha-Me'ati, *Sefer ha-Peraqim* (*Pirqei Moshe*) XXIII.64 (cf. BMMN 227, l. 1; BMMG no. 672).

קְצִידָא (*Aram.*) • **ophthalmia**: Arab. رمد • Ibn Zuhr, *K. al-Aghdhiya* • trans. Nathan ha-Me'ati, *Sefer ha-Mezonot*, fol. 5b: ואם יונח הדק מחלבון הביצה בעין בעלת הרמד ר״ל הקצידא יועילהו (If the powder made from egg white is put on the eye that is affected by ophthalmia, i.e., [Aram.] *qeṣida*, it is beneficial for it). Aram. קְצִידָא is a non-attested parallel term to Hebr. קְצִידָה, a calque of O. Occ. *cassida* ('defluxion of the eyes') featuring in Moses ibn Tibbon, *Perush Aphorismi shel Apuqraṭ* (*Pirqei Abuqraṭ*) III.21 (127) (cf. BCD 248 (NM 3:206); BMCH 1:354, l. 14).

[קצר] • *Nif'al* **נִקְצַר** • **to be constipated, suffer from constipation**: Lat. *constipor* (Arab. انعقال) • Constantinus Africanus, *Viaticum peregrinantis* • trans. Do'eg ha-Edomi, *Sefer Ya'ir Netiv* V.17: ואם לא נמהר לעזור אליו ירזה מאד ועל גופו יהיה נשחת ובטנו יקצר ומהר יסתכן (If we do hurry to treat him, he will become very lean and his body will be worn out; his stomach will be constipated and his life will be quickly in danger). Hebr. [קצר], *Nif'al* נִקְצַר, features in NM 5:179 in the sense of 'to be blocked' in an attestation from Do'eg ha-Edomi, *Sefer Ya'ir Netiv* II.17.1 (cf. IJZ 1–2:645). Moses ibn Tibbon translates the parallel Arab. term انعقال as עוצר (see also the use of Hebr. עוצר הבטן in the sense of 'constipation' (for Arab. احتباس البطن) in Zeraḥyah Ḥen, *Sefer ha-Peraqim* (*Pirqei Moshe*) IX.55 (cf. BCD 212 (NM 1:178); BMMZ 106, l. 14; BMMG no. 782)).

• *Part. Pi'el* **מְקַצֵּר** • **incompetent**: Arab. مقصّر • Maimonides, *Maqāla fī al-rabw* (*On Asthma*) • trans. Joshua Shatibi, *Ma'amar 'al ha-Qaṣeret* XIII.22 (cf. BMA 2:375, ll. 8–11): ודומה לזה תיקר מציאותו בכל מקום ובכל זמן אמנם הרופא המקצר והוא רוב הנמצאים אין ראוי להזיד בו (But such a situation is rare in all places and all times, [so] one should not rely upon an incompetent physician—which is the most common situation). In the sense of 'incompetent,' Hebr. *Part. Pi'el* מְקַצֵּר is a semantic borrowing from Arab. مقصّر and features in BM 6115 in attestations from medieval philosophical literature. Ben Yehuda renders the term as: 'one who does not do what is necessary' (cf. PESHAT:[261] 'one who falls short of realizing a goal'). Samuel Benveniste renders Arab. مقصّر as שאינו שלם and also as חָסֵר (see entry). Anonymous has מְקַצֵּר, just like Joshua Shatibi.

קֹצֶר • **narrowness**: Lat. *angustiae* (Arab. ضيق) • Constantinus Africanus, *Viaticum peregrinantis* • trans. Do'eg ha-Edomi, *Sefer Ya'ir Netiv* VI.16: אולם לפעמים תלדנה בכבדות גם לפעמים אינם יכולות וזה יקרה בסבות רבות ... או בקוצר מעברות דרכי הרחם (Sometimes, however, a woman has a difficult childbirth or cannot give birth [at all], for which there can be many causes ... or because of the narrowness of the passage (birth

261 https://peshat.org/display/peshat_lemmas_00002803 (accessed April 11, 2022).

canal) of the uterus). In the sense of 'narrowness; blockage' (for Lat. *constipatio*), Hebr. קֹצֶר features in NM 5:179 in an attestation from Do'eg ha-Edomi, *Sefer Ya'ir Netiv* III.11. Moses ibn Tibbon translates the parallel Arab. term ضيق as צרות and Abraham ben Isaac has דוחק וצרות.

• **קוצר הנשימה · shortness of breath; dyspnea**: a) Arab. ضيق النفس · Maimonides, *Maqāla fī al-rabw* (*On Asthma*) · trans. Anonymous, *Sefer ha-Qaṣeret* XII.3 (cf. BMA 2:430, ll. 10–12): ואמנם הלעיטות שמנקות הריאה גם כן ומבשלות מה שיש בה ומקילות רקיקתו ומועילות מקוצר הנשימה תועלת נראית והן נלקחות בכל ימי החלי ובאיזה עת שיהיה מהיום והלילה מהן זה (The following are some of the linctuses that also cleanse the lungs, coct [the superfluous humors] in them, ease their expectoration, are clearly beneficial for shortness of breath, and can be taken throughout the disease and at any time during the day or the night). In the sense of 'shortness of breath' (for Lat. *strictura in flatu*), Hebr. קצר הנשימה features in NM 5:179 in an attestation from Do'eg ha-Edomi, *Sefer Ya'ir Netiv* III.7. Samuel Benveniste translates Arab. ضيق النفس as מצוק הנשימה (see entry מָצוֹק) and Joshua Shatibi has צרות הנשימה (cf. BCD 233–234 (NM 4:176) for an attestation from Shem Tov ben Isaac, *Sefer ha-Shimmush* XXVII).

· b) Arab. عسر النفس · Ibn Sīnā, *K. al-Qānūn fī al-ṭibb* · trans. Nathan ha-Me'ati, *Sefer ha-Qanun* II, fol. 123[b]: שיח ... יחתלו במימיו האפר הנקר' רמד בערבי ויתיכנו יועיל מקוצר הנשימה (Wormwood: ... If you foment [the eyes] with its water, it relieves conjunctivitis, called RMD [i.e., *ramad*] in Arab.; it is beneficial for shortness of breath). Zeraḥyah Ḥen translates Arab. عسر النفس as עוצר הניפוש (cf. BCD 212 (NM 1:178) for an attestation from Zeraḥyah, *Sefer ha-Peraqim* (*Pirqei Moshe*) XXIII.79 (BMMZ 227, l. 23; BMMG no. 3344)) and Anonymous has כובד הנשימה (cf. BM 2230 for an attestation from the *Sefer ha-Qanun*).

קרא • גרגיר הקרא → גַּרְגִּיר.

קָרוּחַ (*Pass. Part.*) → [קרח].

קְרוּם • מורסת הקרום → מֻרְסָה.

• *Plur.* קרומים • מורסות קרומי המוח → מֻרְסָה.

קָרוּשׁ • דם קרוש → דָּם.

קָרוּת · **cold**: Lat. *frigiditas* (Arab. برد) · Constantinus Africanus, *Viaticum peregrinantis* · trans. Do'eg ha-Edomi, *Sefer Ya'ir Netiv* VI.1: ואם הקרות והיבשות מושלים בם יהיה הזרע מועט והתאוה נעדרת (If cold and dryness dominate [their temperament], they will have little sperm and no desire [to have sexual intercourse]). In the sense of 'cold,' Hebr. קָרוּת features in BM 6172 in an attestation from Rabb. literature and from medieval linguistic literature, namely from David Kimhi, *Sefer ha-Shorashim*. Moses ibn Tibbon and Abraham ben Isaac both translate the parallel Arab. term برد as קור.

[קרח] • *Pass. Part.* קָרוּחַ · **congealed; coagulated; solidified**: Lat. *congelatus* (Arab. قريض) · Constantinus Africanus, *Viaticum peregrinantis* · trans. Do'eg ha-Edomi, *Sefer Ya'ir Netiv* IV.15: האות הכללי מן דישנטריא הוא העוות והמצוק והבשול הדמי מעורב עם האדומה או עם איזה דבר קרוח לבן (In general, the symptoms of dysentery are colic, pain, [evacuation of] digested food mixed with blood and yellow bile or with white coagulated matter). In the sense of 'congealed; coagulated; solidified,' Hebr. [קרח], *Pass. Part.* קָרוּחַ, does not feature in the current dictionaries. Ben Yehuda refers to the verb קרח in the *Hif'il* conj. (הִקְרִיחַ) in the sense of 'to be frozen, congealed' (BM 6174). Moses ibn Tibbon translates the parallel Arab. term قريض as מכסה המעים הפנימי.

קְרִיסוּת · **acidity**: Arab. حمضة · Maimonides, *Maqāla fī al-rabw* (*On Asthma*) · trans. Samuel Benveniste, *Ma'amar 'al ha-Qaṣeret* IX.15 (cf. BMA 2:276, ll. 8–9): תקח מן החבושים הטובים מעטי החבישה שיש בהם קריסות מועט (Take some fine, slightly astringent, and acidic quinces). In the sense of 'acidity,' Hebr. קְרִיסוּת features in EM 1644 in a reference to this passage, which is quoted as: החבושים הטובים שיש בהם קריסות מועט. Joshua Shatibi translates Arab. حمضة as קביצות and Anonymous has חמיצות.

[קרש] • *Hif'il* הִקְרִישׁ · **to extinguish**: Arab. خمّد · Ibn al-Jazzār, *Zād al-musāfir wa-qūt al-ḥāḍir* · trans. Abraham ben Isaac, *Sefer Ṣedah la-Oreḥim* VI.3: ואם תרצה להקריש תאות התשמיש גם יקל ולהמעיט הזרע קח מזרע קנבס הנק' בלשון ישמעאל שאהדנג' ונקר' חב[262] אלקנב (If you want to extinguish the lust for sexual intercourse [or] to diminish it and to reduce the [flow of] sperm, take seed of hemp, called in Arab. Š'HDNǦ [i.e., *shahdānaj*] and also called ḤB 'LQNB [i.e., *ḥab al-qinnab*, an ancient Arabicized form of Gr. κάνναβις ('hemp'); cf. MIG no. 984]). Hebr. [קרש], *Hif'il* הִקְרִישׁ, does not feature in this sense in the current dictionaries. Moses ibn Tibbon translates Arab. خمّد as [רדם], *Hif'il* הִרְדִּים.

[קשה] • *Hitpa'el* הִתְקַשָּׁה · **to have an erection**: Arab. نعظ · Ibn al-Jazzār, *Zād al-musāfir wa-qūt al-ḥāḍir* · trans. Moses ibn Tibbon, *Sefer Ṣedat ha-Derakhim* VI.1: וימצא מי שיתאוה ולא יתקשה ולא יצא זרע (Many others have sexual lust but have no erection and ejaculate no sperm). Hebr. [קשה], *Hitpa'el* הִתְקַשָּׁה, is not attested in this sense in the current dictionaries. Abraham ben Isaac translates Arab. نعظ as עמד הגיד (see entry עָמַד) and Do'eg ha-Edomi translates the parallel Lat. term *erigor* as *Part.* זוֹקֵף (see entry זָקַף).

• *Hif'il* הִקְשָׁה · **to produce an erection**: Arab. أنعظ · Ibn al-Jazzār, *Zād al-musāfir wa-qūt al-ḥāḍir* · trans. Moses ibn Tibbon, *Sefer Ṣedat ha-Derakhim* VI.1: ומזה תאר מרקחת מחבור בן מאסויה יוסיף במשגל ויקשה (One of these [compound remedies] is the prescription for an electuary composed by Ibn Māsawayh that increases the sexual lust and produces an erection). In the sense of 'to produce an erection,' Hebr. [קשה], *Hif'il* הִקְשָׁה, features as להקשות אבר המשגל in BM 6233 in an attestation from Isaac Pulgar, *Ezer ha-Dat*.

קִשּׁוּא • *Plur.* **קשואים** • **קשואים מרים** · **squirting cucumber** [*Ecballium elaterium* (L.) A. Rich]: Arab. قثّاء الحمار (cf. MIG no. 43) · Ibn al-Jazzār, *Zād al-musāfir wa-qūt al-ḥāḍir* · trans. Moses ibn Tibbon, *Sefer Ṣedat ha-Derakhim* IV.17: ואם הספיק זה והגיע

---

262 חב אלקנב: emend. ed. חבל קוב Ms.

אל הצורך ונשתלשל הבטן טוב ואם לא יוסיף בו עם אלו השמנים והעשבים קולוקינטידא וסחיטת קשואים מרים (If [these remedies] are sufficient and the bowels are emptied, it is well; but if not, one should add these oils and ingredients: colocynth, extract of squirting cucumber …). Hebr. *Sing.* קשוא מר is not attested in the current dictionaries. The regular term for 'squirting cucumber' is קשוא חמור or ירוקת חמור (cf. SHS 1:248 (Yod 1); LF 1549–1550). Do'eg ha-Edomi transcribes the parallel Lat. term *elacterium*, Gen. *elacteri*[*i*] as אלקטרי.

קִשּׁוּט · **cosmetics**: Arab. زينة · Ibn Sīnā, *K. al-Qānūn fī al-ṭibb* · trans. Anonymous, *Sefer ha-Qanun* II, fols. 23b–24a: אס הוא הדס … בקשוט: שמנו וסחיטתו ובשולו מחזק שרשי השער ומונע נפילתו ומאריכו ומשחירו (Myrtle: … [Its use] in cosmetics: The oil, juice, and decoction [prepared from it] strengthens the roots of the hair and prevents it from falling out and makes it grow and darkens it)). In the sense of 'cosmetics,' Hebr. קִשּׁוּט features in BM 6240 in an attestation from the intr. to the *Sefer ha-Refu'ot*. Nathan ha-Me'ati translates Arab. زينة as עֲדִי (see entry) and Zeraḥyah Ḥen has יִפּוּי (see entry).

קְשִׁי • **קושי מתמיד** · **priapism**: Arab. الإنعاظ الدائم · Ibn al-Jazzār, *Zād al-musāfir wa-qūt al-ḥāḍir* · trans. Moses ibn Tibbon, *Sefer Ṣedat ha-Derakhim* VI.2: השער הב׳ בקושי המתמיד (Chapter 2: On priapism). Hebr. קשי מתמיד is not attested in the current dictionaries. A synonym featuring in MD 597 (s.v. *priapism*) is קשוי מתמיד. Abraham ben Isaac translates Arab. الإنعاظ الدائم as כשיעמוד גיד הערוה תדיר (see entry עָמַד) and Do'eg ha-Edomi translates the parallel Lat. term *nimia erectio virgae* as זקיפת האמה ברוב (see entry זְקִיפָה).

קִשְׁקֵשׁ · **to rinse**: Arab. مضمضة · Ibn Sīnā, *K. al-Qānūn fī al-ṭibb* · trans. Zeraḥyah Ḥen, *Sefer ha-Qanun*, fols. 180b–181a: בֶּאדֶאוַרְד … לקשקש בבשולו תשכך כאב השנים (Soldier thistle: … If one rinses one's mouth with its decoction, it alleviates toothache). Hebr. קִשְׁקֵשׁ is not attested in this sense in the current dictionaries. Nathan ha-Me'ati renders Arab. مضمضة as שכשך (cf. BM 7113–7114) and Anonymous has מְצָמוּץ (cf. entry), a noun derived from the verb מצמץ, which features in the sense of 'to rinse one's mouth' (for Arab. تمضمض) in Nathan's *Sefer ha-Peraqim* (*Pirqei Moshe*) XXI.10 and XXII.68 (cf. BMMN 196, l. 26; 217, l. 18; BMMG no. 4867).

קָשַׁר · **to thicken, congeal**: Arab. عقّد · Maimonides, *Maqāla fī al-rabw* (*On Asthma*) · trans. Samuel Benveniste, *Ma'amar 'al ha-Qaṣeret* IV.7 (cf. BMA 2:256, ll. 21–22): ודע שהדברים החמים היבשים מזיקים ביותר לחולי זה כל שכן למזג זה הנזכר מפני שהם מדבקות הלחות שיש בהן דשון ויקשרו ויקפיאו מה שאין בו דשון (Know that the hot and dry ingredients are extremely harmful for this disease [i.e., asthma], especially for the temperament that we mentioned, because they make the fatty humors sticky and thicken and coagulate [those humors] that have no fatness). In the sense of 'to congeal, thicken,' Hebr. קָשַׁר is a non-attested semantic borrowing from Arab. عقّد. For *Hitpa'el* הִתְקַשֵּׁר in the sense of 'to congeal' (intrans.), cf. BCD 253 (NM 3:214) for an attestation from Nathan ha-Me'ati, *Pirqei Abuqraṭ* V.40. Joshua Shatibi does not translate Arab. عقّد, while Anonymous has *Hif'il* הֶעֱמִיד (see entry עָמַד).

ר

רְאָה • בעלת הריאה → **בַּעֲלָה**.

רְאָיָה • *Plur.* **ראיות** · **symptoms**: Arab: دلائل · Maimonides, *Maqāla fī al-rabw* (*On Asthma*) · trans. Anonymous, *Sefer ha-Qaṣeret* XIII.19 (cf. BMA 2:442, ll. 18–20): ואמנם אם ראה שהוא אם היה הדבר בהפך מה שחשב יזיק לחולה הזקה גדולה הוא לא יעשה כפי הקישו ומה שהורו עליו הראיות (But if he concluded that, if the case was the opposite of what he thought, [the purgative] would cause serious harm, [then] he would not act according to his reason nor according to the symptoms). Hebr. *Sing.* רְאָיָה is attested in medieval medical literature in the sense of 'sign' (i.e., symptom) in BCD 255 (NM 3:214) in an attestation from Moses ibn Tibbon, *Perush Aphorismi shel Apuqraṭ* (*Pirqei Abuqraṭ*) VII.41 (393) (cf. BMCH 1:412, l. 12). Samuel Benveniste and Joshua Shatibi both translate Arab. دلائل as הוראות (see entry הוֹרָאָה).

ראש • מלוי הראש → **מִלּוּי**.

• **מורסות הראש** → **מֻרְסָה**.

• **סובין שבראש** → **סֻב**.

• **עורק הראש** → **עֹרֶק**.

• **פלוח הראש** → **פִּלּוּחַ**

• *Plur.* **ראשים • מורסות ראשי האצבעות** → **מֻרְסָה**.

[רבה] • *Inf. Hifʿil* **הַרְבּוֹת • הרבות השתן** · **diuresis**: Arab: إدرار البول · Ibn Sīnā, *K. al-Qānūn fī al-ṭibb* · trans. Zeraḥyah Ḥen, *Sefer ha-Qanun*, fol. 192ᵃ: גָּאוּשִׁיר ... יחליק קשי הרחם ויועיל להטפת השתן וישתה כמו שיעור לוזה[263] ממנו עם המים החמים להרבות השתן (Opopanax: ... It softens the hardness of the uterus and is useful for strangury. A dose of one hazelnut[264] is taken orally with warm water for diuresis). In the sense of 'diuresis,' Hebr. הרבות השתן is not attested in the current dictionaries. Nathan ha-Me'ati translates Arab. إدرار البول as שלשול השתן (see entry שִׁלְשׁוּל) and Anonymous has הגרת השתן (cf. BCD 62 (NM 3:56) for an attestation from Moses ibn Tibbon, *Perush Aphorismi shel Apuqraṭ* (*Pirqei Abuqraṭ*) I.2 (29) (cf. BMCH 1:326, l. 6)).

רִבּוּי • רבוי השתן מבלי רצון · **incontinence**: Arab: كثرة البول من غير إرادة · Ibn al-Jazzār, *Zād al-musāfir wa-qūt al-ḥāḍir* · trans. Moses ibn Tibbon, *Sefer Ṣedat ha-Derakhim* V.18: ולרבוי השתן מבלי רצון יקח רודא יבשה מעט וידוק ויולש בדבש וישתה אותו במים (For incontinence one should take some dry rue, pound it and knead it with honey, and drink it with water). Hebr. רבוי השתן מבלי רצון does not feature in the current dictionaries.

רָגִיל · **experienced**: Arab: دريب · Maimonides, *Maqāla fī al-rabw* (*On Asthma*) · trans. Anonymous, *Sefer ha-Qaṣeret* XIII.30 (cf. BMA 2:446, ll. 6–7): ואמנם שיהיה האיש רגיל

---

263 לוזה: بندقة a.

264 'hazelnut' (Arab. *bunduqa*): I.e., 3.4 grams, cf. IG 164.

בהיותו רואה במעשים ועמד בהם ואף על פי שאין לו חכמה זה שקר (But it is impossible for a person to be experienced [in the medical art] because he observed and saw it being practiced, although he has no [theoretical] knowledge [of it]). Hebr. רָגִיל features in the current dictionaries as 'in the habit of; wont to' (cf. JD 1448) or 'accustomed, used to; versed in' (cf. BM 6409–6411). Samuel Benveniste translates Arab. دريب as בקי and Joshua Shatibi has [רגל], *Part. Hofʿal* מֻרְגָּל (see next entry).

[רגל] • *Part. Hofʿal* **מֻרְגָּל** · **experienced**: Arab: دريب · Maimonides, *Maqāla fī al-rabw* (*On Asthma*) · trans. Joshua Shatibi, *Maʾamar ʿal ha-Qaṣeret* XIII.30 (cf. BMA 2:377, l. 25–378, l. 1): אמנם שיהיה האיש מורגל בראותו המעשים ושמשם גם שלא יהיה יודע זה נמנע (But it is impossible for a person to be experienced [in the medical art] because he observed and saw it being practiced, although he has no [theoretical] knowledge [of it]). Hebr. [רגל], *Part. Hofʿal* מֻרְגָּל, features in the current dictionaries in the sense of 'being accustomed to' (cf. BM 9416–9417). Samuel Benveniste translates Arab. دريب as בקי and Anonymous has רָגִיל (see previous entry).

רֶגֶל • *Dual* **רגלים** • **בעל ארבעים וארבע רגלים** → **בַּעַל**.

• **נכאות הרגלים** → **נְכֹאת**.

רוג׳ה • **רוג׳ה של צבעים** · **common madder** [***Rubia tinctorum*** L.]: Arab. فوّة الصبّاغان · Ibn al-Jazzār, *Zād al-musāfir wa-qūt al-ḥādir* · trans. Moses ibn Tibbon, *Sefer Ṣedat ha-Derakhim* VI.9: בשול השרשים מגיר השתן[265] מספר התועלת לבן מאסויה ערובו יקח רוג׳ה של צבעים (A prescription for a decoction of roots that makes the urine[266] flow abundantly, taken from the *Book of Success* by Ibn Masawayh: Take common madder …). Hebr. רוג׳ה של צבעים (lit., 'dyer's madder') is a compound term, consisting of O. Occ./O. Cat. *roga* for 'madder' (cf. DiTMAO, s.v. *roia*) and Hebr. צַבָּע, *Plur.* צבעים ('dyer;' cf. JD 1259). Abraham ben Isaac translates Arab. فوّة الصبّاغان as פוה הנקרא בלש׳ יון ריזארי (PWH [i.e., Arab. *fuwwa*], called in Gr. RYZʾRY [i.e., ριζάρι]) and Doʾeg ha-Edomi transcribes the parallel Lat. term *rubia* as רוביא.

רוּחַ • **הרוח הנדחה דרך הגרון** · **eructation**: Lat. *ructatio* (Arab. جشاء) · Constantinus Africanus, *Viaticum peregrinantis* · trans. Doʾeg ha-Edomi, *Sefer Yaʾir Netiv* IV.2: אם הוא מן הליחות אין מבושלות יחול מזה חמוץ הרוח הנדחה דרך הגרון (If [lack of appetite] is caused by crude humors, it is followed by sour eructation). Hebr. הרוח הנדחה דרך הגרון is not attested in the current dictionaries. For the synonyms הרוח הנדחה and הרוח הנדחה היוצא מן הגרון featuring in Doʾeg's *Sefer Yaʾir Netiv* II.18.3 (cf. IJZ 1–2:647), resp. III.14, cf. NM 5:184. Moses ibn Tibbon translates Arab. جشاء as Aram. קִבְסָא, which features also as Hebr. קבסה in BCD 236 (NM 3:198) in an attestation from his *Perush Aphorismi shel Apuqraṭ* (*Pirqei Abuqraṭ*) VI.1 (293) (cf. BMCH 1:393, l. 1).

---

265 השתן: الطنث a.

266 'urine': 'menstrual blood' a.

רוּחָנִיּוּת · **flatulence:** Arab. رياح ('winds') · Maimonides, *Maqāla fī al-rabw* (*On Asthma*) · trans. Joshua Shatibi, *Ma'amar 'al ha-Qaṣeret* III.10 (cf. BMA 2:319, l. 26–320, l. 1): ומציצת החבושים אחר האכילה טוב ולא ירבה ממנו לפי שכל הדברים הקובצים כחבושים והשמשניות ועוזרדין יזיקו בזה החולי וכן התפוחים רעים לקביצתם ורוחניותם (To suck quinces after the meal is beneficial, but one should not take too much of them, because all the astringent things such as quinces, [lotus fruits], and common medlars are harmful for this disease; apples are also bad because they are astringent and [produce] flatulence). Hebr. רוּחָנִיּוּת only features in the current dictionaries in the sense of 'spirituality;' cf. BM 6496–6497 and PESHAT:[267] 'quality of something spiritual.' Samuel Benveniste does not translate the sentence وكذلك التفّاح رديء لقبضه ورياحه (apples are also bad because they are astringent and [produce] flatulence) and Anonymous renders Arab. رياح as רוחות.

רוטבה → רֵטְבָּה.

רוע → רֹעַ.

רוֹקֵחַ • *Plur.* רוקחים · **druggists:** Arab. عطّرون · Maimonides, *Maqāla fī al-rabw* (*On Asthma*) · trans. Anonymous, *Sefer ha-Qaṣeret* XII.1 (cf. BMA 2:429, ll. 15–16): אסטוכודוס וזנגביל כנעני והוא הראסן והוא שיודעין אותו הרוקחים במצרים בכנף[268] (Lavender and Syrian ginger—i.e., HR'SN [i.e., Arab. *al-rāsan* ('elecampagne')], which the druggists in Cairo know as *kanaf* [i.e., Arab. *janāḥ* ('wing'); cf. IG 316]). Hebr. רוֹקֵחַ is not attested in medieval medical literature (cf. BM 6731; EM 1700). Samuel Benveniste translates Arab. عطّرون as רופאים and Joshua Shatibi has בסמים (see entry בֶּשֶׂם).

רושם → רֹשֶׁם.

רָחוֹק • ברחוק · **rarely:** Lat. *rarus* (Arab. في الندرة) · Constantinus Africanus, *Viaticum peregrinantis* · trans. Do'eg ha-Edomi, *Sefer Ya'ir Netiv* IV.7: והנה הפוקות יתרפאו בנקל ובקושי כמו אותם הנעשים מהרקה אך אלה כילים? כי ברחוק יבואו (Hiccups can be easy but also difficult to cure, like the hiccups caused by emptying [the body through vomiting], but this occurs only rarely). In the sense of 'rarely,' Hebr. ברחוק is not attested in the current dictionaries. Moses ibn Tibbon translates Arab. في الندرة as בדרך רחוק (see entry דֶּרֶךְ).

• בדרך רחוק → דֶּרֶךְ.

רֵחַיִם · **(lit., 'millstone'); a hard formation in a woman's womb:** Arab. رحى · al-Rāzī, *K. al-Manṣūrī fī al-ṭibb* · trans. Shem Tov ben Isaac, *Sefer Almansur*, fol. 4[a]: פ"ה בחולי הנקרא הרחיים ([Chapter] 85: On the illness called 'millstone' [i.e., a hard formation in a woman's womb]). In the sense of 'a hard formation in a woman's womb,' Hebr. רֵחַיִם features in BCD 260 (NM 1:187; 2:86) in later attestations from the *Sefer ha-Peraqim*

---

267 https://peshat.org/display/peshat_lemmas_00003806 (accessed April 11, 2022).

268 בכנף: بالجناح a.

(*Pirqei Moshe*) XXIII.97 by both Zeraḥyah Ḥen (BMMZ 230, l. 12) and Nathan ha-Me'ati (BMMN 231, l. 9) (cf. also BMMG no. 2058). The same term is used by Abraham Avigdor for the parallel Lat. term *mola*. A synonym of רֵחַיִם, namely אבן הרחים, features in [*Synonima*], Ms. Vatican, Biblioteca Apostolica, ebr. 550, fol. 120[b] (see entry אֶבֶן).

• אבן הרחים → אֶבֶן.

רְחִיצָה • רחיצת בשר · **the water in which meat has been washed**: Lat. *lavatura carnis* (Arab. غسالة اللحم) · Constantinus Africanus, *Viaticum peregrinantis* · trans. Do'eg ha-Edomi, *Sefer Ya'ir Netiv* V.3: וכמו אחרת הנקראת בשול איפטיק ומזה הדם יצא לרוב עם שלשול[269] והוא כמו רחיצת בשר חדש והסבה הוא מאפיסת הכח המבשל הראוי להחליף בכבד מיץ המאכל בדם (There is another [kind of blood resulting from a liver affliction] called 'hepatic diarrhea.' In most cases, the blood emerges [from the body] with diarrhea and looks like the water in which fresh meat has been washed. It is caused by the weakness of the digestive faculty to transform the juice of the food into blood). Hebr. רחיצת בשר is not attested in the current dictionaries. Moses ibn Tibbon translates Arab. غسالة اللحم as רחיצת הבשר.

רֶחֶם • בליטת הרחם → בְּלִיטָה.

• חניקת הרחם → חֲנִיקָה.

• יציאת הרחם → יְצִיאָה.

רְטָבָה • *Plur.* **רוטבות** · **fluids**: Arab. رطوبات · Ibn Sīnā, *K. al-Qānūn fī al-ṭibb* · trans. Nathan ha-Me'ati, *Sefer ha-Qanun* II, fol. 90[a]: יאסמין הטבע הלבן ממנו יותר חם מהמכורכם והמכורכם יותר חם מאשר כגוון הארגמאן ובכלל הוא חם ויבש בשלישית המפעלים והסגלות מרקיק הרוטבות ויועיל לזקנים (Jasmine: Its nature: White jasmine is warmer than its yellow variety. The latter is warmer than the purple variety. Jasmine as a whole is hot and dry in the third degree. Healing effects and specific properties: It rarefies the fluids and is useful for old people). Hebr. *Sing.* רְטָבָה is not attested in the current dictionaries. For the parallel Aram. term רְטָבָא, cf. DAN 402. Zeraḥyah Ḥen and Anonymous both translate Arab. رطوبات as לחויות.

רְטִיָּה • *Plur.* **רטיות** · **unguent; ointment**: Arab. طلاء, *Plur.* أطلية (Gr. κατάχρισμα; cf. UW 335: 'Einreibmittel; Salbe')· Maimonides, *Maqāla fī al-rabw* (*On Asthma*) · trans. Joshua Shatibi, *Ma'amar 'al ha-Qaṣeret* XII.6 (cf. BMA 2:364, ll. 19–20): וכבר אמרנו שמרקי התרנגולים הזקנים יעזרו על הבישול והרקיקה. ואמנם מה שיחזק המוח בזה החולי הנה אבן זהר זכר שהוא מצא העפרים יותר טובים מן הרטיות (We have already said that soups prepared from old roosters are beneficial for the coction [of the crude superfluities] and [for their] expectoration. As for [drugs] that strengthen the brain in this disease, Ibn Zuhr has remarked that he found powders better for this than ointments). Hebr. רְטִיָּה, *Plur.* רטיות, features in the current dictionaries in the sense

269 שלשול: emend. ed. בשול Mss *dissinteria* L.

of 'compress' (BM 6563–6564) and 'emollient; plaster; compress' (JD 1471). Samuel Benveniste and Anonymous both render Arab. أطلية as משיחות. A synonymous term featuring in medieval Hebr. medical literature is רִקּוּחַ, featuring in Abraham ben Isaac, *Sefer Ṣedah la-Oreḥim* I.6.3 (for Arab. طلاء ('liniment')) and I.23.15 (for Arab. لطوخ ('salve')) (cf. NM 5:191–192; IJZ 1–2:546, 580).

ריקוע → רִקּוּעַ.

רַךְ · **fresh**: Arab. غضّ · Ibn al-Jazzār, *Zād al-musāfir wa-qūt al-ḥādir* · trans. Moses ibn Tibbon, *Sefer Ṣedat ha-Derakhim* V.4: ישתה החולה מאיזה מהם שיזדמן שקל במיץ פלנטג״י כתוש סחוט או במי עלי גפנים רכים (Let the patient take one *sheqel*[270] of the [aforementioned] medicines, whichever is available, with juice of broadleaf plantain that has been pounded and extracted or with juice of fresh vine leaves). Hebr. רַךְ features in the current dictionaries in the sense of 'tender; weak; timid; soft; thin' only (cf. BM 6586–6587).

רַכּוּת · **atony**: Lat. *mollicies* (*mollities*) (Arab. استرخاء) · Constantinus Africanus, *Viaticum peregrinantis* · trans. Do'eg ha-Edomi, *Sefer Ya'ir Netiv* IV.13: בשול זה טוב לרכות האסטומכא ולכאב (The following decoction is good for atony of the stomach (gastric atony) and pain [in the stomach]). Hebr. רַכּוּת features in BM 6597 in the sense of 'softness; weakness' without attestations from medieval medical literature. Moses ibn Tibbon translates Arab. استرخاء as רִפְיוֹן (see entry).

רִמּוֹן • *Plur.* רמונים • ורד הרמונים → וֶרֶד.

רִמּוֹנִי · **pomegranate-*N.* (*Adj.*) (from pomegranates)**: Arab. رمّاني · Ibn al-Jazzār, *Zād al-musāfir wa-qūt al-ḥādir* · trans. Moses ibn Tibbon, *Sefer Ṣedat ha-Derakhim* IV.11: ותהיה מזונו תרנגולים קטנים מבושלים בתבשיל רמוני או תפוחי או בסרי (He should eat young chickens cooked in a pomegranate dish or an apple dish or a dish of unripe, sour grapes). Hebr. רִמּוֹנִי features in BM 6610 only in an attestation from Tuviah Katz, *Ma'aseh Tuviah*.

רֹעַ • **רוע הבשול** · **indigestion**: Arab. تخمة (Gr. ἀπέψια) · Ibn al-Jazzār, *Zād al-musāfir wa-qūt al-ḥādir* · trans. Moses ibn Tibbon, *Sefer Ṣedat ha-Derakhim* IV.9: והמקרים המתהוים מרוע הבשול יתחלפו וזה לד׳ סבות (There are four different afflictions caused by indigestion). Hebr. רוע הבשול is attested in BCD 263 (NM 4:195) in a later attestation from Jacob ibn Tibbon, *Hanhagat ha-Beri'ut le-Abu 'Ali ben Zuhr* (cf. RSA 159). Do'eg ha-Edomi translates the parallel Lat. term *fastidium* as אִסְטְנִיסוּת (see entry). Moses ibn Tibbon also uses the term רוע הבשול for Arab. سوء الهضم ('bad digestion; lack of digestion') in *Sefer Ṣedat ha-Derakhim* V.5 (see entry אַיִן).

רָעָב • **רעב עלופיי** · **hunger associated with (causing) fainting**: Lat. *fames syncopalis* · Gerard de Solo, *Practica super nono Almansoris* · trans. Abraham Avigdor, *Ha-Ma'amar ha-Teshi'i le-Sefer ha-Mansuri le-Razi*, fol. 120ª: שער בחולי הנקרא אַפֵּיטִיטוּס

270 Hebr. *sheqel* stands for Arab. *mithqāl*; one *mithqāl* is 4.46 grams; cf. HIM 4–7.

קַנִינוּשׁ: ראוי שתדע שמיני התאוה הבלתי טבעית הם רבים האחד נקרא תאוה כלבית והאחר נקרא בולמוס והאחר נקרא רעב עלופיי והאחר תאוה נפסדת (Chapter on the illness called ʾaPeYṬiṬWS QaNiYNWŠ [i.e., canine appetite]: You should know that there are many kinds of unnatural appetite: One of them is called *taʾawah kalbit* ('canine appetite;' cf. BCD 289 (NM 3:238)), another one is called *bulmos* ('bulimy;' cf. NM 2:110, 127 and entry בּוּלְמוֹס above), another one is called *raʿav ʿilufi* ('hunger associated with (causing) fainting'), and yet another one [is called] *taʾawah nifsedet* ('corrupt appetite')). Hebrew רעב עלופיי is not attested in the current dictionaries. The term עִלּוּפִי on its own features in BM 4509, a.o., in an attestation from the *Sefer ha-Qanun*.

רַעֲבוֹן • חוֹלִי רעבון ← חָלִי.

רְעִיפָה · **nosebleed:** Lat. *fluxus sanguis narium* · Gerard de Solo, *Practica super nono Almansoris* · trans. Abraham Avigdor, *Ha-Maʾamar ha-Teshiʿi le-Sefer ha-Mansuri le-Razi*, fol. 86b: שער ברעיפה (Chapter on nosebleed). Hebr. רְעִיפָה does not feature in this sense in the current dictionaries. The same Lat. term is translated by Abraham Avigdor also as רעיפת הדם and is already attested in Shem Tov ben Isaac, *Sefer ha-Shimmush* XXX.2.55 (for Arab. نزف ('hemorrhage'); cf. BCD 264 (NM 1:115)). Another var. רעיפת הדם מן האף features in Shem Tov's *Sefer Almansur*, fol. 3b. Hillel ben Samuel and Nathan ha-Meʾati use the terms רעיפת דם מן החותם, resp. רעיפת דם מן הנחירים for Arab. رعاف ('nosebleed') in their *Aphorismi*, resp. *Pirqei Abuqraṭ* III.27 (cf. BCD 264 (NM 3:219)).

רַעַם · **intestinal rumblings (borborygmus):** Lat. *gurgulatio* (Arab. قرقرة) · Constantinus Africanus, *Viaticum peregrinantis* · trans. Doʾeg ha-Edomi, *Sefer Yaʾir Netiv* IV.13: ואם יהיה מליחות אדומות ירגיש כאב רב וחום וצמאון ומהרוח הגס מתחלף הכאב ממקום למקום ועושה רעם בחלקים השפלים מהבטן (If [the colic] originates from yellow bile, [the patient] will suffer from severe pain, heat, and thirst. And if it comes from thick flatulence, the pain will change from site to site and cause intestinal rumblings in the lower parts of the stomach). In the sense of 'intestinal rumblings,' Hebr. רַעַם is attested in BCD 264 (NM 1:187–188) in a later attestation from Zeraḥyah Ḥen, *Sefer ha-Peraqim* (*Pirqei Moshe*) VII.55 (for Arab. قرقرة) (cf. BMMZ 84, l. 1; BMMG no. 4080). In addition to רַעַם, Doʾeg translates Lat. *gurgulatio* as הֲבָרָה (see entry). Moses ibn Tibbon translates the parallel Arab. term قرقرة as קִרְקוּר (cf. BCD 251 for attestations from Moses ibn Tibbon, *Perush Aphorismi shel Apuqraṭ* (*Pirqei Abuqraṭ*) IV.73 (210) (NM 3:209–210; BMCH 1:374, l. 3) and Nathan ha-Meʾati, *Sefer ha-Peraqim* (*Pirqei Moshe*) VII.55 (NM 2:84; BMMN 89, l. 10; BMMG no. 4080)).

[רעש] • *Part. Nifʿal* **נִרְעָשׁ** · **suffering from tremors:** Arab. مرتعش · Ibn Zuhr, *K. al-Aghdhiya* · trans. Nathan ha-Meʾati, *Sefer ha-Mezonot*, fol. 7b: וסגלת הארנבת שהיא מפתתת החצץ וסגלת ראשה שאם יבושל עם תפאיה לבנה ויאכלהו הנרעש יועילהו בג״ה ([The flesh of] a hare has the specific property to pulverize [intestinal] stones, and if a person sufferung from tremors eats its head once it has been cooked with white TPʾYH [i.e., Arab. *tafāya*[271]], he will benefit from it, God willing). In the sense of 'suffering from tremors,' Hebr. [רעשׁ], *Part. Nifʿal* נִרְעָשׁ, features in BM 6667 in an attestation from the *Sefer ha-Qanun*.

רַעַשׁ · **trembling; tremor**: Arab. رعشة (Gr. τρόμος; cf. UW 685) · Ibn Sīnā, *K. al-Qānūn fī al-ṭibb* · trans. Zeraḥyah Ḥen, *Sefer ha-Qanun* II, fol. 191ᵇ: גְּנְדַבֵא דֹּסְתַר ... יועיל מן העצבים ויחממם ויועיל מן הרעש והקיווץ הלח והכוז הלח והרפיון והפלג (GoNəDaBe' DoSəTaR [i.e., Arab. *jandubādastar* ('castoreum')[272]]: ... It is useful for the nerves and warms them. It is also beneficial for tremor, 'humid' spasms, numbness, and paralysis). In the sense of 'tremor,' Hebr. רַעַשׁ features in BCD 264 (NM 3:220–221) in an attestation from Do'eg ha-Edomi, *Sefer Agur* VI.26. Nathan ha-Me'ati translates Arab. رعشة as רעישה (cf. BCD 264 for attestations from Shem Tov ben Isaac, *Sefer ha-Shimmush* XXVII (NM 4:196) and Anonymous, *Perush Aphorismi shel Apuqraṭ* (*Pirqei Abuqraṭ*) VI.26 (318) (NM 3:220); BMCH 1:589, l. 3) and Anonymous has רַעַשׁ, just like Zeraḥyah.

רְפָאוּת · **treatment**: Arab علاج · Maimonides, *Maqāla fī al-rabw* (*On Asthma*) · trans. Anonymous, *Sefer ha-Qaṣeret* XIII.20 (cf. BMA 2:443, ll. 3–5): אמר ארסטו בספר ממפורסמי ספריו דברים אלו לשונם אמר: וקודם זה ראוי לנו שנעיין בטבע הבריאות והחלי שלפעמים יטעו רוב הרופאים בזה הכח עד שיהיה סבת המות הרפואה והרפאות (Aristotle has said the following in one of his famous books, and these are his very words: We should first examine the nature [of the patient], both when he is healthy [and when he is] ill. Most physicians are subject to error in [their assessment of] this force, so that the patient dies as a result of their medical treatment). Hebr. רְפָאוּת is not attested in medieval medical literature. Joshua Shatibi translates Arab. علاج as התרפאת and Samuel Benveniste translates الطبّ والعلاج as רפואה.

[רפד] • *Piʿel* רִפֵּד · **to support**: Arab. رفد · Maimonides, *Maqāla fī al-rabw* (*On Asthma*) · trans. Samuel Benveniste, *Ma'amar ʿal ha-Qaṣeret* XIII.8 (cf. BMA 2:299, ll. 22–24): אמר הראזי בפרק אחד מפרקיו וזה פתרונו אמר: בהיות החלי חזק מהכח לא תועיל הרפואה כלל ואם יהיה הכח מתגבר על החלי אין צרך לרופא בשום פנים. ואם היו שוים אז יצטרך לרופא ירפד הכח ויעזרהו על החלי (In one of his aphorisms, al-Rāzī makes a statement with the following meaning: When the disease is more manifest than the strength [of the patient], medicine is of no use at all; and when the strength [of the patient] has the upper hand over the disease, there is no need for a physician in any wise. But when they are equal, then the physician is needed to support and promote the strength [of the patient] against the disease). In the sense of 'to support,' Hebr. [רפד], *Piʿel* רִפֵּד, is

---

271 '*tafāya*': A compound meat dish from the Maghrib consisting of meat, spices, water, maidenhair fern, oil, and salt. The white variety consists of meat that is drier than the green one (cf. D 1:147–148).

272 'castoreum': I.e., a medicament often defined as testicles of a water animal; in fact, it is an excretion derived from the scent glands of the Eurasian beaver [*Castor fiber* Linnaeus, 1758]; cf. MIG no. 183.

poss. a semantic borrowing from Arab. رفد. The Hebr. term is attested in this sense in medieval poetical literature, cf. BM 6675.[273] Joshua Shatibi and Anonymous both render Arab. رفد as סמך.

רְפוּאָה • הרפואה הנקראת מבורך · **the blessed remedy**: Arab. الدواء المسمّى المبارك · Ibn al-Jazzār, *Zād al-musāfir wa-qūt al-ḥāḍir* · trans. Moses ibn Tibbon, *Sefer Ṣedat ha-Derakhim* IV.17: וישתה אחר זה מים שנתבשלו בהם זרעים או תריאק פלוניאה או הרפואה הנקראת מבורך (Then he should drink water in which have been cooked seeds, the philonium[274] theriac, or the blessed remedy). Hebr. הרפואה הנקראת מבורך is a non-attested calque of Arab. الدواء المسمّى المبارك. For this remedy, which strengthens the body and is made from asparagus, milk, butter, pepper, and honey, see Ibn Rabban al-Ṭabarī, *Firdaws al-ḥikma*.[275] Do'eg ha-Edomi transcribes the parallel Lat. term *eulogimen* as אבלוגימרון.

• **רפואה מתירה/מתרת** · **dissolving, dissolvent remedy**: Lat. *medicina dissolutiva* · Constantinus Africanus, *Viaticum peregrinantis* · trans. Do'eg ha-Edomi, *Sefer Ya'ir Netiv* IV.12: וכאשר זה הנפח יבא יאות לעזור אליו ברפואה מתרת רוח הבטן (When the stomach is affected by flatulence, one should treat it with a remedy that dissolves the flatulence of the stomach). In the sense of 'dissolving remedy,' Hebr. רפואה מתירה features in BCD 265 (NM 1:172 (corr.)) in a later attestation from Zeraḥyah Ḥen, *Sefer ha-Peraqim* (*Pirqei Moshe*) XV.25 (cf. BMMZ 156, l. 18). See also entry הסם המתיך (entry סַם).

• **רפואת הקלי** · **a powder consisting of roasted seeds**: Arab. مقلياثا (cf. FAQ 263) · Ibn al-Jazzār, *Zād al-musāfir wa-qūt al-ḥāḍir* · trans. Moses ibn Tibbon, *Sefer Ṣedat ha-Derakhim* IV.15: תאר רפואת הקלי חברתיה לשלשול ועצור (Recipe for a powder of roasted seeds that I prepared for diarrhea, dysentery, ...). Hebr. רפואת הקלי does not feature in the current dictionaries.

• *Plur.* **רפואות • הרפואות המדביקות** · **agglutinant remedies**: Lat. *glutinantes* · Gerard de Solo, *Practica super nono Almansoris* · trans. Abraham Avigdor, *Ha-Ma'amar ha-Teshi'i le-Sefer ha-Mansuri le-Razi*, fol. 87b: המין השלישי הוא הרפואות המדביקות (The third kind [of remedies for a nosebleed] are those that are agglutinant). Hebr. הרפואה המדביקה features in NM 5:189 (for Arab. الدواء الملحم) in an attestation from Nathan ha-Me'ati, *Sefer ha-Peraqim* (*Pirqei Moshe*) XV.56 (cf. BMMN 163, l. 8), where it is translated as: 'a remedy that closes a wound with flesh' (cf. BMW 321). A var.

---

273 Cf. also: Ibn Janāḥ, *K. al-Uṣūl*, 686.

274 'philonium': I.e., Arab. *filūniyā* (Gr. Φιλώνια or (correctly) Φιλώνειος), a remedy invented by Philo of Tarsos, a poet-physician and pharmacist of the late Hellenistic period, which comes in a 'Greek' and a 'Persian' variety (cf. KR 180, n. 66); for Arabic prototypes, see Ibn Sahl, *The Small Dispensatory*, trans. O. Kahl (Leiden 2003), nos. 7–8; see also KR 180, n. 66.

275 Ed. by M.Z. Siddiqi (Berlin 1928), 594, l. 7. I thank Oliver Kahl for this reference.

reading הסם המדביק features in BCD 188 (NM 4:125), s.v. הסם המדביק או המחליק ('the agglutinant or mollifacient remedy') in an attestation from Anonymous, *Sefer ha-Refu'ot ha-Libbiyot*.

• **הרפואות המצרבות** · **drugs that cause blisters**: Arab. الأدوية المقرحة · Maimonides, *Maqāla fī al-rabw* (*On Asthma*) · trans. Samuel Benveniste, *Ma'amar 'al ha-Qaṣeret* XI.2 (cf. BMA 2:283, ll. 10–12): וכבר זכרו הרופאים בתקון קצת מיני החלי הזה והוא המפורסם אצל כל רופא לעשות הרפואות המאדימות על הראש אף כי המצרבות מחשבתם בזה למנוע ההזלות (The physicians have mentioned as part of the treatment of some types of this disease [i.e., asthma]—and it is well known to every physician—the application of rubefacients or even drugs that cause blisters to the head. Their intention with this is the prevention of defluxions). Hebr. [צרב], *Part. Pi'el* מְצָרֵב, does not feature in this sense in the current dictionaries. Joshua Shatibi translates Arab. الأدوية المقرحة as הסמים המנגעים (see entry סַם) and Anonymous has הסמנים המשחינים (see entry סַמָּן).

• **הרפואות המתנגדות למדוים** · **antidotes**: Arab. الأدوية المقابلة للأدواء · Ibn al-Jazzār, *Zād al-musāfir wa-qūt al-ḥāḍir* · trans. Moses ibn Tibbon, *Sefer Ṣedat ha-Derakhim* V.6: תאר מרקחת חברו גלינו' בספר הרפואות המתנגדות למדוים (Composition (recipe) of a remedy composed by Galen in his book *De Antidotis*). Hebr. הרפואות המתנגדות למדוים is not attested in the current dictionaries. Var. readings for the Hebr. trans. of Galen, *De Antidotis* (Arab. الأدوية المقابلة للأدواء) in *Sefer ha-Peraqim* (*Pirqei Moshe*) XXI.32, 50 are הרפואות המקבילות לחליים and הסמים המקבילים לחליים (Nathan ha-Me'ati; cf. BMMN 199, ll. 24–25; 202, l. 2); as well as הרפואה המהפכת לחוליים and הרפואה המנגדת לחוליים (Zeraḥyah Ḥen; cf. BMMZ 197, ll. 17–18; 199, l. 18) (cf. also BMMG 611); and for 'antidote' in general: [נצל], *Part. Hif'il* מַצִּיל (Ibn Tibbon, *Perush Aphorismi shel Apuqraṭ* (*Pirqei Abuqraṭ*) I.1 (27); cf. BCD 178 (NM 3:137); BMCH 1:325, l. 6); and צֳרִי (Anonymous, *Sefer ha-Refu'ot ha-Libbiyot*; cf. BCD 234 (NM 4:176)).

רְפוּאוֹת • **צפרני הרפואות** → צִפֹּרֶן.

רִפְיוֹן · I. **paralysis**: Arab. استرخاء (Gr. παραλύομαι; cf. UW 497) · Ibn Sīnā, *K. al-Qānūn fī al-ṭibb* · trans. Nathan ha-Me'ati, *Sefer ha-Qanun* II, fol. 74ᵇ: גלוז ... יועיל ממכאובי העצבים[276] וגיד הנשה והוא מועיל אל הרפיון (Hazelnut: ... It is beneficial in neuralgia, sciatica, and paralysis). Hebr. רִפְיוֹן features in the sense of 'atonia (atony)' in MD 77; and as 'looseness' (for Arab. تخلخل) in Moses ibn Tibbon, *Perush Aphorismi shel Apuqraṭ* (*Pirqei Abuqraṭ*) V.69 (289) (cf. BCD 266 (NM 3:222); BMCH 1:391, l. 9). Anonymous has רִפְיוֹן as well.

· II. **numbness**: Arab. خدر (Gr. νάρκη; cf. UW 431) · Ibn Sīnā, *K. al-Qānūn fī al-ṭibb* · trans. Zeraḥyah Ḥen, *Sefer ha-Qanun* II, fol. 261ᵇ: פטריות ... מולידים הרפיון והשיתוק (Mushrooms: ... They cause numbness and apoplexy). In his *Sefer ha-Peraqim*

276 העצבים: emend. ed. העצלים Ms العصب a.

(*Pirqei Moshe*), Zeraḥyah translates Arab. خدر throughout as ב(י)טול (cf. BMMG no. 1297). Nathan ha-Me'ati translates Arab. خدر as בטול ההרגש (see entry בִּטּוּל).

• **רפיון האיברים** · **shivers; tetanus**: Arab. كزاز (cf. WKAS 1:166: 'bad cold; shivers; ague;' UWS 2:311, s.v. σπασμός: 'Krampf; Konvulsion;'; 448, s.v. τέτανος: 'Starrkrampf'; DKT 503: 'tetanus') · Ibn Zuhr, *K. al-Aghdhiya* · trans. Nathan ha-Me'ati, *Sefer ha-Mezonot*, fol. 7^b: והוא ערב הטעם ששמנו דק מאד משקיט הכאבים המתחדשים הסבות קרות ומועיל בג"ה מרפיון האיברים ועקום הפה והפלג (And it [i.e, the flesh of the hedgehog] is tasty and its fat is very fine; it alleviates pain caused by cold and it is beneficial—God willing—for shivers (tetanus), paralysis of the facial nerve, and hemiplegia). Hebr. רפיון האיברים features in BCD 266 (NM 2:87) in an attestation from Nathan's *Sefer ha-Peraqim* (*Pirqei Moshe*) XXII.16 (cf. BMMN 211, l. 16; BMMG no. 4371). In his *Sefer ha-Qanun*, Nathan translates Arab. كزاز as התנועה אשר מבלי חפץ (see entry תְּנוּעָה).

• **רפיון האצטומכה** · I. **atony of the stomach (gastric atony)**: Arab. استرخاء المعدة · Ibn al-Jazzār, *Zād al-musāfir wa-qūt al-ḥādir* · trans. Moses ibn Tibbon, *Sefer Ṣedat ha-Derakhim* IV.13: תאר משרה מועיל מרפיון האצטומ' והעוות בה והכאב החזק ערובו (A recipe for a decoction that is good for atony of the stomach (gastric atony), for a colic, and severe pain [in the stomach]). Hebr. רפיון האצטומכה is not attested in the current dictionaries. Do'eg ha-Edomi translates the parallel Lat. term *mollicies* as רַכּוּת (see entry).

רָצוֹן • **הגרת הזרע מבלי רצון** → הַגָּרָה.

• **כשזב הזרע מן הגיד בלא רצון** → [זוב].

• **רבוי השתן מבלי רצון** → רִבּוּי.

רְצוּץ · I. **bruise; bruising**: Arab. وثء (Gr. θλάσμα; cf. UW 297; IJZ 7:97, n. 127) · Ibn al-Jazzār, *Zād al-musāfir wa-qūt al-ḥādir* · trans. Moses ibn Tibbon, *Sefer Ṣedat ha-Derakhim* V.3: ואם יקרה לחולה עם המורסא חום בכבד נשקהו בלבשטיאש ובול ארמיני במיץ פלנטאגי או במיץ מורילא וכל מיני בול יועילו למורסות אשר מדם יקרו בתוך הגוף והרצוץ והחבטה והכתישה ויחבוש בתחבושת צנדל ומה שדומה לזה (If in addition to the tumor the patient suffers from heat in the liver, we should give him rose or blossom of the wild pomegranate, Armenian earth, juice of plantain or of black nightshade. All kinds of earth are good for bodily tumors that originate from blood; [they are also good for] a bruise, shock, and contusion. [The patient] should apply a poultice of sandalwood and the like). Hebr. רצוץ features in BM 6711–6712 in the sense of 'breaking; crushing,' a.o., in an attestation from the *Pirqei Galenus*. In *Sefer Ṣedat ha-Derakhim* VII.15, Moses ibn Tibbon translates the same Arab. term وثء as סדק (cf. IJZ 7:149, l. 3) or רסוק (cf. IJZ 7:165, l. 26; 166, ll. 6, 23; for רסוק, see also BCD 262 (NM 1:68, 115) for attestations from *Sefer Ṣedat ha-Derakhim* VII.25.4 (IJZ 7: 165, l. 26) and Shem Tov ben Isaac, *Sefer ha-Shimmush* XXX.2.89).

· II. **bruise; contusion**: Arab. رضّ · Ibn al-Jazzār, *Zād al-musāfir wa-qūt al-ḥādir* · trans. Moses ibn Tibbon, *Sefer Ṣedat ha-Derakhim* VI.6: ואם תהיה סבת המורסא ההיא מתחלת מחוץ כמו הכאה או רצוץ הנה יספר החולה מה שיגיעהו מזה (If the cause of the tumor [on the testicles] is external, such as a blow or contusion, the patient may tell how he got it). In addition to רְצוּץ, Moses ibn Tibbon translates Arab. رضّ as כְּתִישָׁה (see entry). Subsequently, ר(י)צוץ features in the same sense (for Arab. رضّ) in *Sefer ha-Peraqim* (*Pirqei Moshe*) III.109 by both Nathan ha-Me'ati (cf. BMMN 55, l. 17) and Zeraḥyah Ḥen (cf. BMMZ 48, l. 26) (cf. also BMMG no. 2088). Abraham ben Isaac translates Arab. رضّ as רְצוּץ as well.

• **רצוץ העצבים** · **twisted nerves**: Arab. التواء العصب (Gr. στρέμμα; cf. UW 643) · Ibn Sīnā, *K. al-Qānūn fī al-ṭibb* · trans. Anonymous, *Sefer ha-Qanun* II, fols. 67b–68a: גוז ... עם דבש ורודא לרצוץ העצבים (Walnut: ... [Walnut mixed] with honey and rue [is beneficial] for twisted nerves). Hebr. רצוץ העצבים is not attested in the current dictionaries. Nathan ha-Me'ati translates Arab. التواء العصب as עוות העצבים (see entry עִוּוּת) and Zeraḥyah Ḥen has לפיתת העצבים (see entry לְפִיתָה).

• **רצוץ העצלים** · **muscle tear (rupture)**: Arab. شدخ العضل (Arab. شدخ = Gr. ῥῆγμα (breakage, fracture; laceration, rupture, rent, tear); cf. UW 587, LSG 1568) · Ibn Sīnā, *K. al-Qānūn fī al-ṭibb* · trans. Nathan ha-Me'ati, *Sefer ha-Qanun* II, fol. 122b: ראסן ... יועיל מגיד הנשה ומכאב הפרקים ועקרו[277] אם עושין מעליו תחבשת יועיל מן המכאובים הקרים ומרצוץ העצלים (Elecampane: ... It is useful in sciatica and pain of the joints. If one prepares from[278] its root and leaves a plaster [and applies it] it is useful in cold pains and muscle tear). Hebr. רצוץ העצלעם is not attested in the current dictionaries. Zeraḥyah Ḥen translates Arab. شدخ العضل as הפסד המושקלו and Anonymous has גרידת העצלים. The Hebr. translators probably interpreted the term شَدْخ as derived from شَدَخَ in its general meaning of 'to break, crush, press, squeeze' (cf. Lane 1519) and not in the specific meaning listed above.

רְקוּעַ · **plate**: Arab. صفيحة · Ibn al-Jazzār, *Zād al-musāfir wa-qūt al-ḥādir* · trans. Abraham ben Isaac, *Sefer Ṣedah la-Oreḥim* VI.2: ויקח ריקוע מעופרת ויקשור עליו (He [i.e., a person suffering from priapism] should also take a plate of lead and tie it to his [back]). The term רְקוּעַ features in the Bible in the sense of 'something beaten hammered; beaten flat' (KB 3:1292), in Rabb. literature as 'beaten plate; foil' (JD 1477); cf. BM 6729–6730: 'patch; covering.' Moses ibn Tibbon translates Arab. صفيحة as חתיכה and Do'eg ha-Edomi translates the parallel Lat. term *cingulum* as חגורה.

• *Plur.* **רקועים** • **רקועים ושטחים** · **flakes**: Arab. صفيحة, *Plur.* صفائح (Gr. λέπις; cf. UW 387) · Ibn al-Jazzār, *Zād al-musāfir wa-qūt al-ḥādir* · trans. Moses ibn Tibbon, *Sefer Ṣedat ha-Derakhim* V.14: וימצא בשתן דומה לקלפות ורקועים ושטחים ([Particles] similar to scales and flakes will be found in the urine). Hebr. *Sing.* רקוע ושטח, *Plur.* רקועים ושטחים, does not feature in this sense in the current dictionaries. Without further explication, Ben Yehuda quotes *Plur.* רקועים in an attestation from *Perush Ibn Rushd ʿal Ḥaruzei Ibn*

277 ועקרו אם עושין מעליו: وأصله وورقه ضماد a.

278 'from its root and leaves': Trans. after a.

Sina (i.e., Ibn Rushd's commentary on Ibn Sīnā, *'Urjūza*, trans. Solomon ibn Ayyub (1261)): וכן השמר הדומה לרקועים הוא הנקרא צפאיחי בערב׳ (BM 6730). The synonymous term שטח is not attested in the sense of 'flake' in the current dictionaries. Do'eg ha-Edomi translates the parallel Lat. term *cortices* as סנפירים (see entry סְנַפִּיר).

[רקק] • *Part. Hif'il* מַרְקִיק • סַם → **הסם המרקיק**.

רִשּׁוּם • *Plur.* **רשומים** · **spots [on the body]**: Arab. آثار · Ibn Sīnā, *K. al-Qānūn fī al-ṭibb* · trans. Zeraḥyah Ḥen, *Sefer ha-Qanun* II, fol. 232ᵇ–233ᵇ: לבן חלב ... ומי גבינה יעביר הכלף והרשומים למשוח בו והנה יועיל מהם לשתותו (Milk: ... Whey removes freckles and spots when it is smeared [on the body]. It is also useful to drink it). Nathan ha-Me'ati translates Arab. آثار as רֹשֶׁם (see next entry).

רֹשֶׁם · **I. spots [on the body]**: Arab. آثار · i. Ibn Sīnā, *K. al-Qānūn fī al-ṭibb* · trans. Zeraḥyah Ḥen, *Sefer ha-Qanun* II, fol. 223ᵇ: כַּבְּרִית גפרית ... וכיעורב עם הגומא של הבטם יתלוש הרושם אשר יהיה על הצפרנים (Sulphur: ... When mixed with the resin of the turpentine tree, it removes the spots from the nails). Hebr. רֹשֶׁם is not attested in this sense in the current dictionaries. In philosophical literature, it features for Arab. أثر or تأثير in the sense of 'impact; affection; outcome of an action' (cf. PESHAT[279]). Nathan ha-Me'ati translates Arab. آثار as סִמָּן (see entry), but as רֹשֶׁם as well (see next entry). In addition to רֹשֶׁם, Zeraḥyah Ḥen translates Arab. آثار as רשומים (see previous entry רִשּׁוּם).

· ii. Ibn Sīnā, *K. al-Qānūn fī al-ṭibb* · trans. Nathan ha-Me'ati, *Sefer ha-Qanun* II, fol. 99ᵇ–100ᵃ: לבן ... ומי הגבנה יוציא הכתם ובער׳ כלף והרושם אם מושחים בו וכן אם שותים ממנו (Milk: ... Whey removes freckles and spots when it is smeared or ingested). Zeraḥyah Ḥen translates Arab. آثار as רשומים (see entry רִשּׁוּם).

· **II. scar**: Arab. آثار (Gr. οὐλή; cf. UWS 1:813) · Ibn Sīnā, *K. al-Qānūn fī al-ṭibb* · trans. Anonymous, *Sefer ha-Qanun* II, fol. 68ᵃ: גוז ... הרטוב ממנו תחבשת על רושם ההכאה (Walnut: ... If fresh walnut is put on the scars of injuries, [it is beneficial]). Nathan ha-Me'ati and Zeraḥyah Ḥen translate Arab. آثار as סמנים (see entry סִמָּן).

[רתח] • *Part. Hof'al* מֻרְתָּח • *Plur.* **מורתחים** · **decoctions**: Arab. مغليات · Maimonides, *Maqāla fī al-rabw* (*On Asthma*) · trans. Anonymous, *Sefer ha-Qaṣeret* XII.0 (cf. BMA 2:429, ll. 3–4): אמנם המורתחים שהרצון בהם הבישול וקלות הרקיקה והתנקות הריאה והן שראוי להקד‹י›ם למשלשלים (Decoctions with which one wishes to coct [the superfluities] and to ease expectoration and to clean the lungs, and which should be used before the purgatives). Hebr. [רתח], *Part. Hof'al* מֻרְתָּח, does not feature in this sense in the current dictionaries. Samuel Benveniste translates Arab. مغليات as משקים (see entry מַשְׁקֶה) and Joshua Shatibi has בישולים.

279 https://peshat.org/display/peshat_lemmas_00022412 (accessed February 11, 2022).

ש

שׁבושׁ • שיבוש הגוף · **indisposition; malaise**: Arab. اضطراب البدن · Maimonides, *Maqāla fī al-rabw* (*On Asthma*) · trans. Anonymous, *Sefer ha-Qaṣeret* v.6 (cf. BMA 2:405, ll. 7–9): או כאב הקולנג או כאב הכליות או כאב הטחול או כאב הכבד או כאב החזה או כאב האברים[280] או שיבוש הגוף או קרירות[281] או סמירות או חמימות (Pain in the colon, intestines, spleen, liver, chest, or joints;[282] indisposition; shivering[283] fit; shivering; or fever). Hebr. שיבוש הגוף is not attested in the current dictionaries. Samuel Benveniste and Joshua Shatibi both translate Arab. اضطراب البدن as בלבול הגוף (see entry בִּלְבּוּל).

שְׂבָכָה • השבכה הנפלאת · **rete mirabile**: Lat. *rete mirabili* · Gerard de Solo, *Practica super nono Almansoris* · trans. Abraham Avigdor, *Ha-Maʾamar ha-Teshiʿi le-Sefer ha-Mansuri le-Razi*, fol. 64[a]: ואחר זאת הלחות הזכוכית יש מחיצה אחת נקראת שבכית ותולדתה והתחלתה משבכת המוח הנקראת השבכה הנפלאת (Behind the vitreous humor lies a membrane called 'retina;' its origin and beginning is from the network in the brain called 'rete mirabile'). Hebr. השבכה הנפלאת does not feature in the current dictionaries. The term שְׂבָכָה on its own features in BM 7515 in the sense of 'circulus arteriosus Willisii' (i.e., 'Willis' circle') in an attestation from Meir Aldabi, *Shevilei Emunah*.

שָׁבַר • *Part.* **שׁוֹבֵר** · **diuretic**: Lat. *diureticus* (Arab. فتح السدد) · Constantinus Africanus, *Viaticum peregrinantis* · trans. Do'eg ha-Edomi, *Sefer Ya'ir Netiv* v.11: ואם אותות היבור הקר יתראו שם כמו שאמר גיאלינוס כי רוב תחלואי הטחול יהיו מקרירות ומליחות גסות ואז יאות לתת לו רפואה חזקה גם שוברת היא דִבְרֵיטְקַא (When one sees symptoms of a cold temperament—according to Galen's statement that most diseases of the spleen are caused by cold and coarse humors—one should give [the patient] a strong medicine that also has a diuretic effect; i.e., DiBəReYṬiQa' [i.e., Lat. *diuretica*]). Hebr. שָׁבַר, *Part.* שׁוֹבֵר, does not feature in this sense in the current dictionaries. See also דברים שוברים (entry דָּבָר, for Lat. *diuretica*) in *Sefer Ya'ir Netiv* v.2. Moses ibn Tibbon translates Arab. فتح السدد as פתח הסתומים.

• **דברים שוברים** → דָּבָר.

• *Nifʿal* **נִשְׁבַּר** · **to be amputated**: Lat. *incidor* (Arab. قُطِعَ) · Constantinus Africanus, *Viaticum peregrinantis* · trans. Do'eg ha-Edomi, *Sefer Ya'ir Netiv* v.2: ועוד הסתימה תקרה אל הכבד בשברון האברים האחרים כי אם ישבר היד או הרגל הדם שיהיה רגיל לגדל אותו האבר נשאר בכבד (An obstruction of the liver can also occur because of the amputation of [one of] the other organs, for in the case of an amputation of a hand or foot, the blood that usually nourishes that organ remains in the liver). Hebr. *Nifʿal* נִשְׁבַּר does

---

280 האברים: المفاصل a.
281 קרירות: نافض a.
282 'joints': Trans. after a.
283 'shivering fit': Trans. after a.

not feature in this sense in the current dictionaries. Moses ibn Tibbon translates the parallel Arab. term قُطِعَ as [חתך], *Nifʿal* נֶחְתַּךְ.

שִׁבָּרוֹן · **1. amputation**: Lat. *incisio* (cf. DMLBS 1605) (Arab. قطع) · Constantinus Africanus, *Viaticum peregrinantis* · trans. Do'eg ha-Edomi, *Sefer Ya'ir Netiv* V.2: ועוד הסתימה תקרה אל הכבד בשברון האברים האחרים כי אם ישבר היד או הרגל הדם שיהיה רגיל לגדל אותו האבר נשאר בכבד (An obstruction of the liver can also occur because of the amputation of [one of] the other organs, for in the case of an amputation of a hand or foot, the blood that usually nourishes that organ remains in the liver). Hebr. שִׁבָּרוֹן features in BM 6871 in the sense of 'breaking; breach' and in BCD 268 (NM 3:223) in the sense of 'pain' (for Arab. كلال) in an attestation from Moses ibn Tibbon, *Perush Aphorismi shel Apuqraṭ* (*Pirqei Abuqraṭ*) IV.44 (181) (cf. BMCH 1:367, l. 8). Here, Moses ibn Tibbon translates the parallel Arab. term قطع as חתוך.

שִׁגָּעוֹן • **שגעון כלבי** · **dog mania**: Lat. *mania canina* · Gerard de Solo, *Practica super nono Almansoris* · trans. Abraham Avigdor, *Ha-Ma'amar ha-Teshiʿi le-Sefer ha-Mansuri le-Razi*, fol. 52[a]: וזה השם יאמר בכלל וביחוד. אמנם בכלל הנה היא תורה כל מאניאה קאנינאה ובלשוננו שגעון כלבי ותורה גם כן על מאניאה דִימוֹנִיאַטִיקאה ובלשוננו שגעון שדיי ועל חולי השחורה ובלשונם מאלאינקוניאה (This term [i.e., melancholy] is used in a general and specific sense. In general, it indicates M'NY'H Q'NYN'H [i.e., *mania canina* ('dog mania')], in Hebrew *shiggaʿon kalbi*. But it can also indicate M'NY'H DiYMWoNiY'aṬiYQa'H [i.e., *mania demoniatica* ('demonic mania')], in Hebrew *shiggaʿon shedi*, and 'black bile illness' (melancholy), in Lat. M'L'YNQWNY'H [i.e., *melanchonia*]). Hebrew שגעון כלבי does not feature in the current dictionaries.

• **שגעון שדי** · **demonic mania**: Lat. *mania demoniatica* (read: *demoniaca*) · Gerard de Solo, *Practica super nono Almansoris* · trans. Abraham Avigdor, *Ha-Ma'amar ha-Teshiʿi le-Sefer ha-Mansuri le-Razi*, fol. 52[a]: וזה השם יאמר בכלל וביחוד. אמנם בכלל הנה היא תורה כל מאניאה קאנינאה ובלשוננו שגעון כלבי ותורה גם כן על מאניאה דִימוֹנִיאַטִיקאה ובלשוננו שגעון שדיי ועל חולי השחורה ובלשונם מאלאינקוניאה. (This term [i.e., melancholy] is used in a general and specific sense. In general, it indicates M'NY'H Q'NYN'H [i.e., *mania canina* ('dog mania')], in Hebrew *shiggaʿon kalbi*. But it can also indicate M'NY'H DiYMWoNiY'aṬiYQa'H [i.e., *mania demoniatica* ('demonic mania')], in Hebrew *shiggaʿon shedi*, and 'black bile illness' (melancholy), in Lat. M'L'YNQWNY'H [i.e., *melanchonia*]). Hebr. שגעון שדי does not feature in the current dictionaries.

שָׁדוּף (*Part. Pass.*) → **[שדף]**.

שֵׁדִי • **שגעון שדי** → **שִׁגָּעוֹן**.

[שדל] • *Hitpaʿel* **הִשְׁתַּדֵּל** · **to do promptly, hasten to do**: Arab. بادر · Ibn al-Jazzār, *Zād al-musāfir wa-qūt al-ḥādir* · trans. Moses ibn Tibbon, *Sefer Ṣedat ha-Derakhim* IV.9: ובעבור מה שהקדמנו ראוי למי שנפסד מאכלו ומי שרצה מן האנשים לשמור הבריאות שישמר מכל מסבבי הפסד המאכל וישתדל כאשר מצאהו זה להקיא קודם שישתנה המאכל ויפסד. ואם ימנע הקיא תחכם לשלשל טבעו (Because of what I said before, someone who suffers from indigestion and someone who wants to preserve his health should beware of anything that can cause indigestion; once he is affected he should hasten to vomit before the food changes and putrefies. If he cannot vomit, he should contrive to take a purgative). Hebr. [שדל], *Hitpa'el* הִשְׁתַּדֵּל, is not attested in this sense in the current dictionaries; cf. BM 6914–6915: טרח ועמל ('to make an effort').

[שדף] • *Part. Pass.* שָׁדוּף · **suffering from phthisis**: Arab. مسلول · Ibn Zuhr, *K. al-Aghdhiya* · trans. Nathan ha-Me'ati, *Sefer ha-Mezonot*, fol. 9[a]: המשובח שבחלבים חלב העז בעת שחלבו ואם ישתה בצום ויש בו מזון משובח לגוף עד שחשבו שהוא משמין השדופים (The best milk is fresh goat's milk; if one drinks it on an empty stomach it provides the body with excellent food, so much so that some [physicians] thought that it fattens those suffering from phthisis). In medieval medical literature, Hebr. [שדף], *Part. Pass.* שָׁדוּף, only features in the sense of 'ill' (for Arab. سقيم) in an attestation from Zeraḥyah Ḥen, *Sefer ha-Peraqim* (*Pirqei Moshe*) VIII.14 (cf. BMMZ 88, l. 21; BMMG no. 2409).

שֶׂה • לשון השה → לָשׁוֹן.

[שוב] • שב לישנות · **to become chronic**: Lat. *inveteror* · Constantinus Africanus, *Viaticum peregrinantis* · trans. Do'eg ha-Edomi, *Sefer Ya'ir Netiv* IV.15: יאות למהר לעזור אל החולי הזה כי אם ישוב לישנות ויתחלף בנגעים והמעי יכרת והמות ממהר (One should hurry to treat this illness [i.e., dysentery], for when it becomes chronic and changes into ulcers, the intestine is torn (perforated), and death comes quickly). Hebr. שב לישנות is not attested in the current dictionaries. Hebr. יַשְׁנוּת on its own features as a modern term in EM 701. Moses ibn Tibbon translates the parallel Arab. term تقادم as התישן.

שׁוֹבֵר (*Part.*) → שָׁבַר.

שׁוֹטֶה • עשב השוטה → עֵשֶׂב.

שֻׁוּעָל • ביצי השועל → בֵּיצָה.

שׁוּפַע → שׁפַע.

שׁוֹק · **stem**: Arab. ساق · Ibn Sīnā, *K. al-Qānūn fī al-ṭibb* · trans. Nathan ha-Me'ati, *Sefer ha-Qanun* II, fol. 71[a]: ברשיאושאן ... והוא עשב דק צומח על שפת הנהרות ואגמי מים ובתוך הבורות וידמה אל הכזבורת הלח אך ענפיו נוטים אל האודם ואל השחרות ואין לו שוק ולא ציץ ולא פרח ולא זרע ויאפס כחו מהר (Maidenhair fern: ... It is a thin grass which grows on river banks, near ponds, and inside wells. It resembles fresh coriander but its stalks are reddish with a tinge of blackness. It has no stem and has no blossoms (fruit), flowers, or seeds. It loses its potency quickly). Hebr. שוק does not feature in this sense in the current dictionaries. Zeraḥyah and Anonymous translate Arab. ساق as שוק as well.

שׁוֹקֵט (*Part.*) → שָׁקַט.

שׁוֹרֵץ (*Part.*) → שָׁרַץ.

שָׁחַט · **to press out**: Arab. عصر · Maimonides, *Maqāla fī al-rabw* (*On Asthma*) · trans. Samuel Benveniste, *Ma'amar 'al ha-Qaṣeret* XII.3 (cf. BMA 2:288, ll. 22–23): אחר חזק זכרהו ג'אלינוס: יקח בצל האשקיל וישחטהו וישים עם המים היוצא ממנו כמהו דבש ויעשהו משקה ויקח ממנו כאוקיה לפני האכילה וכמו כן אחריה (Another strong [linctus] mentioned by Galen: Take squill, press it out, add to the juice a similar amount of honey, [thicken it] until it becomes a syrup, and take about one ounce of it before and after meals). In the sense of 'to press out,' Hebr. שָׁחַט is not attested in medieval medical literature; cf. BM 7539; EM 1802. Joshua Shatibi translates Arab. عصر as עָצַר (see entry) and Anonymous has יָצָא, *Part. Hif'il* מוֹצִיא (see entry).

שְׁחִין • שחין דק · ringworm: Arab. قوباء (cf. UW 385, s.v. λειχήν)[284] · Ibn Sīnā, *K. al-Qānūn fī al-ṭibb* · trans. Nathan ha-Me'ati, *Sefer ha-Qanun* II, fol. 91b: כברית ... אם יושם על השרפה[285] והנגע יועיל וימרוק השחין הדק הנק' קובא וקל וחומר עם הדבר הנק' עלך אלאנבאט וקל וחומר עם חומץ וקל וחומר עם נטרון (Sulphur: ... It is useful when it is applied to ulcerated[286] scabies, it purifies (removes) the ringworm called KWB' [i.e., Arab. *qūbā'*], especially so when applied with 'LK 'L'NB'Ṭ [i.e., Arab. *'ilk al-anbāt*, 'mastic;' cf. MIG no. 715], vinegar, and natron). Hebr. שחין דק features in BCD 271–272 in the sense of 'aphthae' (for Arab. قلاع in an attestation from Shem Tov ben Isaac, *Sefer ha-Shimmush* XXVII (cf. NM 4:202)) and 'pustules' (for Arab. بثور in an attestation from *Sefer ha-Shimmush* XXVII and XXX (cf. NM 1:116–117; 4:202)). Zeraḥyah Ḥen only transcribes Arab. قوباء as קובא and Anonymous translates the Arab. term as סַפַּחַת. The latter term also features in Shem Tov ben Isaac, *Sefer ha-Shimmush* XXVII (cf. BCD 194 (NM 4:139)).

[שחן] • *Part. Hif'il* מַשְׁחִין • הסמנים המשחינים → סַמָּן.

שַׁחַק · powder: Arab. دقاق · Ibn al-Jazzār, *Zād al-musāfir wa-qūt al-ḥādir* · trans. Moses ibn Tibbon, *Sefer Ṣedat ha-Derakhim* IV.19: ואם יהיה בו עמק יזרה עליו שחק לבונה (In case [the ulcers] are deep, one should strew upon them incense powder). In the sense of 'powder,' Hebr. שַׁחַק is only attested in modern Hebr. literature (cf. EM 1806). In the Bible, it features in the sense of 'dust' in Is 40:15 (cf. BDB 1007).

שֶׁטַח · space; cavity: Lat. *spatia* (Arab. فضاء) · Constantinus Africanus, *Viaticum peregrinantis* · trans. Do'eg ha-Edomi, *Sefer Ya'ir Netiv* V.5: ובסבה הזאת השטח בין המעים ובין הדף הנקרא שיפק מתמלא (Consequently, the space that is between the intestines and the peritoneum is filled [with that liquid]). Hebr. שֶׁטַח does not feature in this sense in the current dictionaries. Moses ibn Tibbon translates Arab. فضاء as חלל.

• *Plur.* שטחים • רקועים ושטחים → רָקוּעַ.

שיבוש → שִׁבּוּשׁ.

שינה → שֵׁנָה.

שַׁיִשׁ • אבן שיש → אֶבֶן.

שָׁכֵן • העורק אשר על הכף בין האצבע הקטן ושכנו → עֹרֶק.

[שלג] • *Part. Hof'al* מֻשְׁלָג · **ice-cold**: Arab. مثلّج · Maimonides, *Maqāla fī al-rabw* (*On Asthma*) · trans. Samuel Benveniste, *Ma'amar 'al ha-Qaṣeret* VII.3 (cf. BMA 2:267,

---

284 See the extensive discussion of the term قوباء in IJZ 7:105, n. 182, and other translations of the term as: 'eczema; eczema lichenificatum; ichhyosis; lichen.'

285 השרפה והנגע: الجرب المتقرح a.

286 'ulcerated scabies': Trans. after a.

ll. 4–6): אבל המים הקרים אשר לא הגיעו לקוץ בהם האדם לרב קרירותם ואינם מושלגים אלה הם המים המובחרים הראויים לשתותם בעת הצמא וכל שכן למי שמזגו חם (But cold water, which is not so cold that a person shies away from drinking it and which is not ice-cold, is the choicest type of water, which one ought to drink when thirsty—and especially someone with a warm temperament). In the sense of 'ice-cold,' Hebr. [שלג], *Part. Hofʿal* מֻשְׁלָג, is a semantic borrowing from Arab. مثلّج. The Hebr. term features in BM 7119 in attestations from the *Sefer ha-Qanun* and is translated by Ben Yehuda as 'covered with snow.' Joshua Shatibi translates Arab مثلّج as מֻשְׁלָג as well and Anonymous renders the Arab. term as משולג.

שְׁלוּחַ › **diarrhea**: Arab. انطلاق · Maimonides, *Maqāla fī al-rabw* (*On Asthma*) · trans. Samuel Benveniste, *Ma'amar ʿal ha-Qaṣeret* XIII.5 (cf. BMA 2:299, ll. 1–2): ואם קפצת בדברים החובשים ועצרת השלוח הזה ושב הטבע למנהגו ברפואות (And if you hasten to use astringents and thus stop this diarrhea, [your] nature returns to its normal condition by means of medication). Hebr. שְׁלוּחַ does not feature in this sense in the current dictionaries. Joshua Shatibi translates Arab. انطلاق as חֲלָקוּת (see entry) and Anonymous has שלשול.

שִׁלְשׁוּל • **שלשול השתן** › **diuresis**: Arab: إدرار البول · Ibn Sīnā, *K. al-Qānūn fī al-ṭibb* · trans. Nathan ha-Me'ati, *Sefer ha-Qanun* II, fol. 74[a]: גואשיר ... ירכך קשי הרחם ויועיל להזלת השתן וישתה ממנו שיעור לוז[287] במים חמים לשלשול השתן[288] (Opopanax: ... It softens the hardness of the uterus and is useful for strangury. A dose of one hazelnut[289] is taken orally with warm water for diuresis). In the sense of 'diuresis,' Hebr. שלשול השתן is not attested in the current dictionaries. Zeraḥyah Ḥen translates Arab. إدرار البول as הרבות השתן (see entry [רבה]) and Anonymous has הגרת השתן (cf. BCD 62 (NM 3:56) for an attestation from Moses ibn Tibbon, *Perush Aphorismi shel Apuqraṭ* (*Pirqei Abuqraṭ*) I.2 (29) (cf. BMCH 1:326, l. 6)).

• קיא ושלשול יחד → קִיא.

שִׁלְשֵׁל › **I. to act as a diuretic, have a diuretic effect**: Arab. أدرّ · Ibn Sīnā, *K. al-Qānūn fī al-ṭibb* · trans. Nathan ha-Me'ati, *Sefer ha-Qanun* II, fol. 122[b]: ראסן ... תבשיל עקרו ישלשל (Elecampane: ... A decoction of its root acts as a diuretic). Hebr. שִׁלְשֵׁל features in BM 7197–7199 in a variety of contexts, for instance as שלשל את המעים ('to loosen the bowels'). In his *Sefer ha-Peraqim* (*Pirqei Moshe*) IX.71, Nathan translates Arab. أدرّ as [נגר], *Hifʿil* הִגִּיר (cf. BMMN 113, l. 14; BMMG no. 1679). The latter term is also used by Anonymous.

› **II. to purge**: Arab. أسهل · Ibn Sīnā, *K. al-Qānūn fī al-ṭibb* · trans. Nathan ha-Me'ati, *Sefer ha-Qanun* II, fol. 74[a]: גואשיר ... ויועיל מההדרוקן הנקרא קולנג וישלשל התערוב הנא ויועיל מחכוך כיס השתן (Opopanax: ... It is useful for colic called QWLNG [i.e., Arab.

287 לוז: بندقة a.
288 השתן (= Ms Paris, BnF, héb. 1136, fol. 71[b]): emend. ed. השעור Ms.
289 'hazelnut' (Arab. *bunduqa*): I.e., 3.4 grams, cf. IG 164.

qūlanj] and purges raw humors; it is also good for prurigo of the bladder). Zeraḥyah Ḥen and Anonymous both translate Arab. أسهل as שִׁלְשֵׁל, just like Nathan.

• **שלשל דם הוסת** · **to stimulate (induce) menstration**: Arab: أدرّ الطمث · Ibn Sīnā, *K. al-Qānūn fī al-ṭibb* · trans. Nathan ha-Me'ati, *Sefer ha-Qanun* II, fol. 74ª: גואשיר ... ירכך קשי הרחם ויועיל להזלת השתן וישתה ממנו שיעור לוז במים חמים לשלשול השתן[290] ודם הוסת והרחם הקר ופריו כמו כן ישלשל דם הוסת ויותר עם האפסנתין (Opopanax: ... It softens the hardness of the uterus and is useful for strangury. A dose of one hazelnut[291] is taken orally with warm water for diuresis, menstruation, and a cold uterus. Its fruit, especially when taken with absinth wormwood, stimulates menstration). Hebr. שלשל דם הוסת is not attested in the current dictionaries. In his *Sefer ha-Peraqim* (*Pirqei Moshe*), Nathan translates Arab. أدرّ الطمث as הגיר הנדות (XII.10; XVI.2; XXI.66; cf. BMMN 140, l. 1; 165, l. 17; 204, ll. 12–14) and הוסיף הנדות (XVI.2 cf. BMMN 165, l. 20) (cf. also BMMG no. 1681). Zeraḥyah Ḥen translates the Arab. term as הרבה הוסת and Anonymous has משפיע הנדות.

שְׁמִירָה • **שמירה וזהירות** · **diet**: Arab. حمية واحتراس (two synonymous terms) · Ibn al-Jazzār, *Zād al-musāfir wa-qūt al-ḥādir* · trans. Moses ibn Tibbon, *Sefer Ṣedat ha-Derakhim* V.9: ישתה ממנו אוק׳ מי שירצה לשלשל טבעו ממרה אדומה ויוציאה מן הכבד והאצטו׳ וישתה ממנו החזק ב׳ אוקי׳ אחר שמירה וזהירות (He who wants to purge his stools from yellow bile and to expel it from the liver and stomach, should take one ounce of [the mentioned remedy] and ingest it, and if he is strong, he may take two ounces after observing a diet). Hebr. שמירה וזהירות is not attested in this sense in the current dictionaries. Also in the sense of 'diet' (for Arab. حمية), the term שְׁמִירָה on its own features in BCD 278 (NM 1:69) in an attestation from *Sefer Ṣedat ha-Derakhim* VII.17 (cf. IJZ 7: 155, l. 5).

[שמע] • *Nifʿal* **נִשְׁמַע** • **הקול הנשמע באוזן** → **קוֹל**.

שֵׁן • *Dual* **שנים** • **חריקת שנים** → **חֲרִיקָה**.

[שנה] • *Part. Piʿel* **מְשַׁנֶּה** • **הכח המשנה** → **כֹּחַ**.

שֵׁנָה • **גרישת הזרע בתוך השינה** → **גְּרִישָׁה**.

שְׂעוֹרָה • *Plur.* **שעורים** • **שתיתת קלי קמח השעורים** → **שְׁתִיתָה**.

[שער] • *Piʿel* **שִׁעֵר** · **to ordain**: Arab. قدّر · Ibn al-Jazzār, *Zād al-musāfir wa-qūt al-ḥādir* · trans. Moses ibn Tibbon, *Sefer Ṣedat ha-Derakhim* V.16: כשתגיע עת הלידה הטבעית אשר שער אותה ה׳ ית׳ וית׳ יקרה לאשה ההתרה ויתנועע האבר תנועה יותר חזקה שבתנועות לסבת מעוט מזונו (When a woman reaches the time that God—blessed be He—has ordained for natural childbirth, she develops labor pains whereby [the fetus] makes very strong movements because of the little amount of food left for it). Hebr. [שער], *Piʿel* שִׁעֵר, features (for Arab. قدّر) in PESHAT, a.o., in an attestation from Moses ibn

290 השתן (= Ms Paris, BnF, héb. 1136, fol. 71ᵇ): emend. ed. השעור Ms.

291 'hazelnut' (Arab. *bunduqa*): I.e., 3.4 grams, cf. IG 164.

Tibbon, *Qiṣṣur Sefer ha-Ḥush we-ha-Muḥas* in the sense of 'to regulate, measure': ישבח נותן החיים ומשערם יודע החיים.[292] Abraham ben Isaac translates Arab. قدّر as גזר.

שֵׂעָר • השער המתהפך בעפעפים · entropion (inward turning of the eyelid, causing the eyelashes to rub against the eyeball) · al-Rāzī, *K. al-Manṣūrī fī al-ṭibb* · trans. Shem Tov ben Isaac, *Sefer Almansur*, fol. 3[b]: כ״ה בשער המתהפך בעפעפים ([Bk. 9], ch. 25: On entropion). Hebr. השער המתהפך בעפעפים does not feature in the current dictionaries. Abraham Avigdor (fol. 77[a]), has a var. reading השער המתהפך בגבינים העוקץ העין. Note, that he replaces the regular term for 'eyelid' (עפעף) with that of 'eyebrow' (גבין).

שֶׁפֶל • החלקים השפלים מהבטן → חֵלֶק.

שֶׁפַע • שפע הדם · loss of blood: Arab. نزف الدم · Ibn al-Jazzār, *Zād al-musāfir wa-qūt al-ḥādir* · trans. Moses ibn Tibbon, *Sefer Ṣedat ha-Derakhim* VI.10: תאר פתילה תועיל לשפע הדם יקרו (Prescription for a pessary that is good for loss of blood). Hebr. שֶׁפַע features in NM 5:199 in the sense of 'superfluity; residu; superfluous matter' in an attestation from Do'eg ha-Edomi, *Sefer Ya'ir Netiv* III.8.

שׁפַע • שופע נידות · loss of menstrual blood: Arab. نزف · Ibn al-Jazzār, *Zād al-musāfir wa-qūt al-ḥādir* · trans. Abraham ben Isaac, *Sefer Ṣedah la-Oreḥim* VI.10: ואם ירבה לה שופע נידות אז יהיה לה דמות פנים רעים ויתנפחו רגליה ולא יתבשל המאכל באישטומ׳ כי אם בישול חלש (If she loses a lot of [menstrual] blood, her facial color will be bad, her feet will be swollen, her food will only be slightly digested in her stomach). Hebr. שׁפַע is attested in the current dictionaries, esp. as בשפע in the sense of 'abundantly' in later attestations, a.o., from Eliahu de Vidas, *Reshit Ḥokhmah*. Moses ibn Tibbon translates Arab. نزف as שפע only and Do'eg ha-Edomi translates the parallel Lat. term *fluxus* as הזלה.

שִׁפְעָה • שפעת הדם · loss of blood: Arab. نزف · Ibn al-Jazzār, *Zād al-musāfir wa-qūt al-ḥādir* · trans. Moses ibn Tibbon, *Sefer Ṣedat ha-Derakhim* VI.10: השער העשירי בשפעת הדם אשר יקרה לנשים (Chapter 10: On loss of blood occurring to women). Hebr. שפעת הדם is not attested in the current dictionaries. The term שִׁפְעָה alone features in the sense of 'abundance' in BM 7406. Do'eg ha-Edomi translates the parallel Lat. term *fluxus sanguinis* as הזלת הדם.

שִׁקּוּי · dropsy: Arab. استسقاء · Ibn al-Jazzār, *Zād al-musāfir wa-qūt al-ḥādir* · trans. Moses ibn Tibbon, *Sefer Ṣedat ha-Derakhim* V.1: ופעמים שיקרה מפני אלו החלאים חולי יקרא שקוי והנה נזכור כל אחד מאלו החלאים בשער בפני עצמו (Sometimes, these afflictions [of the liver] cause the illness called 'dropsy.' I will mention every single affliction in a chapter on its own). In the sense of 'dropsy,' Hebr. שִׁקּוּי features in BM 7422, a.o., in an attestation from the *Sefer ha-Qanun*. The term also features in BCD 37 (NM 3:63)

292 https://peshat.org/display/peshat_lemmas_00023017 (accessed January 9, 2022).

as בעלי שקוי ('dropsy patients') in an attestation from Hillel ben Samuel, *Aphorismi* VI.27. Do'eg ha-Edomi transcribes the parallel Lat. term *ydropisis* as אידרופיסי.

• **השקוי הבשרי** · **anasarca**: Arab. الاستسقاء اللحمي · Ibn al-Jazzār, *Zād al-musāfir wa-qūt al-ḥādir* · trans. Moses ibn Tibbon, *Sefer Ṣedat ha-Derakhim* V.5: ואולם הכויה הנה תועיל לשקוי הידוע בבשרי ואפשר שיועיל לנודי (Cautery is beneficial for the kind of dropsy known as anasarca and possibly for [the kind known as] tympanites). Hebr. השקוי הבשרי features in BCD 283–284 (NM 2:90) in a later attestation from Nathan ha-Me'ati, *Sefer ha-Peraqim* (*Pirqei Moshe*) XXIII.50 (BMMN 225, l. 3; BMMG no. 2419). Do'eg ha-Edomi transcribes the parallel Lat. term *hyposarca* as איפושיקרא (איפושירקא*).

• **השקוי הנודי** · **tympanites**: Arab. الاستسقاء الزقّي · Ibn al-Jazzār, *Zād al-musāfir wa-qūt al-ḥādir* · trans. Moses ibn Tibbon, *Sefer Ṣedat ha-Derakhim* V.5: ואולם הכויה הנה תועיל לשקוי הידוע בבשרי ואפשר שיועיל לנודי (Cautery is beneficial for the kind of dropsy known as anasarca and possibly for [the kind known as] tympanites). Hebr. השקוי הנודי features in BCD 284 (NM 1:118–119), in a var. reading השקוי הנאדי, a.o., in an attestation from Shem Tov ben Isaac, *Sefer ha-Shimmush* XXX.1.32.

שָׁקַט • *Part.* **שׁוֹקֵט** · **stagnant**: Arab. راكد · Maimonides, *Maqāla fī al-rabw* (*On Asthma*) · trans. Joshua Shatibi, *Ma'amar 'al ha-Qaṣeret* XIII.4 (cf. BMA 2:369, ll. 20–22): וזה שהמדינה לגובה בנינה וצרות דרכיה ורוב מה שיתך משוכניה ומותריהם ומתיהם ונבלות בהמתם ועפוש מה שיתעפש מן מאכלותיהם יהיה אוירה שוקט עכור עב אידיי ענני (In the city—because of its high buildings and narrow streets, the refuse and waste of its inhabitants, their dead and the carcasses of their animals, and the putrefaction of their food—the air becomes stagnant, turbid, thick, misty, and foggy). Hebr. שָׁקַט, *Part.* שׁוֹקֵט, is not attested in this sense in the current dictionaries. Samuel Benveniste and Anonymous both render Arab. راكد as עומד.

שריפה → שְׂרֵפָה.

שְׂרֵפָה • **שריפת השתן** · **(lit., 'burning urine'); a burning sensation during urination (dysuria)**: Lat. *ardor urine* (Arab. حرقة البول) · Gerard de Solo, *Practica super nono Almansoris* · trans. Abraham Avigdor, *Ha-Ma'amar ha-Teshi'i le-Sefer ha-Mansuri le-Razi*, fol. 147[a]: שער ברפואת שריפת השתן: כשימצא החולה שריפה כשישתין וחדוד הרחיקהו מלוח וחמוץ וחריף וזונהו במרקים הרפים והתבשילים הפשוטים (Chapter on the treatment of a burning sensation during urination: When the patient suffers from a sharp and burning urine one should not give him anything salty, sour, or sharp, but feed him with light soups and simple dishes). Hebr. שריפת השתן features in NM 5:200 (for Arab. حرقة البول) in an earlier attestation from Shem Tov ben Isaac, *Sefer ha-Shimmush* XXIX, list 1 (cf. SHS 1:517 (Shin 39)). Shem Tov ben Isaac translates the parallel Arab. term حرقة البول as חריפות השתן (see entry חֲרִיפוּת).

שָׁרַץ • *Part.* **שׁוֹרֵץ** • **הנגעים השורצים** → נֶגַע.

שֹׁרֶר · **navel**: Arab. سرّة · Ibn al-Jazzār, *Zād al-musāfir wa-qūt al-ḥādir* · trans. Moses ibn Tibbon, *Sefer Ṣedat ha-Derakhim* VI.12: ואם תהיה המורסא בפי הרחם ימשך אחר זה כאב

בשרר ובפי הטבעת (If the tumor occurs in the orifice of the uterus, it is followed by pain in the navel and anus). Hebr. שֹׁרֶר features in MD 494, s.v. 'navel.' Abraham ben Isaac translates Arab. سرّة as שֹׁרֶר as well.

שֹׁרֶשׁ • *Plur.* **שרשים • בשול השרשים** → **בִּשּׁוּל.**

• **מורסות שרשי האזן** → **מֻרְסָה.**

• **משקה השרשים** → **מַשְׁקֶה.**

[שרת] • *Part. Piʿel* **מְשָׁרֶת • חולי משרת** → **חֹלִי.**

• **תחלואי המשרתים** → **תַּחֲלוּא.**

שֵׁת • בליטת השת → **בְּלִיטָה.**

שַׁתִּיתָה · **porridge; broth; gruel**: Arab. حسو · Maimonides, *Maqāla fī al-rabw* (*On Asthma*) · trans. Anonymous, *Sefer ha-Qaṣeret* IX.13 (cf. BMA 2:418, l. 27–419, l. 2): וכשתהיה מהבקר יאכל אותו שירצה להקיא קודם שעת המנהג במעט פת מצה במטעמים משונים מהדגים המלוחים והמוריס והאבטיחים והברקוקים אם היה זמנו והצנון והבצל והחציר והדבש ושתיתת הגרישין ושתיתת השעורים בזבלה (The next morning, shortly before the usual [lunch] time, the one who wants to induce vomiting should eat unleavened bread together with different kinds of food—namely, salted fish, *murrī* (a fish or grain-based condiment), melons, apricots when in season, radishes, onion, leek, honey, broth of crushed beans, and barley broth with the husks). Hebr. שַׁתִּיתָה is a Hebraization of Aram. שַׁתִּיתָא (see next entry). Samuel Benveniste translates Arab. حسو as תבשיל and Joshua Shatibi transcribes the Arab. term as חסו.

• **שתיתת קלי קמח השעורים** · **gruel prepared from meal of parched barley (which can be moistened with water or fat)**: Arab. سويق (cf. SDA 1167, s.v. שַׁתִּיתָא: 'Geon. expl.: שיתיתא סויק ... i.e., Arab. سويق, meal of parched barley, wheat, etc. or dried fruits which can be moistened w. water or fat into a gruel;' NTT 477: 'toasted and crushed seeds and grains, mixed with fat and sugar, and stored and used to make drinks, nourishing foods, and thick *khabīs* puddings') · Ibn Zuhr, *K. al-Aghdhiya* · trans. Nathan ha-Me'ati, *Sefer ha-Mezonot*, fol. 2[b]: ואמנם שתיתת קלי קמח השעורים הנקרא סויק הוא המעולה שבמזונות (However, gruel prepared from the meal of parched barley is the best kind of food). Nathan renders Arab. سويق as קמח קלי in his *Sefer ha-Peraqim* (*Pirqei Moshe*) IX.4 (cf. BMMN 103, l. 16; BMMG no. 2566).

[שתן] • *Hifʿil* **הִשְׁתִּין • השתין טפה טפה** · **to suffer from strangury**: Lat. *guttatim urinam facio* (Arab. تقطير في البول) · Constantinus Africanus, *Viaticum peregrinantis* · trans. Do'eg ha-Edomi, *Sefer Ya'ir Netiv* IV.17: וגאלינוס עשה הפרדה בין קוליקא אמיתית ובין כאב הכליות ואמר כי קוליקא כואבת ומחלפת בצדי הבטן לימין ולשמאל מלפנים ומאחור וכאב הכליות לא יזוז לעולם ויעמד במקום אחד וישתין טפה טפה (Galen made a distinction between true colic and intestinal pain and said that [the pain of] a colic moves around in the stomach to the right and to the left, forwards and backwards, while intestinal pain never moves and always stays at the same place and [the patient] suffers from strangury). Hebr. השתין טפה טפה is not attested in the current dictionaries. Moses ibn Tibbon translates Arab. تقطير في البول as הטפה בשתן (cf. BCD 66 for the Hebr.

var. הטפת השתן, a.o., in an attestation from Do'eg ha-Edomi, *Sefer Agur* v.58 (cf. NM 3:64)).

• **השתין בערשו** · **to wet the bed**: Lat. *commingo in lecto* (Arab. بال في الفراش) · Constantinus Africanus, *Viaticum peregrinantis* · trans. Do'eg ha-Edomi, *Sefer Ya'ir Netiv* v.19: יש אשר באין הרגש ישתינו בערשותם (Some people wet the bed without noticing it). Hebr. השתין בערשו does not feature in the current dictionaries. Moses ibn Tibbon translates the parallel Arab. term بال في الفراش as השתין במטה.

שֶׁתֶן • **חגרת השתן מבלי חפץ** → **חֲגָרָה**.

• **חזלת השתן** → **חֲזָלָה**.

• **חריפות השתן** → **חֲרִיפוּת**.

• **יציאת השתן** → **יְצִיאָה**.

• **כיס השתן** → **כִּיס**.

• **מצוקת השתן** → **מְצוּקָה**.

• **עצירת השתן** → **עֲצִירָה**[2].

• **הרבות השתן** → **[רבה]**.

• **רבוי השתן מבלי רצון** → **רִבּוּי**.

• **שלשול השתן** → **שִׁלְשׁוּל**.

• **שריפת השתן** → **שְׂרֵפָה**.

ת

תַּאֲוָה • נפילת תאוה → נְפִילָה.

תֹּאַר • **appearance; looks**: Arab. سحنة[293] (Gr. ἕξις) · Ibn al-Jazzār, *Zād al-musāfir wa-qūt al-ḥādir* · trans. Moses ibn Tibbon, *Sefer Ṣedat ha-Derakhim* VI.9: וכאשר עשה זה בה שב גופה אל תארה הטבעי בימים מעטים (Once he had given her this [treatment], her body regained its natural appearance in a few days). Hebr. תֹּאַר is attested in medieval philosophical literature in the sense of 'attribute; description; quality; adjective; external form; appearance; figure; shape' (cf. HCD 83), or 'attribute used to describe or define something; shape; perceptable shape of a thing' (cf. PESHAT[294]). Abraham ben Isaac translates Arab. سحنة as תוכן הבריאות and Do'eg ha-Edomi translates the parallel Lat. term *figura* as צוּרָה (see entry).

תָּדִיר • כשיעמוד גיד הערוה תדיר → עָמַד.

תּוֹפֵס (*Part.*) → תָּפַס.

תּוֹפֵשׂ (*Part.*) → תָּפַשׂ.

תּוֹצָאָה • *Plur.* תוצאות · **excrements; feces**: Lat. *stercus* (Arab. زبل) · Constantinus Africanus, *Viaticum peregrinantis* · trans. Do'eg ha-Edomi, *Sefer Ya'ir Netiv* IV.16: איליאוש הוא כאב המעים מונע לצאת התוצאות מחלק השפל ולפעמים יתחזק להקיא התוצאות (Ileus is an intestinal pain that prevents the excretion of the feces from below and sometimes it forces [the patient] to vomit them). In the sense of 'excrements; feces,' Hebr. תּוֹצָאָה, *Plur.* תוצאות, features in BCD 292 (NM 3:240–241) in an attestation from Do'eg's *Sefer Agur* IV.83. Do'eg also uses the term תוצאות to render Lat. *egestio*, 'emptying; purgation' (cf. NM 5:202). Moses ibn Tibbon translates the parallel Arab. term زبل as זֶבֶל (cf. NM 5:66 for an attestation from the anonymous trans. of Isḥāq ibn Imrān, *Treatise on Melancholy*).

[תחל] • *Part. Hif'il* מַתְחִיל • סבות מתחילות → סִבָּה.

תַּחֲלוּא • *Plur.* תחלואים • תחלואי המשרתים · **functional illnesses (illnesses that impede the functioning of an organ)**: Lat. *officiales morbi* (cf. DMLBS 2365, s.v. *officialis*: 'of or connected with the performance or function; functional: of organ or part of body; or of ailment or sickness') (Arab. مرض الآلة) · Constantinus Africanus, *Viaticum peregrinantis* · trans. Do'eg ha-Edomi, *Sefer Ya'ir Netiv* V.5: ועוד כי התחלואים הקרובים לכבד אינם יוצאים מכלל שלשה ומהם אמרו הרופאים כי כל איברי הגוף סובלים והם חבור רע תחלואי המשרתים הם הנקראים אופציאלש והפרדת הדבקים ([You should also know that] there are three [kinds] of diseases that affect all the organs, but especially the liver. [These three kinds are]: a bad temperament, functional illnesses called 'WPṢY'LŠ [i.e., Lat. *officiales* [*morbi*]], and dissolution of continuity). Hebr. תחלואי המשרתים

293 The faulty سخنة in BIJS 132, l. 551, should be corrected as سحنة.

294 https://peshat.org/display/peshat_lemmas_00004159 (accessed April 13, 2022).

is not attested in the current dictionaries. Lat. Sing. *morbus officialis* is rendered by Do'eg as חולי משרת (in *Sefer Ya'ir Netiv* v.11; see entry חֳלִי). Moses ibn Tibbon translates the parallel Arab. term مرض الآلة as חלי כליי (see also entry חֳלִי).

תיעוב → תְּעוּב.

תְּכֶלְתִּי · **blue**: Arab. أزرق · Maimonides, *Maqāla fī al-rabw* (*On Asthma*) · trans. Anonymous, *Sefer ha-Qaṣeret* XII.8 (cf. BMA 2:434, l. 16): מקל תכלתי חצי דרהם (Half a *dirham* of blue bdellium). Hebr. תְּכֶלְתִּי features in the current dictionaries as a modern term only; cf. EM 1937. Samuel Benveniste and Joshua Shatibi both transcribe Arab. أزرق as אזרק.

[תמד] • *Part. Hif'il* מַתְמִיד • קושי מתמיד → קֹשִׁי.

תְּמוּנָה · **kind**: Lat. *species* (Arab. صنف) · Constantinus Africanus, *Viaticum peregrinantis* · trans. Do'eg ha-Edomi, *Sefer Ya'ir Netiv* v.5: ואם הלחות הזה יהיה מזער מהרוח ומהעשן אז נולדת התמונה הנקראת היבשה ביבשות עצם הרוח ונקראת טמפניטיש (When there is less moisture than air and vapor, it results in the kind [of dropsy] called 'dry' because of the dryness of the substance of the air. It is also called 'tympanites'). Hebr. תְּמוּנָה does not feature in this sense in the current dictionaries (cf. BM 7791–7792; KTP 4:206–208; BCD 296 (NM 3:245; 4:221)). Moses ibn Tibbon translates Arab. صنف as מין.

• *Plur.* **תמונות** · **kinds**: Lat. *modi* (Arab. أصناف) · Constantinus Africanus, *Viaticum peregrinantis* · trans. Do'eg ha-Edomi, *Sefer Ya'ir Netiv* v.4: הזלת דם הכבד נעשית בענינים רבים והדם יוצא מתמונות משתנות (There are many causes for blood flowing from the liver and the kinds of blood that stream [from the liver] vary). Moses ibn Tibbon translates Arab. أصناف as מינים.

תַּמְרוּק · **deterging property**: Arab. جلاء · Ibn Sīnā, *K. al-Qānūn fī al-ṭibb* · trans. Nathan ha-Me'ati, *Sefer ha-Qanun* II, fol. 75[b]: גבן הוא הגבנה ... ואשר אינו מלוח ישלשל הטבע ומימיו ישלשלו המרה האדומה ויוסיף בו התמרוק אשר בו בעבור הבורקיות אשר בו (Cheese: ... Unsalted [cheese] relaxes the bowels and its water expels yellow bile. It increases the deterging property because of its alkalinity). Hebr. תַּמְרוּק features in BM 7812 in the sense of 'washing; anointment.' In his *Sefer ha-Peraqim* (*Pirqei Moshe*) XIII.6, Nathan translates Arab. جلاء as מרוק (cf. BMMN 146, l. 3; BMMG no. 667). Zeraḥyah Ḥen translates Arab. جلاء as רחוץ (cf. NM 5:185–186 for an attestation from Zeraḥyah's *Sefer ha-Peraqim* (*Pirqei Moshe*) XIII.6 (cf. BMMZ 143, l. 23; BMMG no. 667)) and Anonymous has מרוק, just like Nathan. Shem Tov ben Isaac, *Sefer ha-Shimmush* XXVII, translates the Arab. term as לְטִישָׁה (cf. BCD 137 (NM 4:90–91)).

תְּנוּעָה • **התנועה אשר מבלי חפץ** · **spasm; shivers; tetanus**: Arab. كزاز (Gr. σπάσμα, τέτανος; cf. UW 626–627, 671; WKAS 1:166: 'bad cold; shivers; ague;' DKT 503: 'tetanus') · Ibn Sīnā, *K. al-Qānūn fī al-ṭibb* · trans. Nathan ha-Me'ati, *Sefer ha-Qanun* II, fols. 73[b]–74[a]: גנדבא דסתר ... יועיל אל העצב ויועיל אל הרעישה והקיווץ הרטוב ומהתנועה אשר בלי חפץ הנקרא כזאז הנולדת בעד רוטבה ומהבטול הנקרא כדר והצנון הנקרא פלאג (GNDB' DSTR [i.e.,

Arab. *jandubādastar* ('castoreum')[295]: … It is beneficial for the nerves, and also for tremors, 'humid' spasms, shivers called KZ'Z [i.e., Arab. *kuzāz*] that are caused by moisture, numbness called KDR [i.e., Arab. *khadar*], and paralysis called PL'G [i.e., Arab. *fālij*]). Hebr. התנועה אשר מבלי חפץ is not attested in the current dictionaries. In his *Sefer ha-Peraqim* (*Pirqei Moshe*) VI.48; XXII.16, Nathan translates Arab. كزاز as רפיון האברים (cf. BMMN 72, l. 11; 211, l. 16; BMMG no. 4371); the same term features in his *Sefer ha-Mezonot* (see entry רִפְיוֹן). Anonymous translates the Arab. term as רפיון only, while Zeraḥyah Ḥen transcribes Arab. كزاز as כזז (cf. also the var. readings כוזאז and כזאז in his *Sefer ha-Peraqim* (*Pirqei Moshe*) VI.48; XXII.16 (cf. BMMZ 66, l. 17; 209, l. 1; BMMG no. 4371)).

תָּעַב • תעב המאכל · to suffer from nausea: Lat. *abominationem patior* (Arab. عرض غثيان) · Constantinus Africanus, *Viaticum peregrinantis* · trans. Do'eg ha-Edomi, *Sefer Ya'ir Netiv* IV.10: תיעוב המאכל זהו אבומינסיאון כאשר האדם יתעב המאכל בטרם יקחנו נתבונן כי הליחות הרעות הם באסטומכא (Nausea, i.e., 'BWMYNSY'WN [i.e., Lat. *abominatio*]: When a person suffers from nausea prior to taking food, we should understand that the stomach contains bad fluids). Hebr. תעב המאכל is not attested in the current dictionaries. In the sense of 'to feel nauseous,' the verb תָּעַב features in Rabb. literature (cf. JD 1683). Moses ibn Tibbon translates the parallel Arab. term عرض غثيان as קרה קבסא.

• *Hif'il* **הִתְעִיב • התעיב תעוב · to cause nausea:** Lat. *abominationem facio* · Constantinus Africanus, *Viaticum peregrinantis* · trans. Do'eg ha-Edomi, *Sefer Ya'ir Netiv* IV.10: אבל הליחות הגסות והדבקות מאד באסטומכא יתעיבו תעוב רב (However, the very coarse and viscous humors in the stomach cause severe nausea). Hebr. התעיב תעוב is not attested in this sense in the current dictionaries.

תִּעוּב · nausea: Lat. *abominatio* (Arab. غثيان) · Constantinus Africanus, *Viaticum peregrinantis* · trans. Do'eg ha-Edomi, *Sefer Ya'ir Netiv* IV.17: וזה החולי יש לו מקרים כלליים וקרובים הכלליים הם הקיא והתיעוב כאב רב ועוות גדול בחלק המעי (This illness has general and specific symptoms; the general [symptoms] are vomiting, nausea, severe pain and gripes in part of the intestines). Hebr. תִּעוּב does not feature in this sense in the current dictionaries. Ben Yehuda explains the term as 'a disgusting, loathsome property' (BM 7832). In addition to תִּעוּב, Do'eg translates Lat. *abominatio* as תעוב המאכל (see next entry). Moses ibn Tibbon translates the parallel Arab. term غثيان as Aram. קִבְסָא (cf. BCD 236 (NM 1:66) for an attestation from *Sefer Ṣedat ha-Derakhim* VII.9.4 (cf. IJZ 7:139, l. 15)).

• **תיעוב המאכל · nausea:** Lat. *abominatio* (Arab. غثي) · Constantinus Africanus, *Viaticum peregrinantis* · trans. Do'eg ha-Edomi, *Sefer Ya'ir Netiv* IV.10: תיעוב המאכל זהו

295 'castoreum': I.e., a medicament often defined as testicles of a water animal; in fact, it is an excretion derived from the scent glands of the Eurasian beaver [*Castor fiber* Linnaeus, 1758]; cf. MIG no. 183.

אבומינסיאון כאשר האדם יתעב המאכל בטרם יקחנו נתבונן כי הליחות הרעות הם באסטומכא (Nausea, i.e., ʾBWMYNSYʾWN [i.e., Lat. *abominatio*]: When a person suffers from nausea prior to taking food, we should understand that the stomach contains bad fluids). Hebr. תיעוב המאכל features as תעוב מאכל in BM 7832, s.v. תיעוב, in an attestation from Menaḥem ha-Meiri, *Yoma*. In addition to תיעוב המאכל, Doʾeg translates Lat. *abominatio* as תִּעוּב (see previous entry). Moses ibn Tibbon translates the parallel Arab. term غثيان as Aram. קִבְסָא (cf. BCD 236 (NM 1:66) for an attestation from *Sefer Ṣedat ha-Derakhim* VII.9.4 (cf. IJZ 7:139, l. 15)).

• התעיב תעוב → תָּעַב.

תַּעֲרוּב · **humor**: Arab. خلط · Ibn Sīnā, *K. al-Qānūn fī al-ṭibb* · trans. Nathan ha-Meʾati, *Sefer ha-Qanun* II, fols. 69^b–70^a: בטיך ... ומזונו יותר משובח ותערובו יותר נאות ויאות לאכול אחריו מאכל (Melon: ... It is most nutritious food and it produces most agreeable humors when it is eaten. But that should be followed by eating something [else]). Hebr. תַּעֲרוּב is not attested in the current dictionaries. For a var. reading תַּעֲרֹבֶת, *Plur.* תערובותת, in the same sense, cf. NM 5:204 for an attestation from the anonymous trans. of Isḥāq ibn Imrān, *Treatise on Melancholy*. Zeraḥyah Ḥen and Anonymous both translate Arab. خلط as ליחה.

תַּפּוּחִי · **apple-*N.* (*Adj.*) (from apples)**: Arab. تفّاحي · Ibn al-Jazzār, *Zād al-musāfir wa-qūt al-ḥādir* · trans. Moses ibn Tibbon, *Sefer Ṣedat ha-Derakhim* IV.11: ותהיה מזונו תרנגולים קטנים מבושלים בתבשיל רמוני או תפוחי או בסרי (He should eat young chickens cooked in a pomegranate dish or an apple dish or a dish of unripe, sour grapes). Hebr. תַּפּוּחִי features in EM 1959 in an attestation from modern Hebr. literature only.

[תפס] • *Part.* תּוֹפֵס • כח התופס → כֹּחַ.

[תפש] • *Part.* תּוֹפֵשׂ · **stopping; retaining**: Arab. حبس · Ibn al-Jazzār, *Zād al-musāfir wa-qūt al-ḥādir* · trans. Abraham ben Isaac, *Sefer Ṣedah la-Oreḥim* VI.10: ואם בכל זאת יזוב דמה אז נעשה לה הרפואות המעפיצות והתופשים הדם (If the loss of blood continues nevertheless, we treat her with astringent remedies that retain the blood). Hebr. [תפש], *Part.* תּוֹפֵשׂ, is not attested in this sense in the current dictionaries. Moses ibn Tibbon translates Arab. حبس as עצר. The latter term is also used by Doʾeg ha-Edomi to render the parallel Lat. term *stringo*.

תַּרְדֵּמָה · **I. stupor**: a) Arab. سبات · al-Rāzī, *K. al-Manṣūrī fī al-ṭibb* · trans. Shem Tov ben Isaac, *Sefer Almansur*, fol. 3^b: ה׳ בתרדמה ([Bk. 9, ch.] 5: On stupor). Hebr. תַּרְדֵּמָה features in the sense of, a.o., ‘lethargy; torpor’ (also for Arab. سبات) in BCD 298 in attestations from Moses ibn Tibbon, *Sefer Ṣedat ha-Derakhim* I.16.1 (cf. NM 4:222–223; IJZ 1–2:465) and Nathan ha-Meʾati, *Sefer ha-Peraqim* (*Pirqei Moshe*) XXIII.58 (cf. NM 2:93–94; BMMN 226, l. 4; BMMG no. 2318).

· b) Lat. *stupor* · Gerard de Solo, *Practica super nono Almansoris* · trans. Abraham Avigdor, *Ha-Maʿamar ha-Teshiʿi le-Sefer ha-Mansuri le-Razi*, fols. 34^a–35^a: שער ח׳ דֵי אֵישטוּפּוֹרֵי אֵית טֵירְימוֹרֵי מִינוֹרֵי פָּרַאלִישִׁי: הנה ראוי שתתעורר ותדע בבאור הרובריקאה שזה השם ר״ל אֵישְׁטוּפּוֹר ובלשוננו תרדמה שם משותף לשני ענינים האחת אל

תרדמת המחשבה והוא כאשר יעמוד האדם כאיש נרדם בלתי מדבר ויחשבו אנשים אשר סביביו ביותו טרוד המחשבה בעסקיו ... והענין האחר אשר יאמר בו תרדמה הוא שיהיה האבר נרדם ולא ירגיש הרגשה שלמה (Chapter 8: DeY ʾeYŠṬWuPWoReY ʾeYT ṬeYRəYMWoReY MiYNWoRiY PaRaʾLiYŠiY [i.e., *De estupore et tremore minori paralisi*]: Pay attention and know that the explanation of this heading, i.e., of the term ʾeYŠəṬWuPWoR [i.e., *estupor* ('stupor')], Hebr. *tardemah*, is that it has a double meaning, [it is used to indicate] a lethargic state of mind [lit., 'stupor'], meaning that a person stands still, as if he has fallen asleep, and does not speak and those around him think that his mind is busy thinking about his affairs ..., but it is also used to indicate [the condition of] an organ that is asleep (numb) and has lost part of its sensation).

‣ II. **numbness (condition of an organ that is asleep)**: Lat. *dormitatio* (Arab. خدر) · Constantinus Africanus, *Viaticum peregrinantis* · trans. Do'eg ha-Edomi, *Sefer Ya'ir Netiv* V.12: גם הסובל כאב הכליות ירגיש תרדמה ברגלים (Someone who suffers from pain in the kidneys will also feel numbness in his legs). In the sense of 'numbness,' Hebr. תַּרְדֵּמָה features in BCD 298 in attestations from Moses ibn Tibbon, *Sefer Ṣedat ha-Derakhim* VII.8.2 (cf. NM 1:70; IJZ 7:138, l. 19) and *Perush Aphorismi shel Apuqraṭ* (*Pirqei Abuqraṭ*) V.25 (245) (cf. NM 3:247; BMCH 1:381, l. 10). See also entries צִנּוּן and רִפְיוֹן, and NM 5:205 for the term תרדמת האיברים (Lat. *dormitatio membrorum* (Arab. خدر)) in an attestation from *Sefer Ya'ir Netiv* I.25.

תריאק ‣ **antidote**: Arab. ترياق (Gr. θηριακή, sc. ἀντίδοτος; cf. UW 296) · Ibn Sīnā, *K. al-Qānūn fī al-ṭibb* · trans. Nathan ha-Me'ati, *Sefer ha-Qanun* II, fol. 68[b]: בלאדר ... הוא מכלל הארסים וישרוף התערובים והתריאק שלו חמאת[296] בקר ושמן אגוזים וזה שמשבר כחו (Marking nut: ... It is one of the poisons and burns humors. Buttermilk is its antidote. Walnut oil breaks its toxic strength). In the sense of 'antidote,' Hebr. תריאק is a non-attested calque of Arab. ترياق. Zeraḥyah Ḥen and Anonymous both render Arab. ترياق as תריאק as well.

תַּרְנְגוֹל • תרנגול עוור ‣ **(lit., 'blind rooster'); caltrop [*Tribulus terrestris* L.]** · *Shinnui ha-Shemot ha-Niqra'im Synonimi*, fol. 78[a]: חמסך היא אלשכוהגב והוא תרנגול עוור ונק' בערבי חמץ אלמירי (ḤMSK [read: ḤSK; i.e., Arab. *ḥasak*, 'caltrop;' cf. MIG nos. 229, 343]; i.e., ʾLŠKWHGB [read: ʾLŠKWHG; i.e., *al-shakūhaj*; a Pers. loan word listed by Ibn Janāḥ (MIG nos. 343, 941) among the synonyms of *ḥasak*]; i.e., [Hebr.] *tarnegol ʿivver* [lit., 'blind rooster;' trans. of Rom. **ghālluh jīquh* or **ghālluh jāquh*, corresp. to Mod. Sp. *gallo ciego*; cf. MIG no. 229]; and called in Arab. ḤMṢ ʾLMYRY [read ḤMṢ ʾLʾMYR; i.e., *ḥimmaṣ al-amīr*, lit., 'chickpea of the emir,' a syn. of *ḥasak*, 'caltrop;' cf. DT 2:528 (IV.15): 'Burzeldorn']).

---

296 חמאת בקר: مخيض اللبن a.

• *Plur.* **תרנגלים • תרנגלי יונים** · **young doves**: Lat. *pulli columbarum* · Constantinus Africanus, *Viaticum peregrinantis* · trans. Do'eg ha-Edomi, *Sefer Ya'ir Netiv* IV.17: ויאכל פרדיץ מבושלים עם זרעונים ואניט ותרנגלי יונים גם תרנגלים ישנים מלאים אניט כמון רודא שלגימא מנטא שמן שישמני ונתן לו צף חרדל כתוש עם שמן שקדים ועם חומץ אשקיליטיק (He should eat partridges cooked with chickpeas, dill, young doves; likewise old roosters filled with dill, cumin, rue, salt, mint, sesame oil. We also give him mustard foam pounded with almond oil, and squill vinegar). Hebr. תַּרְנְגוֹל only features in the current dictionaries in the sense of 'cock; hen' (cf. BM 7915–7916).

תְּשׁוּמָה • תשומת מוך · **suppository**: Lat. *suppositoria* · Constantinus Africanus, *Viaticum peregrinantis* · trans. Do'eg ha-Edomi, *Sefer Ya'ir Netiv* IV.17: ונתן לו מיץ חלב עזים הוא שיר עם אלואין רחוץ ועם אשקמוניא מבושלת ונעשה אליו תשומת מוך הוא פשיארי מן ויאולא ומלח ודבש גם אשקמוניא (We administer him [i.e., a colic patient] whey prepared from goat's milk, i.e., [Lat.] ŠYR[WM] with washed aloe, and boiled scammony, and we apply a suppository; i.e., [Lat.] PŠY'RY, of violets, salt, honey, and also scammony). The term תשומת מוך is not attested in the current dictionaries. A var. reading תשומת כלי ממוך can be found in Ms Moscow, Russian State Library, Guenzburg 1481, fol. 102[b]. The term תשומת כלי features in the sense of 'clyster' in *Sefer Ya'ir Netiv* I.18.7 (cf. NM 5:206; IJZ 1–2:621). See also entry מוֹךְ.

• *Plur.* **תשומות** · **vaginal suppositories (pessaries)**: Arab. حمول · Ibn Sīnā, *K. al-Qānūn fī al-ṭibb* · trans. Nathan ha-Me'ati, *Sefer ha-Qanun* II, fol. 61[a–b]: אפסנתין ... איברי נעירה: משלשל השתן ודם הוסת שלשול חזק וקל וחומר כשעושין ממנו תשומות עם דבש וישלשל המרה האדומה (Absinth wormwood: ... Excretory organs: It acts as a strong diuretic or emmenagogue, especially when used as a vaginal suppository (pessary) with honey, and acts as a purgative for the yellow bile). Hebr. *Sing.* תְּשׁוּמָה is not attested in this sense in the current dictionaries. Zeraḥyah Ḥen translates Arab. حمول as סבל (for Arab. احتمل, see also entry סָבַל) and Anonymous has פתילה.

תַּשְׁמִישׁ • חלישות התשמיש → חֲלִישׁוּת.

Bibliography

Afnan, S.M., *A Philosophical Lexicon in Persian and Arabic* (Beirut 1968).

Barkaï, R., *A History of Jewish Gynaecological Texts in the Middle Ages* (Leiden 1998).

Bos, G. (ed. and trans.), *Ibn al-Jazzār on Fevers* (London 2000).

Bos, G. and Kl.-D. Fischer (eds.), *A Glimpse into Medical Practice among Jews around 1500: Latin-German Pharmaceutical Glossaries in Hebrew Characters extant in Ms Leiden, Universiteitsbibliotheek, Cod. Or. 4732/1* (SCAL *15), fols.* 1^a*–*17^b (Leiden 2021).

Bos, G. and R. Fontaine, 'Medico-Philosophical Controversies in Nathan b. Jo'el Falaquera's *Sefer Ṣori ha-Guf*,' *The Jewish Quarterly Review* 90, nos. 1–2 (1999): 27–60.

Bos, G., S. Hajek, and G. Mensching, 'A Fragment of Abraham Avigdor's Translation of Gerard de Solo's *Practica* from the Cairo Genizah: Edition and Analysis with Special Regard to the Old Occitan Elements', *Aleph* 21, no. 2 (2021): 309–357.

Bos, G., S. Lauschus, and F. Savelsberg, 'Substitute Drugs in the Hebrew Tradition' (forthcoming).

Dioscurides, *De materia medica*, ed. by M. Wellmann (Repr. Berlin, 1958); trans. by L.Y. Beck (Hildesheim 2005).

Eisenstein, J.D. (ed.), *Oṣar Midrashim*, 2 vols. (New York 1915).

Ferre, L., *Práctica de Johannes de Parma: Un tratado farmacologico en sus versiones hebreas y catalana* (Granada 2002).

Freudenthal, G., 'The Father of the Latin-into-Hebrew translations: 'Do'eg the Edomite,' The Twelfth-Century Repentant Convert,' in *Latin-into-Hebrew: Texts and Studies*, vol. 1: *Studies*, ed. by R. Fontaine and G. Freudenthal, 105–120 (Leiden 2013).

Freudenthal, G., M.R. McVaugh, and K. Mesler, 'Twelfth-Century Latin Medicine in Hebrew Garb: Doeg the Edomite as a Cultural Intermediary,' *Medieval Encounters* 26 (2020): 226–284.

Hankinson, R.J. (ed.), *Galen on Antecedent Causes* (Cambridge 1998).

Ibn Janāḥ, Marwān, *The Book of Hebrew Roots* (*K. al-Uṣūl*), ed. A. Neubauer (Oxford 1875).

Ibn Rabban al-Ṭabarī, ʿAlī, *Firdaws al-ḥikma*, ed. by M.Z. Siddiqi (Berlin 1928).

Ibn Sahl, Sābūr, *Dispensatorium Parvum* (*Al-Aqrābādhīn al-saghīr*), ed. by O. Kahl (Leiden 1994).

Ibn Sahl, Sābūr, *The Small Dispensatory*, trans. by O. Kahl (Leiden 2003).

Ibn Sīnā, *The Canon of Medicine* (*al-Qānūn fī'l-ṭibb*) (*The Law of Natural Healing*), 5 vols., trans. by L. Bakhtiar (Chicago 2015).

Kahl, O. (ed. and trans.), *The Dispensatory of Ibn at-Tilmīḏ: Arabic Text, English Translation, Study, and Glossaries* (Leiden 2007).

Kahl, O., *The Sanskrit, Syriac, and Persian Sources in the* Comprehensive Book *of Rhazes* (Leiden 2015).

Neubauer, A., *Catalogue of the Hebrew Manuscripts in the Bodleian Library*, and *Supplement of Addenda and Corrigenda*, comp. under the direction of M. Beit-Arié, ed. by R.A. May (Repr., Oxford 1994).

Pormann, P.E., and N.P. Joosse, 'Commentaries on the Hippocratic *Aphorisms* in the Arabic Tradition: The Example of Melancholy,' in *Epidemics in Context: Greek Commentaries on Hippocrates in the Arabic Tradition*, ed. by P.E. Pormann, 211–250 (Berlin 2012).

Richler, B., *Hebrew Manuscripts in the Biblioteca Palatina in Parma: Catalogue*, with palaeographical and codicological descriptions by M. Beit-Arié (Jerusalem 2001).

Richler, B., *Hebrew Manuscripts in the Vatican Library: Catalogue*, comp. by the staff of the Institute of Microfilmed Hebrew Manuscripts (IMHM), Jewish National and University Library, Jerusalem, with palaeographical and codicological descriptions by M. Beit-Arié and N. Pasternak (Vatican 2008).

Richler, B., 'Manuscripts of Avicenna's *Kanon* in Hebrew Translation: A Revised and Up-to-Date List,' *Korot* 30, no. 8 (1982): 145–168.

Shatzmiller, J., *Jews, Medicine, and Medieval Society* (Berkeley 1994).

Steinschneider, M., *Die hebräischen Handschriften der K. Hof- und Staatsbibliothek in München*, 2nd ed. (Munich 1895).

Steinschneider, M., *Die hebräischen Übersetzungen des Mittelalters und die Juden als Dolmetscher* (Berlin 1893).

Steinschneider, M., 'Eine medicinische hebräische Handschrift,' *Magazin für die Wissenschaft des Judentums* 12 (1885): 182–216.

Tanḥum Yerushalmi, *Al-Murshid al-kafi*, ed. and trans. by H. Shy (Jerusalem 2005).

Ullmann, M., *Islamic Medicine* (Edinburgh 1978).

Ullmann, M., *Die Medizin im Islam* (Leiden 1970).

van't Land, K., 'Internal, Yet Intrinsic: Conceptions of Bodily Space and Their Relations to Causality in Late Medieval University Medicine,' in *Medicine and Space: Body, Surroundings, and Borders in Antiquity and the Middle Ages*, ed. by P.A. Baker, H. Nijdam, and K. van't Land, 85–116 (Leiden 2011).

Walker, B.G., *The Woman's Encyclopedia of Myths and Secrets* (San Francisco 1983).

Yassif, E. (ed.), *Sippurei Ben Sira bi-Yemei ha-Benayyim: The Tales of Ben Sira in the Middle Ages* (Jerusalem 1984).

Zonta, M., 'Zeraḥyah: Philosopher and Translator and his Role in 13th Century Rome' (Paper read in Jerusalem, January 1, 2007)

Zotenberg, H. (ed.), *Catalogues des manuscrits hébreux et samaritains de la Bibliothèque Impériale* (Paris 1866).

Used Hebrew Sources

Translator	Title of translation	Original author	Title of original (with English title of ed.)	Ms/ed.
Abraham Avigdor	*Ha-Ma'amar ha-Teshi'i le-Sefer ha-Mansuri le-Razi*	Gerard de Solo	*Practica super nono Almansoris*	Ms Munich, Bayerische Staatsbibliothek, Cod. hebr. 296
Abraham ben Isaac	*Sefer Ṣedah la-Oreḥim*	Ibn al-Jazzār	*Zād al-musāfir wa-qūt al-ḥādir* (*Provisions for the Traveller and the Nourishment for the Sedentary*)	Ms Florence, Biblioteca Medicina Laurenziana, Plut. 88.37 / IJZ 1–2 (I–II)
Anonymous*	*Perush Aphorismi shel Apuqraṭ* (*Pirqei Abuqraṭ*)	Maimonides	*Sharḥ fuṣūl Abūqrāṭ* (*Commentary on Hippocrates'* Aphorisms)	Ms Paris, Bibliothèque Mazarine, 4478 / BMCH 1
	Sammim Libbiyim	Ibn Sīnā	*K. al-Adwiya al-qalbiya*	Ms Munich, Bayerische Staatsbibliothek, Cod. hebr. 280
	Sefer ha-Qanun	Ibn Sīnā	*K. al-Qānūn fī al-ṭibb*	Ms Paris, BnF, héb. 1142
	Sefer ha-Qaṣeret	Maimonides	*Maqāla fī al-rabw* (*On Asthma*)	Ms Jerusalem, The National and University Library, Heb. 8° 3941 / BMA 2
	Sefer ha-Refu'ot ha-Libbiyot	Ibn Sīnā	*K. al-Adwiya al-qalbiya*	Ms Munich, Bayerische Staatsbibliothek, Cod. hebr. 373
David Caslari	*Sefer Ro'a Mezeg Mitḥallef*	Galen	*De inaequali intemperie*	Ms Oxford, Bodleian Library, Opp. Add. Fol. 18 (Neubauer 2083)
Do'eg ha-Edomi	*Sefer Agur*	Hippocrates	*Aphorismoi*	Ms Oxford, Bodleian Library, Opp. 685 (Neubauer 2084)
	Sefer Ya'ir Netiv	Constantinus Africanus	*Viaticum peregrinantis* (*Provisions for the Traveller and the Nourishment for the Sedentary*)	Ms London, British Library, Add. 18969 / IJZ 1–2 (I–II)
Hillel ben Samuel	*Aphorismi*	Hippocrates	*Aphorismoi*	Ms Berlin, Staatsbibliothek Preußischer Kulturbesitz, Or. Qu. 517 (Steinschneider 68)
	Sefer Keritut	Bruno Longobucco	*Cyrurgia Magna*	Ms Oxford, Bodleian Library, Opp. 688

(*cont.*)

Translator	Title of translation	Original author	Title of original (with English title of ed.)	Ms/ed.
Joshua Shatibi	*Ma'amar 'al ha-Qaṣeret*	Maimonides	*Maqāla fī al-rabw* (*On Asthma*)	Ms Munich, Bayerische Staatsbibliothek, Cod. hebr. 280 / BMA 2
Moses ibn Tibbon	*Hanhagat ha-Beri'ut*	Maimonides	*Fī tadbīr al-ṣiḥḥa* (*On the Regimen of Health*)	Ms Oxford, Bodleian Library, Opp. 685 (Neubauer 2084) / BMR
	Perush Aphorismi shel Apuqraṭ (*Pirqei Abuqraṭ*)	Maimonides	*Sharḥ fuṣūl Abūqrāṭ* (*Commentary on Hippocrates'* Aphorisms)	Ms London, British Library, Or. 10526 / BMCH 1
	Sefer Ṣedat ha-Derakhim	Ibn al-Jazzār	*Zād al-musāfir wa-qūt al-ḥādir* (*Provisions for the Traveller and the Nourishment for the Sedentary*)	Ms Oxford, Bodleian Library, Poc. 353, Uri Heb. 314 (Neubauer 2111) / IJZ 1–2 (I–II); IJZ 7 (VII.7–30)
Nathan ha-Me'ati	*Pirqei Abuqraṭ*	Hippocrates	*Aphorismoi*	Ms Paris, BnF, héb. 1107
	Sefer ha-Mezonot	Ibn Zuhr	*K. al-Aghdhiya*	Ms Munich, Bayerische Staatsbibliothek, Cod. hebr. 220
	Sefer ha-Peraqim (*Pirqei Moshe*)	Maimonides	*K. al-Fuṣūl fī al-ṭibb* (*Medical Aphorisms*)	Ms Paris, BnF, héb. 1174 / BMMN
	Sefer ha-Qanun	Ibn Sīnā	*K. al-Qānūn fī al-ṭibb*	Ms Oxford, Bodleian Library, Can. Or. 88
Samuel Benveniste	*Ma'amar 'al ha-Qaṣeret*	Maimonides	*Maqāla fī al-rabw* (*On Asthma*)	Ms Paris, BnF, héb. 1176.1 / BMA 2
Shem Tov ben Isaac	*Sefer Almansur*	al-Rāzī	*K. al-Manṣūrī fī al-ṭibb*	Ms Vatican, Vatican Library, Urb. Ebr. 50 / BMZ (glossary)
	Sefer ha-Shimmush	al-Zahrāwī	*K. al-Taṣrīf li-man 'ajiza 'an al-ta'līf*	Ms Paris, BnF, héb. 1163 / SHS 1 (XXIX, list 1); SHS 2 (XXIX, list 2)
Zeraḥyah Ḥen	*Perush Aphorismi shel Apuqraṭ* (*Pirqei Abuqraṭ*)	Maimonides	*Sharḥ fuṣūl Abūqrāṭ* (*Commentary on Hippocrates'* Aphorisms)	Ms Udine, Biblioteca Arcescovile, 246 ebr. 12 / BMCH 1
	Sefer ha-Peraqim (*Pirqei Moshe*)	Maimonides	*K. al-Fuṣūl fī al-ṭibb* (*Medical Aphorisms*)	Ms Florence, Biblioteca Medicea Laurenziana, Plut. 88.29 / BMMZ
	Sefer ha-Qanun	Ibn Sīnā	*K. al-Qānūn fī al-ṭibb*	Ms Oxford, Bodleian Library, Opp. Add. Fol. 12

Corrections to NM 1–5 and BCD

NM 1:64; 2:179, s.v. עִצּוּר: "Hebr. עִצּוּר only features in the current dictionaries in the sense of 'closing up (of the womb)', and 'obstruction of orifices'": **add** "and 'squeezing; contraction.'"

NM 1:70, s.v. תרדמה: "Arab. خدر 'numbness'; cf. 8.2": **corr.** "Arab. خدر 'numbness'; cf. 9.2".

NM 5:25, s.v. [1]בַּד: "trans. Moses ibn Tibbon, *Sefer Ṣedat ha-Derakhim*, bk. 2, ch. 19": **corr.** "trans. Moses ibn Tibbon, *Sefer Ṣedat ha-Derakhim*, bk. 3, ch. 8".

NM 5:32, s.v. בצל העכבר: "Hebr. בצל העכבר is a non-attested loan translation of Arab. بصل الفأر": **corr.** "In the sense of 'sea squill,' Hebr. בצל העכבר features in BM 584 in an attestation from the *Sefer ha-Qanun*."

NM 5:56, s.v. דֶּשֶׁן: **add** "cf. BCD 60 (NM 2:177) for דשן גפנים ('ash of the grapevine')".

NM 5:85, s.v. חֲשֵׁיכוּת: "(Gr. ἀμβλυωπία) (cf. UW 90)": **corr.** "(Gr. ἀμβλυωπία) (cf. UW 99)".

NM 5:89–90: "[טמטם] • *Part. Pilpel* מְטַמְטֵם • obstructing; closing up": **corr.** "[טמם] (*Aram.*) • *Part. Palpel* מְטַמְטֵם • obstructing; closing up."

NM 5:90, s.v. [טמטם] corr. [טמם]: "Hebr. טמטם features in Rabbinic literature in the sense of 'to thicken into a cohesive mass' and 'to thicken, to obstruct, to blunt the understanding;' cf. tb*Pesaḥim* 42ª: מטמטם את הלב 'obstructs the heart' (i.e., makes a person dull); cf. JD 532. In liturgical literature it is attested in the sense of 'to close [the eyes];' cf. BM 1884": **corr.** "Aram. *Palpel* טַמְטֵם features in Rabb. literature, a.o., in the sense of 'to close (around);'[1] cf. the *Targum* of סָגַר in Ju 3:22 (cf. JD 540, DAN 171)."

NM 5:144, s.v. עֲדוּת: "Constantinus Africanus, *Viaticum* · trans. Do'eg ha-Edomi, *Sefer Ya'ir Netiv*, bk. 1, ch. 17": **corr.** "Constantinus Africanus, *Viaticum* · trans. Do'eg ha-Edomi, *Sefer Ya'ir Netiv*, bk. 3, ch. 11."

NM 5:150, s.v. עָמֵד: "Constantinus Africanus, *Viaticum* · trans. Do'eg ha-Edomi, *Sefer Ya'ir Netiv*, bk. 1, ch. 18": **corr.** "Constantinus Africanus, *Viaticum* · trans. Do'eg ha-Edomi, *Sefer Ya'ir Netiv*, bk. 2, ch. 18."

BCD 18 (NM 1:128), s.v. אדם הביצה: "Maimonides, *Šarḥ fuṣūl Abūqrāṭ* · trans. Zeraḥyah Ḥen (*Pirqei Abuqraṭ*), 2.3: **corr.** Maimonides, *K. al-Fuṣūl fī al-ṭibb* · trans. Zeraḥyah Ḥen (*Sefer ha-Peraqim*), 2.3."

BCD 30 (NM 4:24): "בֶּגֶד • II. papyrus": **read** כאגד; i.e., Arab.-Pers. كاغد ('paper'); cf. WKAS 1:10.[2]

BCD 75 (NM 1:143): "התכי": **corr.** "הַתּוּכִי."

---

1 Cf. the term טִמְטוּם in the sense of 'obstruction' (for Arab. سدّ) in NM 5:89.

2 See also entry כאגד above.

BCD 112 (NM 2:12), s.v. טְחוֹר: "Arab. بواسير": **corr.** "نواسير."

BCD 144 (NM 4:96–97): "מַזְרֵק": **corr.** "מִזְרָק."

BCD 192 (NM 2:167): "סִמּוּר • tremor": **corr.** "shivering fit; rigor."

BCD 123 (NM 3:112): "כאב הצדדים • pleurisy": **corr.** "pleuralgia."

Index of Greek Terms

αἰδοῖον 184
αἱμωδία 186, 187
ἄιτιον: ἄιτιον προηγούμενον 145
ἄιτιον προκαταρκτικόν 146
ἄιτιον συνεκτικόν → συνεκτικόν
ἄνθραξ 22
ἀντίδοτος → θηριακή
ἀπέψια 19, 200
ἀπόζεμα 31
ἀποπληξία 83
ἀχώρ 121, 145, 153

βούλιμος 23, 24

δραχμή 64
δυσουρία 51

ἐκφρακτικός 178
ἕξις 179, 218
ἔναιμος 70, 86
ἐπίθεμα 17
ἐπίσχεσις 18, 54
ἐποχή 18, 54
ἐργαλεῖον 21
ἔριον → πέσσος
ἐσχάρα 190

ἦχος 180, 187

θηριακή, sc. ἀντίδοτος 222
θλάσμα 105, 205

ἴονθος 157

καταντλέω 66
κατάχρισμα 199
κηρίον 90, 121, 128, 145, 153
κολλάω 42
κόλπος 135

λειχήν 211
λέπις 206
λίθος: λίθος σεληνίτης 13

μελικηρίς 90, 121, 128, 145, 153

νάρκη 25, 204
νομή, *Plur.* νομαί 137

ὀρθόπνοια 56, 60, 67, 161, 188
οὐλή 151, 207

παραλύομαι 204
παρωνυχὶα 30, 127, 128
πέσσος 114, 182
πὲσσος δέ ἐστιν ἔριον διεξασμένον 114, 182
πίτυρον 71, 88

ῥαγάς 29
ῥῆγμα 206
ῥῖγος 141

σεληνίτης → λίθος
σπασμός 59, 205
στέφανος 103, 138
στηρίζω 36
στραγγουρία 51
στρέμμα 110, 157, 206
στρόφος 70, 72, 83, 129, 168
συνάγχη 79
συνεκτικόν 145

ταραχή 53
τεινεσμός 163
τρόμος 202
τυρώδης 33

ὑδερικόν [πάθος] 51
ὑποχόνδριον 181

Φιλώνια 203 (n. 274)
Φιλώνειος 203 (n. 274)

φρίκη 150

χαλκῖτις 65

Index of Arabic/Persian Terms

(أدب) تأدّب 89, 90
أدرة 127
أسيلم 126, 170
أصل: أصول ← طبيخ، مطبوخ
أترجّ ← حمّاض
أثر: آثار 151, 207
أذن ← ورم
أصل ← ورم
تأليف 69, 123, 124
أندراني ← ملح
آنك 158
إناء: إناء حنتم 24
آلة ← مرض
آلي ← مرض

بثر: بثور 151, 152, 211
بحوحة: بحوحة الصوت 138, 139
بحران 33, 44, 87
بحراني 33
مبخّر 187, 188
بخور 188
بخار: أبخرة 15
(بدر) بادر 209
بدن ← اضطراب
برد 193
تبريد 57
براز 30, 91, 179
مبارك ← دواء
بسط 177
انبساط 58, 61, 177, 178
بطّ 19
أبطأ 159
بطن ← مراقّ، سهل، طلق، عقل
بقر ← عين
بلادة: بلادة فهم 16
بلغ 135, 136
بلغماني 107
بندق 97
بندقة 51 (n. 62), 107, 108, 196 (n. 263), 212 (n. 287)
بنية 27
بال: بال في الفراش 217
بول ← احتباس، حرقة، إدرار، سلس، عسر، تقطير، كثرة
بول الدم 59
باه ← ضُعْفٌ
أبيض ← شبّ

تخمة 17, 19, 200
ترقوة 165
ترك 24
ترياق 222
تفّاحي 221
تلف 54

ثريدة: ثرائد 86
مثقال ← نصف
مثلّج 211, 212

جبن ← ماء
جبنية 33، 34
جرب: الجرب المتقرّح 37، 38، (211 (n. 285
جرب متقشّر 189
جرادة 39
جوارشن: جوارشن الأفاويه 129
جشاء 34، 197
جفت 97، 106
جلاء 219
(جمد) جمّد 19، 185
جمود 191، 192
جامد 186
جمع 185
جنون 85
جنب ← ذات، وجع
جندبا دستر 25
جوابة 126، 127
أجود 24، 25

(حبّ) حبّب 39، 40
حبّ: حبّ القرع 38
حبس 221
احتباس 18، 20، 54
احتباس البول 164
احتباس الطمث 20، 166، 167
حبل ← عسر
حجاب 93
← ورم
حجر: حجر الرحى 13
حجر المفاصل 13، 59
حجر القمر 13
حدّة: أقلّ حدّة 75، 76
حديد ← خبث
حدبة 24
إحدار 49
حرارة: الحرارة الغريزية 77، 78
احتراس ← حمية
حرقة: حرقة البول 82، 215
حزاز 71، 88، 89
حاسّة: حواسّ 57
حسو 86، 216
حصرمي 27
حصاة 81
انحطاط 139، 140
حفظ 35، 36
حقّ: بحقّ 81
حقن 21، 22، 171، 189
حكّ 177
(حلّ) تحلّل 75، 116، 117
تحلُّل 60
تحليل 116، 117
انحلال: انحلال الفرد 55، 176
محلّل ← دواء
احتلام 37، 39، 127
حمّ 78، 79
حُمّى 78
حمار ← قثّاء
حمضة 194
حمّاض: حمّاض الأترجّ 78
(حمل) احتمل 147، 223
احتمل فتيلة 147
حَمْل 129
← لسان
حمول 223
حمية 123، 213
حمية واحتراس 213

حنتم ← إناء
حنظل ← شحم
اختناق: اختناق الرحم 125
حال: أحوال 16
حيّة: حيّات 139

خبث: خبث الحديد 13, 14
خدر 25, 204, 205, 222
مخدّر 25
خروج: خروج المقعدة 91
إخراج 39
مخرج 115, 142, 173, 174
خراطة 38, 115
خشكراشة 190
(خشن) خشّن 139
خشونة 139, 156
(خصّ) اختصّ 88
خصوصا 87, 102, 189
خفّة 76
متخلخل ← عظم
خلط 221
أخلاط 89
اختلاط: اختلاط الذهن 81
اختلاف: اختلاف دم 163
(خمد) خمّد 194
خنق 124, 125
خانوق: خوانيق 79
تخيّل 180

دبيد 41, 42
(دبر) دبّر 138
داحس 30, 127, 128
(درّ) أدرّ 137, 212
أدرّ الطمث 213
مدرّ ← دواء
إدرار: إدرار البول 51, 196, 212
دربة 57, 68
دريب 28, 29, 196, 197
تدريج: على تدريج 47, 50, 113, 114
درمك 48
دسومة 48, 59, 60
دعا 71
دافع ← قوّة
دقاق 211
دليل: دلائل 51, 196
دلك 66, 122, 130
دم ← بول، اختلاف، إسهال، نزف
دماغ ← ورم
دهن 130
دهني 130
دار: أدوار 146
دائم ← إنعاظ
دون 117
دويّ 180, 187
دوى: أدواء ← دواء
دواء: الدواء المدرّ للبول 44
الدواء المحلّل 149, 150
الدواء المسمّى المبارك 203
الدواء الملحم 203
الدواء الملطّف 149
الأدوية المدرّة 44
الأدوية المقابلة للأدواء 204
الأدوية المقرحة 150, 151, 204
ذبح 64, 79
ذبول 82
ذرور: ذرورات 162, 163

ذَكَر 35, 66
ذهب ← لزاق
ذهبي ← معجون
ذهن ← اختلاط
ذو: ذو الأربعة والأربعين 28
ذات: ذات الجنب 28, 128
ذات الرئة 28
(ذاب) أذاب 84

رئة ← ذات
رئيس 186
ربّ: ربّ عنب 88
أربعة ← ذو
أربعون ← ذو
ربو 35, 183
مربّى 121, 122
رجل ← (صاب)
رجلة (n. 228) 171
رحم ← اختناق، نتوء
رحى 198
استرخاء 200, 204
استرخاء المعدة 205
رضّ 105, 205, 206
رطوبة: رطوبات 199
رعشة 202
مرتعش 201
رغوة 66, 67, (n. 110) 88
رفد 202, 203
رفع 91, 160
مرتفع ← كان
رقّة 178
مراقّ: مراقّ البطن 32
راكد 215
رمد 192
رمكة 148
رمّاني 200
روث 179
ريح: رياح 198
إرادة ← سيلان، كثرة
راض 84
رياضة 84

زبيبية (n. 170) 134, 181
(زحر) تزحّر 165, 172
زحير 64, 73, 123, 163
أزرق 219
زراوند 154
زعف 67
زقّي ← استسقاء
زكام 119
زلق 58, 59
مزمن 18
زائد ← لحم
مزيّن: مزيّنون 154
زينة 90, 156, 195
مزلق ← شيء

سبات 191, 221
سبخة 119
سبخي ← ملح
سَحج 39, 136, 174, 177
سَحْج 56, 136, 137
← إسهال
سحوج 56, 79
سحنة 179, 180, 218
سدّة: سدد 154

← فتح
انسداد 154
سرّة 215, 216
سرسام 128
سعط 140, 171
سعفة 37 (n. 45), 121, 145, 153, (n. 258) 189
ساع ← قرح
سفوف 191
سقوط: سقوط الشهوة 142
استسقاء 214
الاستسقاء الزقّي 215
الاستسقاء اللحمي 215
سلّ 102
مسلول 210
سلس: سلس البول 50, 92
سنّ: أسنان ← تصرير
سهل 124
سهّل البطن 190
أسهل 212, 213
مسهّل 109
إسهال 30, 31, 61
إسهال الدم 31
إسهال طبيعته 143, 144
إسهال وهو سحج 163
سوء: سوء الهضم 17, 200
ساق 210
سويق 216
سيلان 49
سيلان المني 64, 65
سيلان المني من غيرْ إرادة 64

شبّ: شبّ أبيض 17
شتاء 40

شحم: شحم الحنظل 35
شدخ: شدخ العضل 206
شرب 185
شربة 110, 132
شراسيف 181
شرط 103, 104, 148
شريان: شرايين 115, 116
شقّة: شقاق 29, 30, 147
شقيقة 175
شهدي ← ورم
شهوة ← سقوط
الشهوة الكلبية 80
شهواني ← قوّة
شوصة 127, 128
شيء: الأشياء المزلقة 43, 44

صبّاغ ← قوّة
صحيح 72
← دم
صاحب ← طلق
صدر ← ضيق
تصديع 52
تصرير: تصرير الأسنان 82
صغير 157
صفيحة 206
صفائح 152, 206
أصفر: صفراء ← مرّة
صفراوي 14, 15, 103
صفاق 93, 106
صافن 170
صافان 170
(صفا) صفّى 65, 66, 180, 181
صفو 152

مصفاة 120, 121
صَلاَيَّة 13
صِلاَيَّة 13
صنف 179, 219
أصناف 219
(صاب) ← نورة
أصاب الرجل 28
صوت ← بحوحة
صوفة 114, 115, 143, 182
صيف 77, 78

ضربة 52
ضَرَسٌ 186, 187
اضطراب 53
اضطراب البدن 26, 208
ضربان 46, 47, 69
ضُعْفٌ 100, 101
الضعف عن الباه 75, 77
(ضمّ) انضمّ 166
(ضمد) ضمّد 17, 70, 83
ضيق 124, 125, 192, 193
ضيق الصدر 44, 183
ضيق النفس 125, 193

طبيخ: طبيخ الأصول 31, 133
مطبوخ 31, 133
مطبوخ الأصول 31, 132
طبيعة ← إسهال
طبقة: طبقات 104, 105, 124
طبقات المعدة 36
طري 31, 70, 71, 86
مطفأ ← نورة
طلق 53, 62, 172
استطلق بطن صاحب العلّة 143
انطلاق 76, 77, 212
طلاء: أطلية 199, 200
طمث ← احتباس، (درّ)
(طاب) طيّب 104
طيّب النكهة 104
طيب ← ظفر

ظفر: أظفار الطيب 183
ظهر: على ظهره 54

عجم ← منزوع
عجن 157
عجين ← ملح
معجون: معجون يسمّى الذهبي 129
استعداد 60, 61
اعتدال 58
عرض: عرض غثيان 220
عسر: عسر البول 126
عسر الحبل 167
عسر النفس 97, 125, 193
عسلوج: عساليج 108, 190
عشا 20, 109, 152
عصب ← التواء
عصر 91, 167, 171, 210, 211
عصارة 164
عصير: عصير العنب 164
عصفور: عصافير ← لسان
عضل ← شدخ
عضو: أعضاء النفض 14
عطري 31
عطّار: عطّارون 27
عظم: العظام المتخلخلة 121

(عقد) عقّد 160، 195
عقل: عقل البطن 166
عَقْل 164
انعقال 192
عكر 26
علّة ← طلق
معالجة 152، 153
علاج 153، 158، 202
علاجات 121، 153
علق 20، 45، 170
علك 43
علامة 156
استعمال 172
عنب ← ربّ، عصير
عنق: عنق المثانة 179
عانة 33
إعياء 165
عين ← ماء
عين البقر 158

(غثى) أغثى 158
غثي 220
غثيان 220، 221
← عرض
غذاء 34
مغذّ 34
غريزي ← حرارة
غرض 131
(غرا) غرّى 71
غراء 182، 183
تغرية 41
غسالة: غسالة اللحم 199
مغشوش 65

غشي 113
غشاء: أغشية 45
غصن 23
غضّ 200
غلبة 120
غليظ ← معى
مغلي: مغليات 132، 207
(غوط) تغوّط 90، 91، 142
مغيّر ← قوّة

فتح: فتح السدد 208
تفتيح 178
فتق: فتوق 29
فتيلة ← (حمل)
(فجّ) فجّج 173
فرد ← الحلال
مفرد 87
فارسي ← نار
فراش ← بال
إفراط 94
استفراغ 143
فرفري 82، 83
تفرّق: تفرّق الاتّصال 55، 56، 176
فرن 174
فصد 104
مفصل: مفاصل ← حجر
فضل: فضول 89، 94، 95
فضلة 94، 95
فضلات 94
فضلي 95
فضاء 116، 211
فطرة 92
فعل: أفعال 124، 175

فهم ← بلادة
فوّة: فوّة الصبّاغين 197
أفواه: أفاويه ← جوارشن
في 146

قانون: قوانين 48, 147, 168, 169
قبض 18, 69, 70, 162, 184
مقبّض 162
قُبُل 184
قثّاء: قثّاء الحمار 194
(قدر) قدّر 213, 214
قرح: القروح الساعية 137
مقرح ← دواء
متقرّح ← جرب
قرص: أقراص 86
قريض 193, 194
قرطاس 96
قرع ← حبّ
قرقرة 49, 187, 201
قرو 26
متقشّر ← جرب
قشر 190
اقشعرار 150
مقصّر 80, 192
قضيب: قضبان 23, 190, 191
تقطير: تقطير البول 51, 52
قطع 209
قُطِعَ 208, 209
انقطاع 55
قطاة 175
مقعدة ← خروج، نتوء
أقلّ ← حدّة
قلق 53

قلقطار 65
قمر ← حجر
قمع 80
قوباء 153, 211
قوام 161
قوّة 120
القوّة الدافعة 100
القوّة الشهوانية 98
القوة الماسكة 98, 99, 100
القوّة المغيّرة 99, 100
القوّة الهاضمة 98, 99
قيء 57

كابوس 53
كثرة 156, 157
كثرة البول من غير إرادة 196
(كثف) كثّف 84, 85
كحل: أكحال 100
كحّال: كحّالون 101, 154 (n. 211, 212)
مكترز 119
كزاز 205, 219, 220
كشك 104
إكليل 103, 138
كلبي ← شهوة
كلف 105, 157
كمّية 103
(كمد) كمّد 83
كهبة 52, 53, 54
كان: كان مرتفع 90, 159, 160
كاو 97, 98
كيفية 16

(لثم) التثم 42
لبن ← مخيض
لثة 47, 101, 102
لحج 154
(لحم) ألحم 42
ملحم ← دواء
لحم ← غسالة
لحم زائد 32
لحمي ← استسقاء
لذيذ 85
لذع 115
تلزّز 41, 184, 185
لزوجة 41
(لزق) ألزق 42
لزاق: لزاق الذهب 43
لسان: لسان الحمل 111, 112
لسان العصافير 32, 111
(لطف) تلطّف 72, 73
ملطّف 169
← دواء
لطيف 46, 47
لعوق 36, 108, 109, 111
لفافة 109
لقوة 110, 140, 157, 168
لهاة 169
التواء: التواء العصب 110, 157, 206

ماهية 114
مثانة 101
← عنق
مخيض: مخيض اللبن 77
تمدّد 46, 59
امتداد 46, 59

مرّة: المرّة الصفراء 15
(مرأ) استمرأ 17
(مرخ) تمرّخ 123
مرض: مرض الآلة 74, 218, 219
المرض الآلي 74
ماسك ← قوة
مضمضة 36, 126, 195
مفصل: مفاصل ← حجر
معدة ← استرخاء، طبقة
معى: أمعاء 47
الأمعاء الغلاظ 122
مغص 70, 72, 83, 129, 168
مقلياثا 203
(مكن) تمكّن 36
ملة 23, 74
ملح: الملح الأندراني 119
ملح سبخي 119
ملح العجين 119
مني ← سيلان، وعاء
ماء ← نورة
ماء الجبن 118
الماء النازل في العين 117
ميبختج 88

نتوء: نتوء الرحم 26, 92
نتوء المقعدة 26, 27
ندرة: في الندرة 47, 198
منزوع: منزوع العجم 143
نزف 201, 214
نزف الدم 214
نازل ← ماء
نزلة: نزلات 52
نسخة 138

ناسور: نواسير 32، 84
انتشار 61
انتصاب ← نفس
انتصاب النفس 56، 57
ناصور 135
نصف: نصف مثقال 22
نطل 66
تنطيل 57، 140
نعظ 68، 160، 194
أنعظ 194
إنعاظ: الإنعاظ الدائم 67، 68، 160، 195
انتفاخ 142
منفذ: منافذ 175
نفس ← ضيق، عسر، انتصاب
نفس الانتصاب 60، 67، 161، 188
نفض ← عضو
نافض 141، 150 (n. 202)، 208 (n. 281)
نقرس 140، 141
نقوع 133
تنقّل: التنقّل 20، 174، 175
ناقه: ناقهون 120
نكهة ← (طاب)
نمش 157
نملة 74
نمى 42
نهم 38
(نها) انتهى 37
منتهى 54
نوبة 131، 132
نار: النار الفارسي 22
نورة: نورة غير مطفأة 148، 149
نورة لم يصبها ماء 149

مهراس 118
هضم 181
← سوء
هاضم ← قوّة
هطل 44، 45
هامّة: هوامّ 169
هيضة 49، 188

وثء 105، 205
وجع: وجع الجنبين 96
(ورث) أورث 94
ورد 63
ورم: أورام 181، 182
أورام أصل الأذن 129
أورام حجب الدماغ 129
الأورام الشهدية 90، 128
وشم 103، 105، 106، 151
وصف 19، 154
صفة 85، 133، 134، 161
إتّصال 43
← تفرّق
وطئ 131
وعاء: أوعية المني 46، 101، 102
وقع 142
أوقع في 142
(ونى) توانى 71
وهن 69

يبس 19
يرقان 50

Index of Latin/Romance Terms

ablatio 20, 54, 167
abominatio 220, 221
  abominationem facio 220
  abominationem patior 220
abstinentia 123
acceptio 185
accipio 185
aduno 186
aetas → *venio*
agallocha 188
agnus: agnus castus 16
alienatio: alienatio mentis 81
alumen 18
anas 19
angustia 124
  angustia urine 126
angustiae 192
antecedo: Part. *antecedens* 145
anus → *exitus*
apostema, Plur. *apostemata* 181
  Plur. Acc. *apostemas* 181
apozema, Plur. *apozemata* 31
  Plur. Acc. *apozemas* 31
  → *apozima*
apozima → *apozema*
  apozima de radicibus 31, 132
appetitivus → *virtus*
appetitus 80, 81
  appetitus caninus 80
  neque appetitus minoratur 142
ardor 115
  ardor urine 82, 215
argalia 21
  → *ergalium*
arsura 115
ascaris: ascarides et cucurbini 38
asma 183
avis → *lenga, linga, lingua*

bombicinus → *carta*
bulimus 74, 75

calx: calx viva 149
caninus → *appetitus, mania*
carentia 54
caro: caro superflua 32
  → *lavatura*
carta: carta bombicina 96
castus → *agnus*
catarticum → *do*
catharacta 117
chirurgia 73
cingulum 206
circa 146
clistere → *facio*
coagulatus 186
  → *sanguis*
coagulo 19, 185, 186
cogo: cogor 71
cohabito 28
coitus 131
colamenta 156
colatura 152
colera: colera rubea 15
colericus 14
collum: collum vesicae 179
colocontida 35
  → *coloquintida*
coloquintida 34
  → *colocontida*
columbar → *pullus*
commingo: commingo in lecto 217
communis → *sal*
congelatio 191
coniunctivus: coniunctiva 70, 117
constipatio 124, 164, 193
constipo: constipor 192
constringo 166
contentivus → *virtus*
cortex 152, 190
  → *crusta*
  Plur. *cortices* 152, 207
crassus → *intestinum*
crepatura 29
  → *crepitura*
crepitura 29
  → *crepatura*
crisis 44, 87
crus, Plur. *crura* → *vena*
crusta 152
  → *cortex*
cucurbinus, Plur. *cucurbini* → *ascaris*
cupula, Plur. *cupulae* 106

cura 158
curo: curor 158

declino 139
defectio 101
deficio 21
  deficior 21
demoniacus → *mania*
demoniaticus → *mania*
denarius 64
dens → *stridor*
desiderabilis → *virtus*
diacrisis 129
diaphragma 93
diaroma 129
dies: dies prenunciata 87
diffinio 35
digestio 30, 181
  digestio sanguinis 31
disenteria 163
dissolutivus → *medicina*
diureticum, Plur. *diuretica* 44, 208
diureticus 44, 208
do: do catarticum 84
dominatio 120
dormitatio 222
  dormitatio membrorum 222
dysenteria 79

effusio: effusio spermatis in somno 39, 127
egero 90
egestio 30, 218
eiectio 39
elacterium 195
  Gen. *elacteri*[*i*] 195
eminentia 26
emitto 40
epithema 17
erectio: nimia erectio virgae 67, 160, 195
ergalium 21
  → *argalia*
erigo 67, 161
  erigens 68
  erigor 68, 160, 194
escrupulus 22
  → *scrupulus*
eulogimen 203
excoriatio 56
excorio, Part. *excorians* 177
exitus: exitus ani 26, 27
expressio 53, 172
expulsivus → *virtus*
extractio 171, 172
extremitas, Plur. *extremitates* 76

facio 138
  → *abominatio, guttatim*
  facio clistere 190
fames: fames syncopalis 200
farmacia, Plur. *farmacie* 15
fastidium 19, 200
ferrugo 13
festino 71
figura 179, 218
flatu → *strictura*
flegmaticus 107
fluxus 51, 214
  fluxus sanguinis 214
  fluxus sanguis narium 201
frenesis 128
frico 123
  fricor 123
frigiditas 193
fumigo 188
furcula, Plur. Acc. *furculas* 166

gema → *sal*
gibbositas 24
gibbus 24
gingiva, Plur. *gingivae* 101
glutino, Part. Plur. *glutinantes* 203
gonorrhea 64
  → *gonorrhoea*
gonorrhoea 50
  → *gonorrhea*
gravitas 123
gurgulatio 49, 201
guttatim: guttatim urinam facio 216

hypochondria 181
hyposarca 215

ictericia 50, 51
ignis: ignis sacer 22
imaginatio 180
incendo 107
incido: incidor 208
incisio 209

incisus 55
incubus 53, 109
index → *vena*
indigestibilitas 17
inferior: inferiores ventris 32, 76
inflatio 141
intentio 131
intestinum: intestinum crassum 122
invetero: inveteror 210
iunctura → *separatio*

lavatura: lavatura carnis 199
laxativus 109
lectus → *commingo*
lenga: lenga avis 111
→ *linga avis*
lenificantium, Plur. *lenificantia* 43–44
lenis 75
levitas 76
libra 169
licoricie → *sucus*
licorucie → *sucus*
linga: linga avis 111
→ *lenga avis*
lingua: lingua avis 111
lingua ocelli 111
lingua ucelli 111
liquefacio 84
lubrica → *urina*
lubricatio 58, 59
lumbus, Plur. *lumbi* → *ulcus*
lupia 153 (n. 210)

mania: mania canina 75, 209
mania demoniaca 209
→ *mania demoniatica*
mania demoniatica 75, 209
→ *mania demoniaca*
mascara 109
matrix → *suffocatio*
medicina: medicina dissolutiva 203
medicino 158
melanchonia 75, 209
→ *melancolia*
melancolia 75
→ *melanchonia*
membrum, Plur. *membra* → *dormitatio*
mens → *alienatio, stupor*
mictus: mictus sanguinis 59
minoro → *appetitus*
mirabilis → *rete*
mitigo, Part. *mitigans* 169
modus, Plur. *modi* 219
mola 199
mollicies 200, 205
→ *mollities*
mollities 200
→ *mollicies*
morbus: morbus officialis 73, 74, 219
officiales morbi 74, 218
morphea 23
multitudo 156
mutabilis → *virtus*

naris, Plur. *nares* → *fluxus*
nascale 143
→ *nastare*
nastare 143
→ *nascale*
nates 143
neglego 24
nimius → *erectio*
nodus 14, 183
nutrimentum 34
nutritivus 34

ocello, Plur. *ocelli* → *lingua, ucello*
odiferus 31
officialis → *morbus*
Plur. *officiales* 55, 74
→ *morbus*
opilatio 154
os, Gen. *oris* → *tortura*
ovum → *vitellus*
oxiregimina 34

panaric 30
panaricium → *panaric*
patior: patior subeth 191
→ *abominatio*
pecten 33
pellicula: pelliculae stomachi 45
Plur. Acc. *pelliculas* 93
peripleumonia 28
pleuresis 28
polipus 84
pollex → *vena*
pollutio 37, 39, 127

pondus 123, 163, 174
pondus tenesmon 162
potestas 120
prenunciatus → *dies*
primitivus: primitiva 146
principalis 186
proprius 88
pruna, Plur. Acc. *prunas* 159
pullus: pulli columbarum 223
pulsatio 47
pulvis 191
punctura 70, 168
purus 72

qualitas 16
quantitas 103

radix → *apozima*
ranula 14(, 183)
rarus 48, 198
rasura 38, 39
reiectio 39
ren, Plur. *renes* → *ulcus*
rete: rete mirabili 208
rhagas, Plur. *rhagades* 147
rheuma 119
rubeus → *colera*
rubia 31, 197
ructatio 197
Rx 69, 123

sacer → *ignis*
sal: sal communis 119
sal gema 119
→ *salgema, salgemma*
salgema 119
→ *sal gema, salgemma*
salgemma 119
→ *sal gema, salgema*
salsugo 120
sanguis: sanguis coagulata 20, 45
→ *digestio, fluxus, mictus*
sanguisuca 170
sapa 88
saporatus 85
scarificatio 39, 103, 148
scarifico 104
scrupulus 22
→ *escrupulus*
secessus 91
separatio: separatio iuncture 55, 176
serum 118
significatio 156
signum 156
sinapi → *spuma*
siphac 93
solidatio 42
solido 42, 71
solutio 61
solutio ventris 143
solutus 143
solvo: solvo ventrem 144
somnus → *effusio*
spatia 211
species 179, 219
sperma → *effusio, vasa*
spuma: spuma sinapi 182
squinantia 79
status 37, 54
stercus 218
stomachus → *pellicula*
stranguria 164
strictio 164
strictura: strictura in flatu 193
stridor: stridor dentium 82
stringo 221
studeo 72
studeamus ut sudet 73
stupor 221
stupor mentis 81
suavis 169
subeth → *patior*
subtilitas 178
sucus 114, 133
sucus licoricie 114
→ *sucus licorucie*
sucus licorucie 114
→ *sucus licoricie*
sudo → *studeo*
suffocatio 124
suffocatio matricis 79, 125
suffumigatio, Plur. *suffumigationes* 57, 140
superfluus → *caro*
supinus 54
suppositorium, Plur. *suppositoria* 223
syncopalis → *fames*

techinatio 46
techinositas 46 (n. 60)
tenesmos: tenesmon → *pondus*
tenesmus 73
tensio 46
tortura 72, 130
  tortura oris 73, 140, 168
trociscus, Plur. Acc. *trociscos* 86
tunica, Plur. *tunicae* 93
turbulentia 26

ucello, Plur. *ucelli* → *lingua, ocello*
ulcus: ulceres lumborum et renum 176
unctuosus 130
urina: lubrica urina 50, 92
  → *angustia, ardor, guttatim*
uvula 169

vasa: vasa spermatis 46, 101, 102
vena: vena que est inter pollicem et indicem 126, 170
  ambas venas in cruribus 170
venio: venio ad aetatem 135, 136
venter → *inferior, solutio, solvo*
vesica → *collum*
virga → *erectio*
virtus: virtus appetitiva 98
  virtus contentiva 98, 99, 100
  virtus desiderabilis 98
  [*virtus*] *expulsiva* 100
  virtus mutabilis 99
vitellus: vitellus ovorum 15
vitreus 65
vivus → *calx*
vomitus 15
vulneratus 37

ydropisis 215

www.ingramcontent.com/pod-product-compliance
Lightning Source LLC
LaVergne TN
LVHW092117300926
849161LV00002B/162
9789004534407